The Medical School's Mission and the Population's Health

Kerr L. White   Julia E. Connelly
Editors

The Medical School's Mission and the Population's Health

Medical Education in Canada, The United Kingdom, The United States, and Australia

Proceedings of a Conference Sponsored by
The Royal Society of Medicine Foundation, Inc., and
The Josiah Macy Jr. Foundation
December 9–12, 1990, Turnberry Isle, Florida

With 20 Illustrations

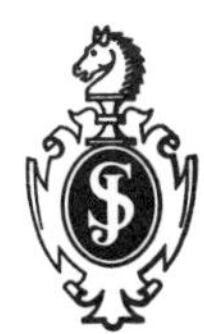

Springer-Verlag
New York Berlin Heidelberg London Paris
Tokyo Hong Kong Barcelona Budapest

Kerr L. White
(Retired Deputy Director for Health
Sciences, The Rockefeller Foundation,
New York)
2401 Old Ivy Road, #1410
Charlottesville, VA 22901-3470 USA

Julia E. Connelly
Associate Professor of Medicine
University of Virginia Medical Center
Charlottesville, VA 22908 USA

Library of Congress Cataloging-in-Publication Data
The Medical school's mission and the population's health : medical
    education in Canada, the United Kingdom, the United States, and
    Australia / Kerr L. White, Julia E. Connelly, editors.
            p.   cm.
    Based on a meeting organized by the Royal Society of Medicine
Foundation and the Josiah Macy, Jr. Foundation, Dec. 9–12, 1990 at
Turnberry Isle, Fla.
        Includes bibliographical references and index.
        ISBN 0-387-97733-3. — ISBN 3-540-97733-3
        1. Medical education—Congresses.   2. Medical education policy-
    -Congresses.   3. Public health—Congresses.   I. White, Kerr L.
    II. Connelly, Julia E.   III. Royal Society of Medicine Foundation.
    IV. Josiah Macy, Jr. Foundation.
        [DNLM: 1. Public Health—education—Australia—congresses.
    2. Public Health—education—Canada—congresses.   3. Public Health-
    -education—Great Britain—congresses.   4. Public Health—education-
    -United States—congresses.   5. Schools, Medical—Australia-
    -congresses.   6. Schools, Medical—Canada—congresses.   7. Schools,
    Medical—Great Britain—congresses.   8. Schools, Medical—United
    States—congresses.   W 19 M4913 1990]
    R735.A2M43   1992
    610'.71'1—dc20
    DNLM/DLC
    for Library of Congress   91-5154

Production coordinated by Chernow Editorial Services, Inc. and managed by Christin R. Ciresi;
Manufacturing supervised by Jacqui Ashri.
Typeset by Edwards Brothers, Inc., Ann Arbor, MI, USA.
Printed and bound by R.R. Donnelley & Sons, Harrisonburg, VA, USA.
Printed in the United States of America.

9 8 7 6 5 4 3 2 1

ISBN 0-387-97772-4 Springer-Verlag New York Berlin Heidelberg (softcover)
ISBN 3-540-97772-4 Springer-Verlag Berlin Heidelberg New York (softcover)
ISBN 0-387-97733-3 Springer-Verlag New York Berlin Heidelberg (hardcover)
ISBN 3-540-97733-3 Springer-Verlag Berlin Heidelberg New York (hardcover)

Foreword

Medical schools exist as part of a complex educational and health care system with affiliations to universities, teaching hospitals, outpatient clinics, students, and communities.

Those of us who serve as trustees and volunteers on boards and committees of medical schools carry obvious responsibilities for the performance of the institution with regard to those affiliations, including those that relate to the community.

By what criteria, and by what standards, do we as trustees assess that performance? For trustees of medical schools, I suggest that the most important criteria are those concerned with the purpose for which the school was originally established and those that relate to the community that supports it and is served by it.

For a medical school performance criteria should be defined in a statement of purpose: the "mission" of the school. This mission statement should provide trustees with direction on such vital matters as the following: What does the medical school seek to accomplish? Whom does it serve? Where is it going? What is the relationship to the geographic region or other community that it may seek to serve?

Such questions are stated more easily than they are answered, but they should be asked. For trustees who are responsible for the education of students, the management of faculty, and the stewardship of funds they are a matter of serious concern.

Is there a "community" or "population" to be served by the medical school? If so, how is it to be defined? No doubt, as an educational institution, the medical school is concerned with the education and training of its students. At the same time, as part of the health care system, is the school also to be charged with any responsibility for understanding and meeting the health care needs of the population or its "community"?

This volume is the outcome of a meeting organized by the Royal Society of Medicine Foundation and the Josiah Macy Jr. Foundation to discuss that question. Those who participated had, for the most part, already concluded that some responsibility does exist. They came together, therefore, to examine how medical schools in the United States, United Kingdom, Canada, and Australia can profit from each other's experience in organizing medical education, so that faculty and students recognize more fully their responsibility for understanding and meeting the health needs of the community. The 37 participants from the four countries represented perspectives in medical education, clinical practice, epidemiology, and government.

In their planning, the organizers of the meeting were guided by a series of questions they believed to be relevant in all four countries. How should physicians be educated to respond most effectively to the anticipated health care needs of the population as well as to the needs of individual patients? To what extent is the "social contract of medicine" at odds with or in harmony with the value of diversity in medical education? How do medical schools determine their collective responsibilities and activities? How do medical schools individually and collectively view their obligations for the health of the public? To what extent can medical schools be held accountable for critical problems in health care (e.g., escalating costs, overspecialization, accessibility), and how should they respond when a community is beset by huge problems (an epidemic such as AIDS) and a need to find a system of health care that will provide coverage for all its citizens?

I was delighted to have participated, as President of The Royal Society of Medicine Foundation, in the lively discussion of the excellent papers and critiques presented at the meeting. We commend this volume to you as an important contribution to a vital part of the national debate on health care policy. Hopefully, it will assist you in framing your own questions, or, at least, shaping your beliefs as to the role and mission of the medical school in contributing to the health of the community.

Arthur J. Mahon
President
The Royal Society of Medicine Foundation

Preface

William G. O'Reilly, Executive Director of the Royal Society of Medicine Foundation, Inc., New York (the North American arm of the Royal Society of Medicine), and Thomas H. Meikle, Jr., M.D., President of the Josiah Macy Jr. Foundation, New York, conceived the idea for the Conference resulting in this volume; the latter Foundation financed it. The two sponsors perceived urgent problems facing medical schools in four countries that have similar approaches to medical education, research, and patient care. In their view the present situation warranted an exploration of common themes underlying the malaise besetting medical educators in these countries. Of greater importance was the prospect of collaborating in the search for fundamental changes needed in the preparation of physicians to cope with society's health problems. The Planning Committee for the Conference consisted of

Mutya San Agustin	David S. Greer	David H.H. Metcalfe
Sir Douglas Black	Thomas S. Inui	Victor R. Neufeld
Sir Christopher Booth	Lionel E. McLeod	William G. O'Reilly
Julia E. Connelly	Thomas H. Meikle, Jr.	Robert S. Spasoff
	Kerr L. White (Chair)	

To generate fruitful discussion during the Conference, this Committee, meeting in June 1989, prepared a statement of its principal objectives. These included the need to develop strategies for expanding the medical school's mission to embrace the population perspective, in addition to the biomedical and individual patient–physician perspectives that now dominate most of Western medical education. To this end the Planning Committee drafted five recommendations. In addition to these recommendations, the statement of objectives included possible mechanisms for ensuring their enforcement through examinations, certification, accreditation, and licensure. Such measures should reassure the public that medical schools are indeed being responsive to concerns about its health status and health services. Promulgation of a mission statement by each medical school should relate the faculty's educational, research, and patient care commitments to the present and projected health needs of the populations they serve, and should define the population-based competencies required to accomplish the mission.

The Planning Committee selected the authors and participants; all the first choices accepted. Papers and topics were chosen on the basis of the five possible recommendations drafted by the Committee. The authors and topics selected for the Conference were designed to provide theoretical discussions, illustrative data, and practical examples of approaches to meeting the population's health needs as reflected in the five draft recommendations. The authors' outlines for the papers were reviewed by all members of the Planning Committee and comments returned to them; the first drafts of the full papers were similarly reviewed. Final versions of all the papers, together with three additional written discussions, were circulated to all participants three weeks prior to the meeting. These arrangements assured ample time for informed debate by the 37 participants from the four countries over the four days of the Conference at Turnberry Isle, December 9–12, 1990.

Several authors revised their papers slightly following the meeting and we have edited them by removing most laudatory and redundant passages, maintaining reasonable consistency of style, and using American spelling. The basic messages, together with the three discussants' comments for each contribution, should have survived intact. From reports prepared by eight rapporteurs the editors have distilled, without attribution, additional comments on the issues raised.

The final sets of definitions and recommendations reflect a strong consensus among the Conference Participants; not everyone will agree with every element of each statement but as a body they all endorse the general thrust of the ideas recounted in Chapter 9. If these ideas generate further debate within each of the four countries, and, more importantly, within individual medical schools, this exercise will have achieved its objectives.

Timely cooperation by everyone enabled the editors to prepare the manuscripts for rapid publication. With this and other tasks William O'Reilly, his assistant Betty Chase, and Julia E. Connelly's assistant Dale Vandervoort, provided most effective support. We are grateful to all of them, as well as to our colleagues in this endeavor. We trust our collective efforts will contribute to an international debate about *how*, not *whether*, medical education must change.

Kerr L. White
Julia E. Connelly

Contents

Contributors

ROBERT D. COHEN, M.D.   Professor of Medicine, London Hospital Medical College, University of London, Whitechapel, London El 1BB, England

JOHN D. HAMILTON, M.D.   Dean and Professor of Medicine, Rankin Drive, University of Newcastle, Newcastle, NSW 2308, Australia

THOMAS S. INUI, M.D.   Professor and Head, General Internal Medicine and Professor of Health Services, School of Medicine, 105A Harborview Hall, University of Washington, Seattle, WA 98104, USA

MICHAEL G. MARMOT, M.B., Ph.D.   Professor of Community Medicine, 66-72 Gower Street, University College and Middlesex School of Medicine, London WCIE 6EA, England

DAVID H.H. METCALFE, M.B., B.S.   Professor and Chairman, Department of General Practice, Rusholme Health Centre, Walmer Street, University of Manchester Medical School, Manchester M14 5NP, England

VICTOR R. NEUFELD, M.D.   Director, Centre for International Health and Professor of Medicine and Clinical Epidemiology, HSC-3N44B McMaster University, Hamilton, Ontario L8N 3Z5, Canada

MUTYA SAN AGUSTIN, M.D.   Director, Department of Ambulatory Medicine, North Central Bronx Hospital, 3424 Kossuth Street, Room 4M-08, Montefiore Medical Center, Bronx, NY 10467, USA

ROBERT A. SPASOFF, M.D.   Professor and Chairman, Department of Epidemiology and Community Medicine, 451 Smythe Road, University of Ottawa, Ottawa, Ontario K1H 8M5 Canada

ANTHONY B. ZWI, M.B., Ch.B.   Department of Epidemiology and Public Health, 66-72 Gower Street, University College and Middlesex School of Medicine, London WC1E 6EA, England. Present address: London School of Hygiene, Keppel Street, London WC1E 7HT, England

1
Redefining the Mission of the Medical School

KERR L. WHITE and JULIA E. CONNELLY

I. Introduction

Organizational and institutional turbulence and shrinking academic budgets are buffeting medical schools in both industrialized and developing countries. Current political and public scrutiny is focused on escalating health care expenditures and on the large unexplained variations within and among countries in the rates for use of services and the appropriateness of many interventions.

In spite of medicine's breathtaking advances and a spate of efficacious interventions, societal unrest has increased, both with the medical profession's performance and with the seemingly insatiable demand for resources. Canada, the United Kingdom, the United States (Blendon 1989), and Australia are experiencing a crescendo of public dissatisfaction with their health care arrangements and implicitly with medicine's leadership. Examples of this dissatisfaction include the call for redistribution of health priorities and services in the 1978 WHO/UNICEF Declaration of Alma Ata (Director-General of WHO and Executive Director of UNICEF 1978), the renaissance of primary care and growth of "alternative medicine" movements in response to demands for early care and preventive services, the documentation of wide disparities in health status and use of health services among social classes in Britain (Black 1980), and the publication by the Organization for Economic Co-operation and Development (OECD) of international comparisons of health statistics showing huge variations in expenditures, services, and outcomes (OECD 1990).

Few weeks pass in which the popular press, radio, and television in Canada, the United Kingdom, the United States, and Australia do not carry stories about the inadequacies or costs of their respective health services. Other detailed pieces cover two divergent perspectives of health and disease that confuse the public and lead to unattainable expectations. At one extreme, high technology, now or in the near future, is touted as the source of all efficacious interventions for most bodily ills, if not "answers" for every patient's "problems." At the other extreme, emphasis is placed on the dangers of environmental exposures, and on the need for behavioral or "life-style" changes, adequate exercise, and improved nutritional habits in the interests of disease prevention and health promotion. Balanced presentations that relate the two views are scarce.

In Canada, most provinces recently have established commissions to examine their health care arrangements in response to inequitable distribution of services and rapidly increasing costs. For example, the Saskatchewan Commission on Directions in Health Care has called for a "Consumer-Controlled Health Care System" with local Councils of laypersons determining priorities and allocating resources. It recommends much greater emphasis on "Community and Supportive Living Services," and creation of "an autonomous Health Analysis and Development Commission to monitor and analyze health programs and practices." This new entity is to report directly to the Provincial legislature and to local Health Councils (Saskatchewan Commission on Directions in Health Care 1990). A project entitled "Educating Future Physicians of Ontario" aims "to change medical education . . . so that it is relevant to the requirements of society. The primary objectives are

- To define the future roles of physicians in Ontario in relation to community needs, and to translate these role descriptions into educational objectives for undergraduate medical education in Ontario;
- To prepare educators in Ontario's five medical schools for helping medical students achieve the stated objectives; and
- To design new assessment tools and systems for determining the achievement of the competencies[1] of future Ontario physicians, to be used in Ontario medical schools (Task Force on the Staffing and Funding of Clinical Academic Units 1990).

In the United Kingdom, the Conservative government moving to contain costs has legislated draconian reforms designed to encourage greater efficiency by means of competition among hospitals, tighter fiscal management, and provision of global budgets for large group practices. These measures have the potential for dismantling much of that country's 40-year-old National Health Service, long held in high regard by the general public. The medical profession's traditional autonomy is to be drastically reduced with the government setting the contractual rules and standards. Henceforth there is to be less talk about "inputs" and "activities"; accountability will be determined on the basis of "clinical outcomes" (Klein 1990). All of this is to be accomplished in the absence of an adequate, population-based information system and accompanying analysis (McLachlan 1990).

Commissions spawned by the United States Congress and other bodies have advanced proposals for dealing with national health care arrangements

---

[1]*Competencies: knowledge, skills, and attitudes.* A term used in evaluating outcomes of educational and training endeavors.

in serious disarray. Problems with the United States' "system" have resulted in social tragedies that are rapidly becoming politically intolerable. They include the 15% or more of American citizens who have no health insurance and little access to appropriate medical care, failure to provide long-term insurance and care for the aged, and inadequate community care for the mentally ill. At the same time, the wisdom of recent attempts to improve so-called "health care delivery systems" is being called into question. These measures have included aggressive competitive market strategies, prepayment, capitation, and "incentive" bonus schemes, health maintenance organizations, and myriad other corporate innovations. More specifically, in response to gross imbalances in the provision of generalists and specialists, the majority of training funds in New York state have been shifted from specialty to primary care residencies as recommended by the State Council on Graduate Medical Education (New York State Council on Graduate Education 1988).

In Australia, the Federal government has launched a major review of its health services following recent reviews of medical (Doherty et al. 1988) and public health (White 1986) education.

The problems of health care in each of these countries have multiple origins. Society's expectations, political views on the role of government, vested interests, administrative strategies, and professional intransigence all contribute. Erosion of public trust and confidence in the medical profession are the unhappy consequences; collective disenchantment appears to be at an all-time high. For this state of affairs, the academic branch of the profession must assume much of the responsibility and now has the opportunity to provide renewed leadership. The contributions that follow, therefore, are designed to stimulate discussion and provide concrete examples of strategies for reversing these trends by responding to the public's concerns.

Loss of interest by medical faculties in the health of populations is a twentieth-century phenomenon. In the latter half of the nineteenth century, the London Epidemiological Society, consisting largely of prominent clinicians, numbered among its members such academic luminaries as Richard Bright, Sir Charles Hastings, and T. Clifford Albutt. The titles of papers read before the Society attest to the organization's broad interest in the population's health: "On the Geographical Distribution of Health and Disease in Connection Chiefly with Natural Phenomena," "Suggestions for Utilizing the Statistics of Disease Among the Poor," "On the Diseases and Injuries of Artisans and Labourers, Traceable to Their Respective Occupations," and "On the Present Position and Prospects of Epidemiological Science" (Epidemiological Society of London 1901).

In 1832, a group of America's foremost physicians with postgraduate training in France founded the Society for Medical Observation, which, like the London Society, was modeled after a similar entity organized in France by Pierre-Charles-Alexandre Louis (1787–1872), the brilliant clinician who originated the *méthode numérique*. This society foundered shortly after creation in 1908 of the American Society for Clinical Investigation, largely by physicians whose training was in German bacteriological laboratories. A subtle "paradigm shift" occurred at this juncture. Medicine's broad perspective encompassing populations and the environment, as well as individuals, was supplanted by a much narrower reductionist approach dominated by preoccupation with bacteria and the "germ theory" of disease.

Meticulous clinical observation and use of quantitative methods were superseded rapidly by intense obsession with laboratory investigations to unravel disease processes and mechanisms in individual patients. This undeniably successful strategy resulted in the biomedical revolution that eventually ensued and great benefits have accrued to society. There have been unintended negative perturbations, however, as academic medicine lost touch with the common medical problems that plague most populations. Many argue that too much of medicine's efforts have been directed at conditions of relatively low frequency. In the meantime, the study of group phenomena and of patterns surrounding the occurrence of disease in populations has waned. It is now time to redress the balance and restore the broader vision that once informed the missions of the profession and its medical schools.

For at least two decades, national and international bodies have documented inequalities in health status and health services within and among countries. They have called for "more involvement with primary care," have proposed that medical education be more "community oriented" and "population based," and have urged medical faculties to establish closer associations with "the community's health problems" and conduct more "essential health research" (Royal Society of Medicine and Josiah H. Macy Jr. Foundation 1973; Gastel and Rogers 1988; World Federation for Medical Education 1988; Commission on Health Research for Development 1990). Yet the problems persist. Grafting onto the curriculum a few lectures on statistics, epidemiology, and the environment, or hiring a few social scientists has not worked; the grafts have not taken. A much more intensive and focused effort is needed to facilitate the kinds of change that will improve the health and health care of the public. The place to start is by redefining the mission of the medical school.

II. Opportunities and Challenges

Realistically, medical schools today have little choice but to respond constructively to the population's needs; yet few elect to do so. Some schools continue to debate whether or not their faculties and students should embrace a balanced, broad view of the health enterprise that includes the population perspective[2] as well as the individual patient–physician and biomedical perspectives. All three, but especially the individual patient–physician and population perspectives, are frequently linked through population medicine.[3] Others, however, have moved on to questions about the most useful strategies for achieving a balanced set of goals. If medical schools and their affiliated institutions are to provide appropriate types and numbers of physicians to meet the population's health needs, what assumptions should govern the choices, what principles should be considered, and what information is needed? How are these needs to be identified and their relative importance measured? Who should do this? What are the respective roles of universities (and their medical faculties), professional organizations (colleges, accrediting bodies, specialty societies, and certifying boards), licensing authorities, and governmental entities in making these choices? In particular, what institutional and professional competencies are required to make medical graduates—and future physicians—more responsive to the citizens' perceived individual and collective needs? Such questions provide the rationale for the contributions that follow.

The four countries' major medical bodies, i.e., the American, Australian, British, and Canadian Medical Associations, are dominated by practitioners—often generalists. Their influence on educational policy varies within each country but is, for the most part, modest. In the United States especially, and in Canada, but to a lesser extent in Australia and Great Britain, academics determine research agendas and provide leadership for most professional colleges, specialty organizations, and associations. More often than not, academic specialists and subspecialists control virtually all the nodal points at which critical professional decisions are made. As a consequence, decisions by faculty members and representatives of medical schools, teaching hospitals, and diverse credentialling bodies drive the profession's collective response to the people's health problems and health services. And how are the health needs of the population now identified? How are the research, educational, and clinical service agendas of the medical profession now set? All too often these tasks are defined narrowly by the faculties' limited experiences within tertiary care hospitals. Rarely, at least until comparatively recently, have medical schools begun to assess the health needs of the populations surrounding them. Rarely have their faculties deliberately attempted to design appropriate strategies to ensure that those needs are met (Eisenberg 1990).

---

[2]*Population Perspective: The capacity to appreciate the determinants, ranges, and variations of health status and disease in the entire community.* Terms such as Population Health, Health of Populations, and Public Health also employ the Population Perspective as an organizing concept.

Population Medicine: The application of those concepts and methods embodied in such largely quantitative disciplines as epidemiology, economics, demography, and statistics, and in such behavioral sciences as cultural anthropology, sociology, and social psychology. Population-based medicine is an analogous term.

To whom should members of a community turn when they are not satisfied with, for example, their health status, their relationships with physicians, the excessive use of technology to prolong life in defiance of the wishes of patients and their families, widespread disparities among different populations in the rates for common, and not-so-common, surgical procedures and medical prescriptions, aggressive investigative searches for low-probability conditions, inequities in the availability of health care, and the unjust allocation of scarce resources? Some look to health departments or equivalent statutory entities, while others look to medical societies and professional colleges, or to local consumer advocacy groups concerned with health matters. Pressure to attend to these problems now is increasingly directed to medical schools and their faculties.

Every physician has some responsibility to provide leadership. Academic physicians in particular have unique opportunities to assume these roles on behalf of all physicians. It is the faculty who select the students to become the physicians of the future; it is they who supervise medical education; it is they who help to shape the values and viewpoints of medical students; it is they who recruit housestaffs. Teachers' attitudes, values, and behavior, whether by intent or not, can be used to guide, broaden, or narrow their students' perspectives. As a result, each faculty member's viewpoints, priorities, and examples can support or detract from students' interest in the full range of health problems and issues society expects the profession to address.

Today, the opportunity has never been greater for medical schools and the medical profession as a whole to regain the public's trust and confidence in responding to all their medical needs and in assisting society to solve its many health problems. As a first step in understanding the origins of the profession's mandate, we need to understand that an implicit social contract exists between medicine and the public it serves. The notion of the social contract, fostered by Locke and Rousseau and expanded by Jefferson, covers many of society's unwritten agreements with those who seek to serve it. Welcome or not, medical schools are among the institutions on which the social contract is binding.

For its part, society endows the medical profession, and particularly its academic component, with enormous influence, substantial resources, unequalled status, and generous financial rewards. In turn, the profession, led by its medical faculties, can reasonably be expected to help identify, understand, and ameliorate the population's individual and collective health problems. These relationships are based on a social contract; no other profession has this mandate or these expectations. The latter's very existence seems unknown to many, as others challenge its validity.

To the extent that a social contract has existed in the minds of the medical profession's leaders, it has gradually unraveled in all four countries since World War II. Bismarck's introduction of social insurance in Germany a century ago, one of the contract's earliest tangible expressions, should have alerted the profession to its responsibilities as a major beneficiary of this innovation. Instead, there has been a long history of resistance to governmental control of medical care payment mechanisms. But in every confrontation the profession has had to retreat sooner or later and public dissatisfaction with the profession has increased. It follows, then, that the first step in any strategy for change should be to promote collective understanding of the nature of the contractual relationship the profession has with society. Everything else follows from that. Medical faculties should accept fully society's mandate to foster more effective relationships with patients and the populations they serve. In the Chapter 2 this implicit social contract is subjected to extensive scrutiny.

Medicine, together with law, following the example set by their professional schools, must surely be one of a diminishing number of "service" professions and social enterprises that responds to the public's expectations with what some take to be an "elitist" approach. Other successful service organizations start with "market" and demographic surveys, to use commercial jargon, with opinion polls, to use political language, or with population-based or catchment area surveys, to use epidemiological terminology. A helping profession seeking to serve the people should start with careful analyses of the public's individual and collective problems, especially when it is they who do the suffering and pay the bills. The definition of the population served (for example, the municipality, county, district, province, state, nation, region, or the world) and assessment of its health problems are prerequisites for determining priorities and planning medical education, clinical research, and health services.

III. Limitations of Traditional Approaches

In most biomedical research—especially that done in clinical departments—the prevailing approach can be expressed as the unspoken right of each investigator to decide the important questions based on his or her own curiosity and interest. Granted, the investigator's curiosity drives all successful research. But, especially in clinical (as contrasted to fundamental or basic) research, should not the importance of the health problem to the population also be a major consideration? Today, in contrast to the days of the London Epidemiological Society, for example, the community's health and social problems attract the interests of far too few physicians and health care institutions, especially medical schools. There is no reason to believe that institutional responses to social need and investigator responses to scientific curiosity are mutually exclusive. Achievement of coordination and balance, however, does require that each school develop an explicit mission statement.

Medical faculties too often tend to adopt a "top-down" approach in structuring their educational, research, and service agendas. If this view is to be superseded by more person-oriented and community-based perspectives each faculty will need to consider how the relative importance of society's health problems is to be determined. Measures will be needed for the extent of pain, suffering, and disability together with their personal and monetary costs. And each medical school will need to determine how best to use this information for setting educational, research, and service priorities. The community's health and related social problems demand much more attention than they are currently accorded by medical schools if medicine is to fulfill its part of the social contract. All this needs to be done with population-based numbers.

A wide array of population-based health statistics available internationally, nationally, and locally now enable the public and politicians to question both the authoritative and authoritarian aspects of the medical profession's role. As illustrated in Chapters 3 and 4 most of these statistics cover the nature and distribution of health problems and services. Others assess the outcomes of interventions in relation to types and appropriateness of health services. Much more information is on the way. This exponential increase in credible "health intelligence" about the relative benefits, risks, and costs of medical interventions is being published in the lay press as well as in professional journals. The notion that the medical school alone is the last court of appeal and the keeper of the "gold standard" for the profession is being challenged by those who prefer to invoke other sets of "facts" about the population's health. This shift recognizes that it is no longer valid to give greater credibility to anecdotes about "individuals"—the medical profession's patients—than to "numbers" that aggregate the population's collective problems, experiences, and health status. The numbers, or health statistics as they are known in medical circles, in the memorable words of the late Major Greenwood, the eminent British statistician, "represent people with the tears wiped off." As numeracy catches up with literacy, numbers become just as vivid indicators of the human condition as accounts of individual suffering.

The profession now has an opportunity to use this vast array of information to guide medical education and research, to design strategies for improving the health of the public, and to attend to their pressing health care needs. Balance is required both between society's needs and investigators' curiosity and between academicians' preoccupations and the duty to provide medical students with appropriate skills for coping with the full range of society's medical problems. To achieve this balance, each Faculty will need to redefine its mission, realign the tasks of its members, and, perhaps, change its composition.

The helping and caring functions of the physician have been adumbrated temporarily by the proliferation of technological procedures—many of dubious efficacy. The unquestioning trust of many patients in their personal physicians has helped to bolster the profession's belief that the public collectively has remained confident and supportive. In addition, medical schools have come to assume and expect the public's undiluted confidence and trust; they have tended to believe that they derive from this an almost limitless authority. To restore the public's trust, medicine must reestablish itself as the public's advocate. This will require the reintroduction into medical education of population-based concepts and skills to balance those required in traditional patient–physician relationships. Such measures are most likely to foster constructive attitudes and broader perspectives in future physicians. Achievement of these objectives involves not only redefining the mission of the medical school but practical changes in the context in which medical education takes place, as well as in the priorities assigned to each component of the content. Some schools have adopted innovative, population-based, problem-oriented approaches to understanding and responding to the health and medical needs of the local citizenry and society generally. Practical examples of these strategies are discussed in Chapters 4 and 5.

IV. Contemporary Developments Favoring Change

In spite of our current problems, there are grounds for optimism. If social, financial, and political pressures are deemed insufficient, five contemporary developments in medicine are allies in the urgent quest for needed change (White 1991). Although many medical school faculties are contributing to these developments, few have formally taken inventory of those bits and pieces that presage the need for major shifts in institutional perspectives and priorities. This is especially true for the medical curriculum.

First, there is the *information revolution*. Information comes from many sources, such as observations, experiments, analyses, syntheses, books, journals, bibliographies, and statistics. All are essential if the profession is to respond appropriately to individual and collective health needs, but filters are required to do this effectively and efficiently (Hardin 1985). One filter involves the skills of critical appraisal. Based on statistical and epidemiological concepts and methods, these skills should be applied vigorously and rigorously to evaluate most types of information, especially those involving interventions and maneuvers designed to do "good." Computer searches of the medical literature, analyses of databases, and exposure to the scientific and popular media provide professionals and the public alike with ready access to medical advances and information. An avalanche of publications threatens the health enterprise with distracting noise that drowns out the few nuggets of credible knowledge and the even rarer glimpses of wisdom. In turn, it can scarcely be overemphasized that newspapers, popular magazines, radio, and television regularly carry extended pieces on medical matters. Increasingly well-informed populations ask probing questions about the efficacy, risks, availability, appropriateness, and costs of medical care.

Another filter also uses epidemiology and statistics (especially health statistics, in contrast to biostatistics) to illuminate the nature, extent, and locus of health problems. There is growing familiarity on the part of clinical faculty with the statistical methods applied to laboratory studies, but much less familiarity with the use of statistical concepts, especially probabilistic thinking, in setting goals and objectives for education, research, and service. Health statistics are based on the adequacy and accuracy of clinical information, including diagnostic labels at all levels of care. These data elements are aggregated into the health statistics that are essential for guiding equitable resource allocation and for evaluating and managing health services.

Suitable filters can array a population's health statistics to show, for example, the rank order of population-based rates by diagnostic or problem labels and by age, sex, and occupational groupings of such measures as days in pain, days in bed, disability days, hospital days, work or school days lost, tests, prescriptions, procedures, etc. By this means, rates for both small and large geographic areas can be compared over time and place. Institutional and educational goals can then be set to respond to the target population's health problems in a timely and reasonably objective fashion. Medical faculties can now replace rhetoric and precedence with quantitative evidence as the basis for defining the school's mission. The *information revolution* is bound to extend and strengthen the scientific base of the health enterprise and hasten the need for redefining the medical schools' mission to include appropriate attention to the population's collective health problems.

The second ally is our increasing awareness that just as "information" concerns the message, "communication" concerns the messenger. Both are important—hence the need for wider and better *communication*. Reading, writing, and talking face-to-face or through computers, videos, telecommunications, and "hard copy" are means of communication. So are listening, observing, touching, counselling, and explaining. Interpersonal transactions are the core of most communication in the health field at both the individual and population levels. There is renewed interest in the patient–physician relationship and growing recognition that effective diagnosis, treatment, and management require meaningful bilateral communication. This must include physicians' awareness of the ubiquitous power of two phenomena that present-day medicine, in contrast to commerce and industry, largely ignore. The first is the Placebo Effect, i.e., the capacity of a physician's ministrations, or of any non-specific intervention, to evoke subjective and physiological responses in patients. The second is the Hawthorne Effect, i.e., the behavioral responses of patients and others to institutional or organizational "caring" in many different dimensions. Both are prerequisites for fulfilling the tasks of all health professionals. Through exposure to the humanities, many student physicians whose medical education is technologically oriented become familiar with the therapeutic powers of "hope" and "caring." They also become familiar with the extraordinary diversity of the human condition and its expression on a continuum extending from "health" to "disease." There seems little doubt that both individuals and the public are insisting that the medical profession respond more sensitively and sensibly to their perceived personal and collective needs. The prospect of improved *communication* of all types is bound to require medical schools to redefine their missions to include concerns for populations as well as for the individuals comprising them.

The third ally is our growing knowledge of genetics and the immune system—the era of *molecular biology*. The vast (and controversial) enterprise to map the human genome is regarded as the contemporary equivalent for health of the Manhattan Project. A full assessment of the medical and social impacts of such a quantum leap in our knowledge of where we start, how we are circumscribed by our inheritance, and how we must live to achieve the potential of our "talents" is not appropriate here. Nevertheless, the implications of this project are truly revolutionary, not only for medical interventions, but also for behavioral, educational, nutritional, occupational, and especially environmental modifications. Physicians, employers, educators, the public, and politicians all will need to cope with this potentially promising new penetration into the origins, boundaries, and potentials of life itself.

To understand the genetic heritage that characterizes individual and collective health risks a population-based perspective is essential. As the human genome is mapped, molecular biology must surely turn increasingly to the study of populations. Genetic surveys of families and communities whose health status may be at risk for certain diseases will need to be conducted if the nature, extent, and prospects for prevention are to be appreciated fully. Assessment of "vulnerability factors" such as inheritance of oncogenes or genetic predisposition to major mental illnesses are examples of important applications. Further advances will mean that we can move from describing disease processes to understanding the substrate from which "good" and "ill" health arise. Of equal concern will be societal and professional debates on, for example, the ethical aspects of fetal research and genetic engineering to determine what action we take based on this accumulating knowledge. These considerations alone are bound to involve surveys of the public's views, the relative, costs, risks, and benefits of interventions as well as population-based estimates of the prevalence of the conditions under discussion.

We have long talked about host, environment, and agent, but in spite of Pasteur's pioneering efforts, the bulk of that talk in medical circles during the past half-century has been about the agents—bugs and worms. During recent decades interest has turned much more to the other two components of the triad. In addition to our genetic inheritance, there is the matter of exposure to a wide variety of animate and inanimate stimuli that condition each individual's reactions to subsequent exposures. Appreciation of the way he or she perceives and responds to these exposures and experiences may become more important than identifying the exposures themselves.

The powerful new field of psychoneuroimmunology (an unfortunately cumbersome term), aided and abetted by the neurosciences and the behavioral sciences, is now codifying both the characteristics of diverse stimuli and the pathways through which they are mediated. The nature, frequency, and perception of these stimuli are being studied at the individual level. Similarly, stimuli affecting groups of individuals, including poverty, unemployment (or the threat of it), natural disasters, occupational stress, managerial style, domestic strife, and even the utterances of charismatic leaders, need to be measured and factored into the establishment of health priorities. "Training," and perhaps learning to "control" the immune system, is likely to increase in importance as knowledge of the factors governing it grows, but we are only at the threshold of untold possibilities. The rapidly unfolding insights provided by *molecular biology* are bound to require clarification of the medical school's mission so that studies of individual patients are related to problems experienced by entire populations and subgroups of those populations.

The fourth ally is the growing societal and political concern with the state of the *environment*—locally, regionally, and globally. There is not only increasing awareness of the environment's impact on the public's health, but recognition that the environment is probably the most malleable of all possible points for intervention. The potential for changes in our genetic heritage will remain limited, at least during the foreseeable future. Human behavior, unquestionably the most important factor to change, is also the most difficult. For some time we have known that occupational and general environmental hazards are major determinants of health status. The range of known factors extends from exposure to toxic substances, shift-work, and job insecurity, through air, water, food, radiation, and even visual and auditory pollution, to global warming. Social planning to modify and improve the *environment*, as well as to protect the vulnerable, should include the medical profession's active participation. This will undoubtedly require that medical schools redefine their missions to include study of the wide range of environments to which populations and patients are exposed.

The fifth ally is the *managerial era* now being imposed on virtually all health services; the days of the solo practitioner are over. The emphasis has shifted from concerns about "inputs" of resources and reports of "activities" such as numbers of visits to doctors, X-rays taken, and tests ordered to measures of results achieved based on medical audit, quality assurance, functional outcomes, and value for money. These changes have spawned new types of "corporate" practice that include group practices, health centers, consortia, networks, foundations, "systems," and other organizational configurations. Governments at all levels, as well as small clusters of practicing professionals, are now believed to require "managers" responsible for deploying resources and assessing clinical and financial performances. Their activities, in turn, are guided and governed by relatively new fields such as health services research, health systems research, clinical epidemiology, technology assessment, medical audit, outcomes research, and cost–benefit, cost–effectiveness, and decision analyses. All these use quantitative methods and population-based concepts. All are concerned with greatly increased professional accountability and what the seventeenth-century Oxford Professor of Anatomy, founding father of epidemiology and economics, Sir William Petty (1623–1687), called "political arithmetic."

In this new era the individual practitioner no longer has access to unlimited resources and unexamined professional freedom. Rules, regulations, public accountability, supervision, and management—all based on "information"—now define and constrain the environment in which physicians will operate in the future. If medical graduates are to participate responsibly in both shaping this climate and cooperating effectively with colleagues in the *managerial era*, medical schools will have to redefine their missions. For responding to society's calls for help they will need to guide the medical enterprise by means of continuing assessment of the population's health status and priorities.

V. Conclusions

These five developments, accompanied by renegotiation of medicine's social contract with the public, have great potential for expanding the perspectives of the biomedical sciences. They will also alter the contemporary paradigm constraining the profession's vision. This, in turn, requires medicine to expand its horizons to encompass not only cells, organs, and individual patients, but entire populations and the circumstances in which they live, become ill, recover, or die. This new vision will need to be shared widely among physicians, administrators, politicians, and society as the medical school proceeds to redefine its mission. Cooperation among all the interested parties is a prerequisite for achieving balanced and integrated systems of medical education, research, and services. Without such vision and cooperation, fragmented, divergent, and unbalanced strategies for all three modalities are likely to persist, thereby obstructing appropriate professional responses to the full array of society's health needs.

For example, in the United States, and to a lesser extent in Canada, there is growing awareness that the imbalance between generalists and specialists limits the access of all citizens to early, compassionate, science-based, cost-effective care. Many more appropriately trained general physicians are required to sort out patients' initial symptoms and complaints. These physicians should be competent to manage 90–95% of the initial problems presented to them without resorting to costly and often unproductive investigations. There is critical need for earlier recognition of such common conditions as potentially chronic or disabling cardiac and respiratory disorders, accident proneness, masked depression, and childhood behavioral problems. Countless visits involve somatic complaints—backaches, headaches, and other musculoskeletal disorders—that, more often than not, have some association with psychological, occupational, or domestic stress requiring early attention. Loneliness, alcoholism, drug dependency, child abuse, sexual ignorance and dysfunction, to name the more commonplace, abound in general populations. Both the appropriateness of training and the ratios of generalists to specialists determine the profession's capacity to respond to such problems.

In Australia and the United Kingdom, where the general practitioner is the backbone of the National Health Service, the ratio of generalists to specialists is about three to one; in the United States the situation is the reverse; and in Canada it is about one to one. In all four countries, the attitudes of faculty members, the teaching venues, the content of education, and the conceptual context in which education, research, and care take place determine the mix of doctors entering the profession's ranks each year. Every medical school will be faced with questions about its priorities for educating generalists *vis-à-vis* specialists—and then for determining the mix of specialists. Political and governmental incentives—often financial—for training generalists and help from the media to enhance their image could help to shift the distribution dramatically. But in all this a resort to population-based information should enlighten the debates and inform these decisions as the medical school redefines its mission.

What then is the mission of the medical school? It was Albert Einstein who observed that the greatest difficulty confronting the twentieth century revolved around the persistent ambiguity of our "goals" even as we perfect the "means" to achieve them. Preoccupation with mechanisms of disease and the processes of health care, particularly the advent of each new technology, seems to overshadow the ability to set goals designed to meet the public's needs. Fresh ways of thinking about the problems and new institutional and individual competencies will be demanded of both faculty and students. Recognition of the population's needs provides the justification for Chapters 7 and 8 and their specific proposals for redefining the mission of the medical school to encompass concerns for the entire population's health.

Rudolf Virchow (1821–1902) asserted that "medicine is a social science, and politics nothing but medicine on a large scale." Redefining the mission of the medical school will require political activity—in the best sense of the term—on several fronts. This includes medical school politics, as well as local and national politics. Individual medical schools can take initiatives to prepare and promulgate specific mission statements; public pressure through the media can be brought to bear on those institutions that fall short of societal expectations; political and governmental influence can be directed toward achieving the shared vision that is essential for success. Leverage also can be exerted through institutional requirements set by bodies such as the General Medical Council in Britain, the Accreditation Committee of the Australian Medical Council, and the Liaison Committee on Medical Education of the American and Canadian Medical Associations, the Association of American Medical Colleges, and the Association of Canadian Medical Colleges. In addition to the latter two organizations, the National Board of Medical Examiners in the United States, all the Royal Colleges in Britain, Australia, and Canada, and the various medical specialty boards and societies can set examination and entrance requirements that ensure the attainment of specified competencies. Finally, the British Parliament, the Australian, and Canadian Parliaments and the respective State and Provincial Legislatures, the United States Congress and State Legislatures can hold hearings, legislate, and use the power of the purse. In all of this, medical schools should remember that in every previous renegotiation of the social contract with the profession, society has always won. There is every reason to believe that in resolving the problems and issues we have raised, society will win again.

Acknowledgments. The authors gratefully acknowledge the helpful criticisms of the Planning Committee members, and Eugene C. Corbett, Jr., David S. Fedson, and Marcia Finney.

References

Blendon, R.J. 1989. Three systems: A comparative survey. *Health Management Quart* **11**:2–14.

Black, D. 1980. *Inequalities in Health*: *Report of a Research Working Group*. (*The Black Report*). London: Department of Health and Social Services; or Townsend, P and Davidson, N. 1982. *Inequalities in Health*: *The Black Report*. Harmondsworth: Penguin Books.

Commission on Health Research for Development. 1990. *Health Research*: *Essential Link to Equity in Development*. New York and Oxford: Oxford University Press.

Director-General of the World Health Organization and Executive Director of the United Nations Children's Fund. 1978. *Primary Health Care*. Geneva and New York: WHO and UNICEF.

Doherty, R.L., et al.. 1988. *Australian Medical Education and Workforce into the 21st Century. Report of the Committee of Inquiry into Medical Education and Medical Workforce*. Canberra: Australian Government Publishing Service.

Eisenberg, L. 1990. From circumstance to mechanism in pediatrics during the Hopkins century. *Pediatrics* **85**:42–49.

Epidemiological Society of London. 1901. *The Commemoration Volume*: *Containing An Account of the Foundation of the Society and an Index of the Papers Read at its Meetings Between 1855–1900*. London: Shaw and Sons.

Gastel, B., and Rogers, D.E. (Eds.). 1989. *Adapting Clinical Medical Education to the Needs of Today and Tomorrow*: *Proceedings of the Josiah Macy, Jr. Foundation National Seminar on Medical Education*. New York: New York Academy of Medicine.

Hardin, G. 1985. *Filters Against Folly*. New York: Penguin Books.

Klein, R. 1990. From status to contract: The transformation of the British medical profession. Paper presented at the Anglo-American Symposium, University of North Carolina, May 17–19.

McLachlan, G. 1990. *What Price Quality? The NHS in Review*. Rock Carling Fellowship 1990. London: Nuffield Provincial Hospitals Trust.

New York State Council on Graduate Medical Education. *First Annual Report*. 1988. Albany: State Health Department.

Organization for Economic Co-operation and Development. 1990. *Health Care Systems in Transition: The Search for Efficiency*, OECD Social Policy Studies No.7. Paris: OECD.

The Royal Society of Medicine and the Josiah H. Macy Jr., Foundation. 1973. *The Greater Medical Profession: Report of a Jointly Sponsored Symposium*. New York: The Josiah H. Macy Jr., Foundation.

Saskatchewan Commission on Directions in Health Care. 1990. *Future Directions for Health Care in Saskatchewan*. Regina: Saskatchewan Department of Health, Public Affairs Branch.

Task Force on the Staffing and Funding of Clinical Academic Units. 1990. *Conceptual Framework for Clinical Academic Units in Ontario Faculties of Medicine and Affiliated Teaching Hospitals/Academic Health Centres*. (Working Draft) Toronto: Ministry of Health.

White, K.L. 1986. *Australia's Bicentennial Health Initiative: Independent Review of Research and Educational Requirements for Public Health and Tropical Health in Australia*. 1986. Canberra: Commonwealth Department of Health.

White, K.L. 1991. *Healing the Schism: Epidemiology, Medicine, and the Public's Health*. New York and Heidelberg: Springer-Verlag.

World Federation for Medical Education. 1988. *World Conference on Medical Education Report (7–12 August, 1988)*. Edinburgh: World Federation for Medical Education.

Discussion

David S. Greer

"Redefining the Mission of the Medical School" is a call for revolution in Canada, the United Kingdom, the United States, and Australia. Its strength is in the accurate and incisive identification of current problems; its weakness is in the forces it identifies as available for the struggle against the formidable defenders of the status quo. In the final analysis, it relies on the rationality and civility of the establishment that, in the presence of better information and improved communication, will see the error of its ways and reform from within; history provides little support for such optimism.

The historical review that comprises the first half of the chapter apparently inspires confidence in the authors that the time is now ripe for change. I find it depressing; it is an account of opportunities shunned, pressures resisted, and humanitarian needs ignored by a self-centered academic-professional elite. I find no basis for the authors' statement that, "Realistically, medical schools today have little choice but to respond constructively to the population's needs." Indeed, a broad view of the profession in 1990 reveals little consensus on the role of academic faculties and practitioners in addressing those needs. Some argue that the problems are fundamentally economic, social, cultural, or political and therefore outside the purview of medicine; education in these areas is often regarded as "political" or ideological and therefore inappropriate in an "objective" scientific community.

It is therefore significant that the authors omit political or economic pressure from their list of potential solutions and rely, instead, on "contemporary developments" that they perceive as "allies in the urgent quest for needed change." To me, they appear to be weak allies, if indeed they are allies at all.

The Information Revolution has certainly expanded and improved the population database. But sufficient information to document societal need has existed for decades without substantial response from the academic or professional sectors. Self-interest has generally triumphed over communal altruism, as it does in most human endeavors.

Improved communication, the authors' second ally, is a two-edged sword: trumpeting the latest "miracle cure" derived from reductionist biological research may more effectively mobilize the support of the masses than appeals to their communal instincts, particularly in these days of relative atrophy of the latter tendencies.

It seems odd to me that authors' count molecular biology as an ally. Granted its value, I had always thought of it as the enemy, not to be destroyed but rather to be constrained. To make molecular biology an ally, somewhat strained second-order thinking is required that relates it to societal issues. I have detected no tendency to such extension of the field among molecular biologists or its advocates. Similarly, the interest of the academic community in environmental issues, the authors' fourth ally, has been primarily focused on biological aspects; there is a notable absence of career physicians in environmental programs and advocacy agencies, and the environment is almost totally unrepresented in medical school curricula except as it relates to disciplinary interests, e.g., passive exposure to tobacco smoke in cardiology and pulmonology.

Finally, the managers of health services that I know have minimal interest in "population-based concepts," except as they may affect market share and profit. Managers, by definition, make neither policy nor revolutions. They respond to the needs of their sponsors, in this case the profession, and at best they compromise those needs only as a means to the achievement of their sponsors' ends; thus, the focus on consumer satisfaction as important to the welfare of the providers.

I do not fault the authors for their reluctance to face the unpleasant and inevitably stormy consequences of their call for revolutionary change. It is difficult to develop successful revolutions, to feel confident that the strenuous methods required will produce the desired improvements rather than chaos and retrogression. Despite the authors' assertions to the contrary, this may be a particularly bad time to effect radical change in our four countries: the dominant mood seems egocentric, individualistic, complacent, and antirevolutionary to many observers. Where will the self-sacrificing leadership come from? In Leon Eisenberg's words, "Rudolf Virchow: Where Are You

Now That We Need You?" How does one generate successful revolutions and dedicated revolutionaries? And, if those appeared, would they inspire or frighten us?

John D. Hamilton

Abraham Flexner in his report on Medical Education in the United States and Canada spent much of his time establishing the prime importance of a scientific foundation for medical education, for the involvement of teachers in research, and for students to learn from the direct experience of the care of patients in teaching hospitals. Then right at the end of the section on the proper basis of medical education he extends the scope of a doctors' role in this interesting commentary:

Scientific progress has greatly modified his ethical responsibility. His relation was formally to his patient—at the most to his patient's family; and it was almost altogether remedial . . . but the physician's function is fast becoming social and preventive, rather than individual and curative. Upon him society relies to ascertain, and through measures essentially educational enforce, the conditions that prevent disease and make positively for physical and moral well-being. It goes without saying that this type of doctor is first of all an educated man.

I have, on occasions, used that 1910 quotation without at first defining its source. It has been acclaimed as a fine and modern perception of medicine.

White and Connelly have correctly identified several new spheres of learning and technology that underpin an expansion in the role of medicine to the health of the population. The new role has some affinity with the role defined by Flexner. While this volume has to do with the role of the medical school, that is subservient to the role of medicine and of doctors within it. And here is necessarily a major challenge:

* The reorientation and expansion of the scope of medicine has to confront the issue of whether all of these new skills can be encompassed within a single profession. Alternatively, should the profession develop streams of expertise not only in final career paths (itself poorly developed and a problem in its own right) but also in the undergraduate sphere. We are familiar with selective experience through electives, but by and large medicine has stuck to the principle that there is one comprehensive, basic medical education. There are exceptions: for instance the People's Republic of China trains a Public Health doctor in parallel with a clinical doctor. Unfortunately the Public Health doctor is regarded as second best and the same might happen to a Population Health doctor. But it might be managed otherwise by admissions criteria, career path, and distinction of the degree.
* While doctors may well need an awareness of management, information science, health statistics, and health economics, should they become experts in these fields? It is more likely that other professions will carry the

main burden of the technical, if not the policy, roles built on these disciplines. So should there be an interlocking between the training of those professions and the training of doctors? We talk about this as between the traditional health professions although we do not make much of a fist at it. If we are to attempt the same with this much broader sweep of professions we will have to build quite different links within our universities. The World Health Organization called for universities to play a comprehensive role in primary health care, recognizing the importance of management, environmental sciences, and the social sciences. The list of professions and disciplines relevant to health and welfare is almost endless. If well-founded and sufficient medical education were to require both interrelations with the other professions and also a substantial academic base and practical experience in these wider fields then the length of the course, the complexity of relations with other disciplines and the size and profile of the medical faculty would have to expand greatly. Flexner stressed the need to go to the reality of experience to learn medicine—to the laboratory and bedside. So for these wider fields, students would need comparable experience in management information systems and the analysis and change of the physical and social environment of society. Both the academic and the logistic requirements of this are enormous and for small schools the resources may just not be available. Flexner consigned many small schools to the wall for just that reason.

- The authors speak of the opportunity of medicine to seize again a leadership role. Perhaps they have underestimated the role of those outside of the profession in the shaping of medicine. Abraham Flexner, Aneurin Bevan, and Florence Nightingale are striking examples. Maybe our consciousness of our professional role and its tendency to introversion stops us from liberating ourselves for the future.
- We may have become hidebound by our prescriptions for a basic medical qualification and its preparation for the gate-way internship. Should we be more creative and seek the appropriate background for these new roles in Population Health. Perhaps we should look to select for medical school those who already have management and other basic experience. Or perhaps we should reorder the sequence of medical education. The challenge of real management and real data analysis occurs only after a graduate has taken responsibility for patients. Maybe that is the time to concentrate on the new skills; and not just for those going into medical administration but for all doctors irrespective of their individual professional aspirations.
- And that leads to a final point that all plans will wither if there is not a clear-cut career pathway or a career profile that will allow these new skills and priorities to be realized. Careers must include academic as well as service careers and they must be founded on intensive research and scholarship. These are the old principles of Flexner brought to a new context. Perhaps if he had more time, he may have written this himself.

David A. Shaw

None will argue with the general thrust of the statement by the authors of this chapter. None will deny that the medical profession has an obligation to meet as best it may the needs of the society that it serves and by which it is supported. In teasing out the threads of the arguments on which the statement is based it is important that its coherence should not be diminished. But it raises a number of interesting and fundamental questions that are worthy of exploration. Some relate to definitions and divisions of responsibility and others to educational concepts and principle.

It is self-evident, although readily forgotten, that the quality of tomorrow's health services will depend in large measure on the students of today—on their selection, their education, and their attitudes. It will depend also on the scope and success of today's research, much of it undertaken in or in association with medical schools, and its translation into the clinical practice of tomorrow. The responsibility of the medical schools is thus paramount and the need for them to respond to the changing circumstances and expectations of society is undeniable. But their capacity to take responsibility for the political and financial manipulation of social change is less certain and probably differs in the four countries. In the United Kingdom the setting of priorities in health care and the allocation of resources are the business of the National Health Service (NHS) rather than the faculties of medicine and the NHS has a major role in the funding of postgraduate and continuing medical education. That is not to deny the growing recognition of the importance of a firm partnership between the NHS and the medical schools both in educational matters and in service provision.

Of more fundamental importance is the view that a medical school takes of itself as a seat of learning for the promotion of scholarship, for the encouragement of liberal and creative thinking, and for the provision of opportunities for curiosity-led research. Education that is utilitarian, emphatically vocational, and sensitive to short-term manpower requirements does not reflect the traditional concepts of a university. These concepts are, of course, under serious threat and at least partial surrender to pragmatism and commercialization has been inevitable.

As regards research, while there is much to be said for the development of a strategic approach to research in methods of health service provision, the notion of directed research in other areas is highly controversial. In such a program, it is possible that the benefits of molecular biology, rightly seen as a contemporary development of outstanding importance, might have eluded us.

Implicit in the argument for a more "population-based" medical education is a plea for increased emphasis on prevention. Attention is drawn in the chapter to the relative neglect of epidemiological research and it is justifiably attributed to the counterattractions of other areas of science, many involving exciting and challenging technological developments. There are the additional reasons that epidemiological research is often slow in its returns and problems of funding may prove a disincentive. But perhaps more important is the uncertainty of outcome in terms of practical application. Some would argue that interventions are justifiable only when the experimental evidence on which they are based is beyond dispute and their effectiveness is clearly demonstrable. Such high standards of proof are not required by all and some would justify the introduction of prevention programs on "the balance of probability" in the belief that scientific certainty is seldom if ever achievable. There is the added deterrent that in our present state of knowledge success in bringing about change in patterns of human behavior in absence of immediately obvious gain is highly problematical. Controversies in the field of coronary heart disease prevention and in various screening programs illustrate these dilemmas.

There can be no argument about the need for medical education to become more aware of and receptive to the needs of sufferers from a wide range of conditions, many of them stress-related and hitherto regarded as banal. The combination of ignorance of their mechanisms and inadequacy in their management has led to a lamentable degree of neglect by the medical profession and the flourishing of therapeutic programs administered by others. The manipulation of populations, however, raises problems of a different order and when the initiative comes from the doctor rather than the patient, the ancient injunction *primum non nocere* is surely paramount.

General Discussion

There was agreement that are too many mismatches between what medical schools do and what is needed or expected by society with respect to health services and the mixes of physicians. The roles of medical schools should be understood within the broad context that includes all the health professions (including medicine), the health care system, societal trends and values, and the prevailing political arrangements. Although there are substantial differences among the four countries, there appeared to be common goals, and even means, that are applicable to most of their medical schools. The mission of the medical school requires redefining but of greater importance than what we *say* is what we *do*; this imbalance should be addressed.

There was less agreement about the need for *all* medical schools to undertake a major commitment to assuring that all faculty members and students appreciate the *population perspective*. Perhaps only some should do this; but who is to say which should and which should not? Is there a set of "core competencies" bearing on the population perspective that should be required of *all* medical graduates, or just of some? How realistic is it to expect all physicians to undertake all the roles proposed for them?

Do medical schools have within themselves, the energy, motivation, and capacity to undertake needed changes or must the impetus, even demand, come from external social, economic, and political forces? How broad a mandate should medical schools assume, in addition to being the "filter" for selection and preparation of future physicians? For example, should the faculty assume responsibility for influencing physician payment systems to achieve better balance in the provision of health services?

Several suggestions for facilitating both local and more general changes were advanced:

- Establish or negotiate social contracts with defined communities; learn from the experience of institutions around the world that have done this;
- Undertake an institutional self-study that requires discussion of input from a broad range of "stakeholders" including community leaders, government officials, students, professional organizations, voluntary agencies, consumers' groups, patient advocates, etc.;
- Systematically examine the mechanisms by which a continuing "dialogue with the community (ies)" can best be undertaken using pilot projects, board memberships, councils, and exchanges of experience;
- Establish sustainable and dynamic interactive "partnership systems" involving the medical school (and the university), informal and formal community leaders, and governmental agencies for developing and monitoring an agenda for population-based research and cooperative service activities. These partnerships could be a vehicle for influencing the medical curriculum;
- Dedicated funds could be sought for innovative interdisciplinary research bearing on high priority health problems in the community and for educational experiments related to societal needs and expectations;
- Faculty development programs are needed to prepare present and future medical faculty members with the "new skills" required for such undertakings as: academic strategic planning, restructuring (social) organizations, becoming a constructive partner with communities and governments, etc., and curriculum planning to incorporate the population perspective and related skills; and
- Create opportunities for students, and especially faculty members, to work in community settings (sometimes referred to as "community-based experiential learning") and make this activity an integral part of the academic reward system.

2
The Social Contract and the Medical School's Responsibilities

THOMAS S. INUI

I. Introduction

This is a chapter with a point of view. In brief, since medical care is a social good, medical schools have "social responsibilities" that can and should be manifest in their mission and activities. Our exploration of this thesis will begin with an examination of the origin of the medical school's mission in the notion of "social contract," go on to a description of the legitimate roles of physicians, ask next how (or if) we prepare physicians for these roles, and finally review the opportunities for (and sources of resistance to) mission-driven change in medical schools. I do not seek to denigrate medical schools. They are the communities in which I live and work. I admire their accomplishments as bastions of biomedical science and worry about the focus and quality of their other activities. These are the loving and serious criticisms of a native son.

II. The Medical School's Mission

The medical school's central responsibility is for the education of physicians. In this simple, declarative form the statement seems almost tautologic. Most of the physicians will go on to careers of medical practice, and a smaller proportion will devote themselves principally to research, teaching, or both. The cumulative experience of the past 50 years in medical science, medical education, and medical practice suggests that all, no matter what the dominant activities of their careers, need to be prepared for lifetimes of continued scholarship, since a considerable fraction of the body of knowledge and skills physicians acquire in medical school is subject to obsolescence and/or decay well before the end of their careers (Manning and DeBakey 1987).

Many would think this a too-narrow construct for the medical school's mission, however, particularly in North America where medical schools do not generally exist as stand-alone institutions but are, instead, part of a nexus of institutions referred to as the "academic medical center." The academic medical center may be located on or near the general university under whose aegis the medical school was founded, and often includes the "health sciences schools" other than medicine (pharmacy, nursing, public health, social work, for example), ambulatory care facilities, and the academic/teaching hospital of the university and medical school. Each of these institutions has an administrative head, its own central missions, training programs, and public constituencies. While coexisting under the general university's academic administrative structures, each institution also adheres to independent, external standards for academic program accreditation at graduate or undergraduate levels. The university hospital and ambulatory care facility are also in the business of providing medical care, ranging from primary care for nearby populations to true subspecialty services for referred populations.

To further complicate matters in the United States, all of the institutions within the academic medical center may be in competition with peer institutions pursuing similar missions. In our metropolitan environments, health sciences schools compete for reputation, trainees, research grants, and other scarce resources. Specialists at university hospitals acknowledge (with equal measures of pride and chagrin) the extent to which they "train their own competition," since the alumni/ae of the university-based medical and surgical subspecialty programs are recruited to practices in the communities where they complete training.

External competition aside, within the academic medical center the school of medicine and other constituent entities may or may not be able to act in concert with other elements of the institution. The medical school's desires for educational experiences for its students may conflict with the university hospital's perceived need for time-efficient medical clinic practice, for example. Even within the school of medicine, departments of medicine, surgery, and psychiatry may espouse different points of view on such matters as the need for expanded programs in primary care for their city's homeless populations versus the need for a liver transplantation program. Debates of this genre are resolved only after detailed and sometimes heated discussions of the institution's missions in education, research, and clinical care, and then only by reference to such nonacademic issues as "niche" in the marketplace, competitive advantage, and the need for preservation of extended referral networks for subspecialty services (*cf.* Ludmerer 1985, 255–280). In the academic medical center's ecologic environment, then, even the medical school's "narrow mission" for the education of physicians gets complicated.

Further complexity emerges when we observe that the activities of effective medical practice and scholarship (the aforementioned principal foci of the physicians' future careers) are not *ends* in themselves but *means* for the maintenance of health of the populations served by the medical school and its academic medical center. What we choose to adopt as our working construct for "health," how preeminent we consider medical care services to be among the general social resources for health, on what grounds we assess the effectiveness and appropriateness of medical practices and the productivity of medical research—all these are questions for many parties, not just for those in medical academe. Other parties with a stake include the public (who are themselves patients at academic medical centers, parents of children who may seek education at medical schools, and taxpayers whose remittances constitute the general revenue fund), various professional organizations (with representational, credentialling, and accrediting responsibilities), and governmental bodies at state, regional, or federal levels that fund medical care and medical education.

Indeed, if influence were directly proportionate to magnitude of funds in determining whose perspective has greatest weight when developing a construct for health, effective medical care, and the medical school mission, the general public and the governmental institutions that represent the public would have the final word in any such discussion, not the professionals who work in academic medical centers. Medical schools and academic medical centers in the United States derive a majority of their support from public funds (Schroeder, et al. 1989). Public sources are in the majority not only in state-supported medical schools, but also in our "private" institutions, where they arrive as grants and contracts for research, reimbursement through governmental programs for medical care services, supplementary funding ("educational adjustment") to federally funded medical care, and direct federal support for graduate medical education in primary care fields (among others). Under these circumstances, the financial viability of the medical schools and their academic medical centers can fairly be said to be founded on service to the public. Here, then, is an alternative construct for the medical school's mission—the medical school as an educational institution in service to the public's health. In this mode of thinking, the medical school, whether a "private" or "public" institution, may be viewed as a social resource, medical care as a social good, and the school's responsibility to the public as a social contract. A full explication of this last notion serves as the foundation for all that follows in this chapter and could take one of several forms.

First, a relatively complete argument can be made for the existence of a social contract, if a medical school is a public institution operating under the aegis of elected government. The University of Washington, for example, is the only medical school for the populations residing in the states of Washington, Alaska, Montana, and Idaho. In this geopolitical area, four state legislatures annually appropriate funds from their general revenues in support of medical education activities at the University of Washington School of Medicine (UWSM). The extent to which the UWSM, therefore, serves the needs of the people of these states can also be evaluated by the legislatures at whatever frequency they see fit to do so, on whatever measures or constructs of health they deem appropriate, and with direct implications for the appropriations process they conduct. Where the dialogue between the school and the legislature does not produce consensus, the opinion of the legislature prevails. In Washington, for example, the state and the UWSM do not concur on the level of support for the school of medicine from the state budget. The magnitude of state support per medical school graduate at the UWSM is at least one order of magnitude less generous than comparable support to other state institutions of arguably equivalent reputation in the United States. From the UWSM's perspective, this is reason enough to request increased state support to the school. Pacific Northwest legislators, however, argue that lesser investments are needed in our medical schools because the in-migration of competent practitioners to the "attractive environment" of the Pacific Northwest adjusts for any shortfall we might experience in the indigenous production of medical manpower.

Even in the case of medical schools not operating under the aegis of government, however, we could observe that requisite financial conditions are present for positing the existence of a "contract" between the general public (or its governmental representatives) and medical schools/academic medical centers. By accepting a substantial proportion of institutional income from public sources, the medical school and its academic leadership implicitly enters into contracts to serve the public. The terms of their responsibility are not to be found solely in the cumulative documentation available for all of the individual grants, contracts, medical care reimbursements, and other categorical sources of public support to the institution. A social historian would contend that these categorical programs had been developed *seriatim* in response to perceived problems of general social significance in health and medical care, such as inadequate access, manpower maldistribution, and "medical indigency." While each of the programs was established in a general policy context that did have certain implications for medical education at a graduate or undergraduate level, many were not developed explicitly to reform medical education (Starr 1982, 352–378). For this reason, no adequate interpretation of a medical school's responsibility to the public trust could be limited to an examination of the specific conditions for receipt of public funds. Instead, the inquiry would have to move beyond this literal examination of the "terms of the contracts" to a more abstract consideration of intended effects of these social policies on the "public good" *and* to specific, substantive assessments of the institution's performance in these respects.

An alternative approach to explicating the notion of "social contract" is closer to a Rawlsian theory of justice and social utilitarianism than to political history or legal analysis (Daniels 1985). In this alternative tradition of reasoning and speaking we replace the notion of an "implicit contract" derived from the receipt of public funds with the notion of health as a scarce and necessary resource (at some level) for all persons in society, if they are to have an opportunity to be productive. Health, we say, is such an important prerequisite for productivity that we, as a society, act through our political mechanisms to assure its maintenance for all, for the same reasons we seek to assure "adequate" education, housing, nutrition, and clothing. The just society would not permit the systematic underprovision of medical care to vulnerable segments of the general public and, therefore, uses income redistribution measures to provide effective medical services, including provision of special support to medical schools, source of new knowledge, and medical manpower. In this line of reasoning, medical schools are one of the important mechanisms for maintaining a just society.

A third approach to conceptualizing the notion of "social contract" emerged from the twentieth-century libertarian tradition (Ackerman 1980). In this context, social theorists construe the institutions and procedures of government as those which support a dialogic process through which the distribution of scarce resources is arranged. The basic right of a citizen in this society is to equity—no individual's needs and desires are to be valued above any other's, because no individual is intrinsically more worthy than any other. Central problems in the libertarian theory are to provide for equity, in spite of uneven distribution of genetic or other inheritable resources affecting capacity and intergenerational competition for resources among vulnerable populations (between children and the elderly, for example). In this context, education and health are construed as enabling resources necessary for full participation in the dialogic process. Because illness itself erodes each affected individual's capacity for active participation, medical services (preventive or curative) should be available to all. Academic medical centers, and the medical schools within them, are "enabling resources" for the citizens of the liberal state, whether or not they operate under the aegis of government or receive public funds.

However one chooses to argue the point (as a contractarian, utilitarian, or libertarian), the medical school has a social responsibility to the population it serves. The central responsibility is for the educational preparation of effective physicians and, through the actions of these persons, for the maintenance of the public's health. The ways in which physicians serve the public and make their contributions to health are diverse, a diversity which (in turn) has implications for the medical schools' curriculum, pedagogy and content alike.

III. The Physician's Contributions to and Responsibilities for Health

In this section I argue that practicing physicians, the "principal product" of all medical schools from a health personnel perspective, can affect the health of the population for whom they assume responsibility in two principal modes of action, one referred to as "clinical" and the other as "societal." Acting in the clinical mode, clinicians directly render services to individual patients and/or other affected members of patient's families. When acting in a "societal mode," physicians use their special knowledge for the benefit of their patients but act through other helping institutions to maintain health. I wish, of course, to avoid broadening physicians' roles to all those kinds of work any may undertake. I acknowledge that physicians may, like other members of a free society, turn to careers in politics, art, or philosophy, and in these alternative careers add to the general good. These career transitions, however, are remote enough from the central responsibilities of physicians (to prevent, cure, or ameliorate ill health, preserve function, avoid harm, and always to attend in knowledge and appreciation), as to be distinguishable under most circumstances from "physician's work." My attempt is to denote the legitimate domain of physician's professional work, work requiring the knowledge and skills of physicians and inherently tied to societal notions of health and well-being for which physicians share responsibility.

There are five distinguishable roles for the physician acting in a *clinical mode*.

- The physician may act as a *"preventionist,"* identifying threats to the maintenance of his/her patient's health and acting to prevent conditions that would subsequently erode functional capacity, longevity, or both. In this role, the physician may act largely on the basis of epidemiologic information regarding the prevention of disease, disability, and untimely deaths (Battista and Lawrence 1988). The quality of evidence for specific actions varies from one health threat to another, and physicians must decide, in concert with the patients they see, what constitutes "prudent" behavior. Some clinical preventive care is clearly unusual in clinical practice, even though it would constitute an effort to avoid major causes of disability and untimely deaths in the United States (Committee on Trauma Research 1985). Injury prevention activities that clinicians might undertake to limit the sequelae of automobile injuries, disability and deaths from household fires, and firearms injuries are not highly prevalent in clinical settings, for example.
- The physician may serve as a *"provider"* of curative and ameliorative services for patients and their families, an interpreter of symptoms, a rational diagnostician who recommends proper treatments for the diseases once found. This is the now familiar paradigm of modern medicine, in some respects the "core responsibility" for biomedical practitioners. In a broader construct but within the same rational model are the activities of the "biopsychosocial" clinician (Engel 1977) who engages in problem solving with the affected persons and families, themselves operating within illness systems that may never be properly resolved to "diseases" in a biomedical context (Gordon 1988).
- Physicians act as *"case managers"* for patients under certain circumstances. In this capacity she/he may coordinate medical services, invoke or request needed nonmedical helping services (vocational rehabilitation, homemaking, and personal care, for example), and serve as an advocate for the patient in interactions with other helping systems (when evaluating and providing information on disability, for example).

- The physician may also serve as a *"gatekeeper"* or *"rationer"* of scarce resources for a patient as a member of an enrolled population of patients, all of whom must depend on the physician to preserve resources that must be available when any one of them is in clear and present need. In this capacity, the physician is called on to act simultaneously as a technical expert, a prudent advocate of a particular patient's best interests, and as a parsimonious protector of the commons (Eisenberg 1986, 57–86). These are not "public health" responsibilities in a classic sense, since they do entail actions on behalf of particular patients by the responsible physician as the means by which the patient's needs, as a sick person and as a representative of a larger class of persons, are met. They do, however, invoke precisely the kind of lived conflict between serving as a patient's "perfect agent" and serving the public good with which persons working within the public health system have always been familiar.

- Finally, physicians serve as *"health watchers,"* observers of sentinel events, persons who may accumulate the experience of practice in an effort to monitor the state of their population's health, the problems of health care, and the sources (biomedical or not) of disease, distress, disability, destitution, and untimely death which prevail (cf. Pickles 1972). Using "information systems" as technologically unintensive as paper-and-pencil logs, chart reviews, and registries, individual practitioners can acquire an appreciation of the phenomena with which they work in order to detect special hazards in their patients' microenvironments, practice more intelligently, reorder their differential diagnoses, recalibrate their Bayesian prior probabilities, focus and direct their own programs of continuing education, and choose topics for patient education. Special attention to nonbiomedical risk factors for ill health will be increasingly important, if we are to be appropriately vigilant when working with members of vulnerable subpopulations (Bunker et al. 1989), detecting and intervening in domestic violence (Kellerman 1990), participating effectively in the social management of drug abuse, and detecting work-related illnesses (Cullen et al. 1990).

  In their role as health watchers, clinicians are clearly using the methods of epidemiology but acting within a clinical population, blurring the distinction between clinician and epidemiologist, as many have chosen to do with good effect in the development of the field of clinical epidemiology (Sackett et al. 1985). Using these population-based strategies within practice settings as a source of intelligence for clinical decision making, public health education, and continuing medical education are basic approaches within what has been espoused as "community oriented primary care" (Kark 1981; Nutting 1987). Certain observations on the health of enrolled practice populations and population-based measures of the completeness of preventive care services may even become a basis for compensation of general practitioners in the United Kingdom (Iliffe and Haines 1989).

There are three readily identifiable roles for the physician acting in a *societal mode*. The physician's objective in each is to improve the health of the public she/he serves by participating actively and competently with representatives of his/her community, its organizations, and institutions. These are all actions in which the physician makes use of his/her special expertise in health and medical care, as well as the physician's knowledge of how she/he works in a clinical mode. In these activities, however, the physician must also clearly act as an advocate of the general public's health and is not drawn into these activities directly as the advocate or agent of a single patient. The physician may act as a

- *Citizen-advocate* for health concerns when participating in the work of non-clinical public institutions that, by dint of their authorities, resources, and actions, have an impact on the health of the community. These institutions or organizations include some within the general health sector itself, such as those which finance, regulate, plan, review, and assure the quality of health services. Other organizations and institutions that affect health, however, include those in public education (school health education programs, for example), those which deal with the general welfare of the public (housing, food, special transportation, and other social support services for disabled and elderly), those that monitor and provide information on occupational and environmental threats to health, and the courts that provide for the resolution of grievances arising in a medical care context. Acting beyond the confines of his/her immediate community, but as a physician-citizen of the nation and member of the global community, the health-advocate may legitimately choose to create a "medical presence" for arms control activities and surveillance of human rights violations.
- *Socially responsible member of professional organizations.* While professional organizations of physicians certainly exist to promote the interests and serve the needs of the physician members themselves, most organizations of this nature also sponsor activities in which a physician may serve as a protagonist for the public's health. To the extent that the physician is an active participant—locally, regionally, or nationally—of his/her professional organization's activities in public education, policy analysis from the public's perspective, and professional surveillance of other elements of the medical–industrial complex, she/he is acting as a socially responsible member of these professional organizations. Such physicians may also be proactive in their organizations, influencing them from within to act on issues that are beyond the strict bounds of membership self-interest, but important to the health of the public. Activities and concerns of this kind may even focus on matters of scientific interest, insofar as agenda for research funding, for example, are shaped by social and political influences which may, or may not, serve the public's health needs.
- *Participant, in a societal mode, in management and governance of provider organizations* such as hospitals, group practices, and others. These activities can take place on a salaried or pro bono basis and range from full-time to part-time commitments. In such contexts, physicians may as-

sist institutions to make decisions on the assumption of responsibility for provision of health services to particular populations (the poor, the chronically mentally ill, persons with AIDS, those in need of trauma services, etc.), the price of services, the spectrum of services available for those unable to defray the costs of care, and other policies substantially affecting the content, quality, and effectiveness of medical care.

I readily admit that this spectrum of roles and responsibilities for physicians is, perhaps even within the clinical mode, a broader portfolio of activities than some in medicine would identify as innately part of the physician's tasks (Seldin 1981). If medical care is a "social good," and medical schools have social responsibilities, however, then the use of a "social construct" for health and the healer's responsibilities seems a more appropriate standard than relatively more limited professional constructs (White 1988, 4–46). Furthermore, modern medicine may be experiencing "the best and worst of times" presently, a situation from which it will be extricated only by the adoption of a social construct, whether this occurs as the result of movement within medicine or of external forces. Biomedicine has never been in a better position to produce detailed, powerful information, while, paradoxically, causing such dismay, distrust, fear, and financial distress (Kolata 1990). Just as biomedicine seems to be on the verge of its final flowering, characterized as an ability to understand and intervene in the molecular biologic processes of disease, physicians may be losing their special niche in society, capacity to heal, and place in their culture (Inui 1988).

Charles Odegaard (1986) and others have cautioned us that physicians—if they choose to ignore the social constructs for health, healing, and effective medical practice—do so at their peril and may lose an opportunity for participation in a general social reconstruction of medicine that must occur in our time. Escalating expenditures alone may drive the reconsideration of medicine as a social resource in the United States, but the potential for healing and improvement in health status may also be greater if we broaden or reform the underlying model of medicine on the basis of social constructs (DeVries 1981). Within those broader constructs, all the physician actions alluded to above are certainly considered to be legitimate, perhaps even necessary to the maintenance of the fiduciary relationship between patients and physicians. If this be the case, do the educational processes in medical school and postgraduate training activities of physicians provide the requisite knowledge base, attitudes, and skills to produce competence among practitioners for these tasks?

IV. To What Extent Are Medical Schools Preparing Physicians for Their Roles and Responsibilities?

Before offering impressions of the adequacy of preparation for the kinds of roles and responsibilities we have alluded to above, I must publicly regret the absence of adequate data, even descriptive survey research, that would permit statements to be made about the presence or absence of courses of particular types in the medical curricula in Canada, United States, the United Kingdom, and Australia. The approach taken to characterize certain attributes of the medical school activities in Europe (Walton 1985) would have served as a point of departure for discussion, but was not applied to North America. Even these data, however, might not have been adequate to the task at hand, since course availability is a necessary but not sufficient criterion for adequate preparation. Furthermore, course titles would certainly not serve as an adequate taxonomy for desirable elements of the curriculum. Studying the syllabi of courses produces a greater appreciation of content and purpose but is clearly less feasible. At the University of Washington, we have found it necessary to devise a key word abstracting and indexing system. When a course is first described for this system, students submit key words after each lecture and at the end of the course to describe course content. Student data are catalogued by course and session, entered into a microcomputer database, updated annually by course instructors, and are available for retrieval. Using this database, one can finally ask *where* in the curriculum (in what courses) content pertinent to clinical prevention, for example, is being presented. The actual comprehensiveness, coherence, and scientific validity of the information itself cannot be known with certainty at present. Furthermore, we are unable to say whether the pedagogical approaches used to present the material produce lasting impressions, appropriate skills, opportunities to practice those skills, appropriate attitudes, and appetites for continued learning. All of these elements would be necessary in an effective curriculum to produce competent practitioners.

- *We may be force-feeding too much biomedical science.* On the basis of our students' performance on standardized exams taken during and after the medical school experience in North America, we can contend that the knowledgeable biomedical science-centered provider is the principal product of our medical school educational process. This is certainly no mean accomplishment, but substantive criticisms of the medical school experience are being articulated with increasing frequency in recent years (Ebert and Ginzberg 1988; Gastel and Rogers 1989; Panel on the General Professional Education of the Physician 1984; Schroeder et al. 1990; World Conference of Medical Education 1988). Many attributes of the curriculum are focal points for criticism, including the massive commitment to rote memorization of a huge body of information from the classic basic sciences of anatomy, microbiology, and pathology, as well as an increasingly prodigious effort to accommodate the burgeoning domain of molecular biology, which now underpins such basic sciences as physiologic chemistry, pathophysiology, immunology, genetics, and pharmacology. Under present circumstances it is difficult to decide how much biomedical information is too much, and (a second question) how much of what can be taught is really pertinent to the tasks of the physician?

- *We may be failing to nourish students' interpersonal skills.* Simultaneously, criticisms are being levied at medical education in its nonbiomedical aspects, now referred to by some as the "humanistic dimensions" of medical education. The concern is a substantial one—physicians may have become so immersed in molecular biology, other new science, and its attendant technology that they have lost touch with the human dimensions of healing. This concern about the so-called "nontechnical skills" of physicians has been fueled from outside the profession of medicine and academic medical centers by general perceptions that medicine in the United States is held in less high regard than may have previously been the case (Kolata 1990, for example). Certifying boards, such as the American Board of Internal Medicine, have sufficient concerns about the "humanistic skills" of their examination candidates to have developed systematic suggestions for residency program directors to use when evaluating these capacities among their trainees (American Board of Internal Medicine 1985).

  Encouragingly, important new efforts have emerged in the United Kingdom, Canada, and the United States to reorient and reinvigorate research, teaching, and practice in clinical communication (Stewart and Roter 1989; Pendleton et al. 1984). Astonishingly, this most basic of clinical competencies has fallen into educational doldrums. Talking with patients has come to be construed as interviewing for symptoms of disease, not dialogue to appreciate the story of an illness (Cassell 1985). Under these circumstances, it is certainly not difficult to imagine why patient satisfaction with medical care and the medical care system suffers as pressures for "productivity," service intensity and velocity, and patient expectations for the fruits of the new science all escalate. The need for understanding "patient-centered" medical care, family dynamics, and the clinician's role in illness systems all become paramount, but loom large only in the primary care fields in medical academe. While we can and should take note of our ability to produce biomedically knowledgeable graduates, we clearly need to reexamine the effectiveness of these educational and training processes on the other capacities of our trainees. They may be "effective" technical practitioners in a clinical mode but are often not as effective as healers in the patient's lived world. This lack of competence will adversely affect clinicians in all their tasks, since communication and empathetic appreciation are critical to all varieties of care, case management, rationing of scarce resources, and health advocacy.
- *We are teaching students medicine in the wrong locales.* In the clinical years of medical education in the United States, criticism is focused on the still preeminent positions of the inpatient experiences in the required clerkships of medicine, surgery, psychiatry, pediatrics, and so on. Especially as hospitals in the United States have decreased the length of stay in all patient areas substantially, the heuristic significance of the inpatient "case" now seems diminished, and the pace of activities in the inpatient service too frenetic to comfortably accommodate the student's paced and

reflective participation. The inpatient stay, furthermore, always a minor portion of the natural history of most patients' illnesses, now constitutes an even smaller portion and no longer includes some of the most important activities of diagnostic evaluation and acute treatment. New instrumentation, both diagnostic and therapeutic, permits increasing proportions of human illness and some classic diseases with heuristic importance to be dealt with effectively and economically on an ambulatory care basis altogether.

Finally, the emphasis on inpatient experience has serious opportunity costs, including the students' lack of exposure to primary care and ambulatory, autonomous patients receiving their medical care while carrying on with their usual activities and responsibilities to others. For a Faculty member who tries to teach students something about medicine and healing in a social context, it is akin to teaching surgery without ever going to the operating room.

- *We continue to ignore the clinical relevance of population-based information and perspectives.* While this may not be as problematic an issue in the United Kingdom, Australia, and Canada as it is in the United States, I believe that practitioners in general have inadequate preparation to acquire and use information about the health of their communities, even their practice populations. In the United States, this may have to do with the now-historic split between the fields of "public health" and clinical medicine, now institutionalized in our separate schools of public health and medicine, as well as public health departments distinctly separated from the personal health care system. We have failed to produce the public information systems that would support practitioners in the "health watcher" role and leave them without adequate training today to devise their own. The microcomputer may be nearly ubiquitous in United States' physicians' offices today but appears doomed to such restricted applications as billing for services rendered and the occasional automated search of the medical literature.

Today's clinician-in-training has even less preparation for his/her work in a societal mode, for discharging his/her "social responsibilities." In the United States, these legitimate physician's roles are certainly not unimportant *or* arcane. Physicians should be trained to work competently when providing information for legal proceedings. They should know how to perform disability evaluations of persons seeking social support, should know something about the difference between disability and functional evaluation and the usual history and physical examination for the discovery of disease processes.

Students of medicine might also be better prepared for the tasks of public education, a different activity than individual patient counselling, in order to contribute more effectively to public service announcements and open community debates (on such matters as homelessness, air quality, fluoridation of water, and public funding of abortions). They should have had an introduction to their opportunities for participation in the activities of community boards or councils with institutional oversight responsibilities, and in the development of curricula in health-related topics for schools, churches, or other organizations. With their peers and representatives of the practitioner community, they should have considered their own affinity, capacity, and preparation for such important, disparate physician–citizen activities as participation in the legislative process (Bergman 1986), the general effort of humankind to assure human rights (Geiger et al. 1989), the work within organizations of medicine to assure the quality of medical care and the primacy of the public's interests (Winkenwerder and Ball 1988), and the heroic efforts of "social rescue" programs that tackle head-on some of the thorniest problems we see as health care practitioners (Schor 1988). Though I would accept without objection comments that suggested the presence of substantial United States–Canada–United Kingdom systematic variations in the frequency and severity of these problems, I expect they are nevertheless substantial and important in all of our settings.

- *Is there too little or too much time in medical school?* One irony in all current discussions of reform in medical education is the juxtaposition of opinions suggesting that no room remains in the curriculum for new content and other perspectives suggesting that the fourth year of medical school is an educational wasteland. During that last year, considerable time is committed to subspecialty elective experiences in many curricula in the United States, and even to elective experiences in the hospital(s) where students want to acquire their residency training (the so-called "senior year audition"). These latter experiences seem unnecessary, given the extensive experience to be acquired in these same settings during the internship and other postgraduate residency years.

  Whether or not the fourth year is available for a new curriculum, the challenge is to identify ways and means, in the course of medical school, residency, and continuing medical education, to offer sufficient exposure and opportunities for physicians to enhance their knowledge, attitudes, and skills in these expanded domains of competence. The educational and training process should at least produce a basic appreciation of these roles and varieties of work, while also making available more extensive opportunities for deeper learning, skill acquisition, and practice for those who elect advanced training.

The mechanisms for progressive change in these educational domains are best characterized, I believe, as the use of internal "management by increment" strategies to effect medical school curricula and postgraduate training activities. At least in the United States, it seems unlikely that major external forces can be expected in the near term to produce coherent, comprehensive change at the medical undergraduate and postgraduate training levels. Indeed, it has been argued that one of the principal problems with the preparation of physicians for their careers is the dissociation of educational responsibility for medical school and postgraduate experiences. From the disparate perspectives of the external testing, accrediting, and funding entities that influence medical education, it is difficult to imagine how a consensus to support preparation for such a diverse set of competencies might ever appear. In fact, activities devoted to learning more about successful public education approaches, for example, are likely to be viewed as a direct subtraction from the already too-scarce faculty and student effort for learning basic sciences.

The advantages of working from within an institution include the opportunity to make constructive use of the institutional sense of "academic community" as a dependable centripetal force when reacting to external change, debating divisive issues, negotiating differences, and arriving at consensus through friendly persuasion (or other varieties of legitimate power). Additionally, within the medical school, the regular recurrence of certain discussions, decisions, and actions constitutes opportunities for progressive, incremental change. These include discussions and decisions about the mission of the school, who is enrolled, how, where, and what the faculty teaches, who the faculty are, and how educational programs are evaluated.

V. Identification of the Medical School's Mission as an Opportunity for Change

The leaders of many medical schools in the United States believe their institutions to have a national responsibility for contributions to medical knowledge and practice. Since their student body is admitted from more than one geographic area and, on graduation, is distributed to a national pool of residency programs, they make the *res ipse loquitur* argument for a "national mission." This kind of thinking has historically prevailed in many of the institutions in which a *prima facie* case for regional or areal responsibility could also be made, for example, at those state medical schools that receive a portion of their funding from state governments. Furthermore, to the extent that highly subspecialized, reference institutions of national reputation actually do serve local populations in the near region as a primary resource for inpatient and outpatient care, they too have community responsibilities. In fact, it seems reasonable to ask of all medical schools whether there are specific catchment areas, communities, governments, subsegments of the general population, or other entities with which the school is *de facto* affiliated (Koska 1990). If there are such relationships, especially if a particular subpopulation is dependent on the medical school and its affiliated hospital for primary medical care, a series of other questions become pertinent to the school's mission and, once addressed, may provide the stimulus for change in the school's activities. These questions include the following:

- What do we (the medical school leadership) know about the health status and medical care needs of this population?
- What are the services we render to this population, either directly or through our affiliated institutions?
- Is the mix of these services—prevention, care and cure, case and resource management, health watching, socially responsible health advocacy—a good match to the needs of the population for services?
- Do we have mechanisms in place that will permit us to monitor and assure the quality, effectiveness, and equitable distribution of these services?
- Do the determinations of need, appropriateness, quality, effectiveness, and equity reflect the views of the population served as well as our professional views?

This list of questions could clearly be expanded. My purpose is to illustrate the need for institutional discussion, not to develop the complete agenda. When examining its institutional culture and elaborating its mission, the medical school has an opportunity to deal with the population it serves responsibly, not as a substrate for educational activities (the population served as "teaching material") nor as a captive population important to the institution's financial health (part of the institution's market "niche"). The dialogue on mission always needs to include medical school insiders and representatives of community organizations—political, religious, industrial, educational, or other. In fact, whether a "primary care relationship" between the school and specific subpopulations exists at all is a question that may only be addressed in dialogue and answered on the basis of bilateral expectations, not by either entity alone.

This kind of discussion, carried on at least through the questions outlined above, would have implications for a number of decisions affecting the functions of the medical school. Should clinical teaching activities be based in community settings, how much financial risk can be assumed by the school to provide unfunded care to local populations, whether or not the medical school should enter into joint ventures with community clinics, long-term care facilities, specific employers, or worker populations—all these decisions would clearly be better informed if placed in the general context of the dialogue on mission.

Finally, the medical school's research emphases may also be affected by the dialogue on mission. Many of us who now conduct research in medical schools consider ourselves to be entrepreneurs and free agents in the choice of topics, methods, "laboratories," information dissemination, and in all other matters pertaining to our research. Nevertheless, we all make conditioned choices at some level, choices that the medical school can influence. Whether or not common technical instrumentation, laboratory space, special libraries, and other enabling resources are available to us does affect our competitiveness for research funding and may influence our choice-making within the universe of all possible, interesting, and important research activities.

The medical school can influence directly the availability of "bench research" ("wet lab") space versus the development of office areas for research most appropriate to epidemiology, clinical research involving interviewing, or other "dry lab" activities. The school may also provide in-kind or even monetary "seed" resources for developing specific research programs. Sponsoring symposia, guest faculty in residence, the work of interest groups, and cross-disciplinary teaching programs may directly stimulate the development of research.

In all these research-related matters, management of institutional resources might be informed, or even driven, by affiliations, sites of care, knowledge of a population's health needs, mismatches between needs and available resources, and the direct requests of the public. If "venture capital" is used to stimulate additional activities, these kinds of incentives and rewards could be put in place without directly penalizing existing programs. Because new research activities are likely to produce additional collaborative opportunities for existing faculty now working in investigator-initiated programs, the appearance of interdisciplinary research programs responsive to the needs of a defined population is likely to augment the activities and opportunities for all, rather than constraining the opportunities of traditional investigators. This certainly is the experience of the Occupational Medicine Program, for example, at the University of Washington. This program is based both in the School of Medicine and the University of Washington School of Public Health and Community Medicine (SPHCM). Its research activities are in major part a function of the interests and expertise of the faculty within Occupational Medicine, but some of the topics for field research are in fact chosen from an agenda for work that the State Department of Labor and Industries, State Legislature, or major employers may (and do) make known to the program through the Department of Environmental Health (SPHCM). The investigator-initiated activities, such as chemoprevention trials for lung cancer among shipworkers with significant asbestos exposure, identification of risk factors for pulmonary injury and the natural history of such injury among fire fighters, and laboratory toxicology and clinical surveys to understand the consequences of solvent exposure among airplane assembly workers using volatile materials in closed spaces, or pesticide exposure among agricultural workers, are all topics that address special health needs of local (Seattle-area) populations served by the UWSOM affiliated clinical programs. Work on these topics and others clearly provides new opportunities for basic researchers in environmental toxicology, neurology, nutritional science, and other disciplines within the UWSOM and SPHCM.

VI. Enrollment Choices as Opportunities for Change

In the United States, each medical school devises and implements its own program for screening and admitting students, submits institutional preference lists for candidates in the matching programs for postgraduate training, and "markets" continuing medical education programs. The health needs and medical care service requirements of the medical school's population can inform all of these decisions. The need for additional primary care manpower in the rural regions of Washington, Alaska, Montana, and Idaho (WAMI) has shaped the University of Washington WAMI program directly, not only as *raison d'être* for the WAMI program at its inception, but also in the annual selection processes that bring medical students to the central campus at the University of Washington in Seattle either directly or through decentralized first-year programs for the medical curriculum based in Anchorage (Alaska), Missoula (Montana), and Moscow (Idaho). Epidemiologically, students beginning in the latter sites are more likely to return to these specific states in rural locations or to comparably underserved areas after finishing medical school and residency training (Adkins et al. 1987).

The same kind of information about the geographic distribution of manpower deficiency areas in the Pacific Northwest also figured in the original decision to commit one-third of the slots annually in the University of Washington's internal medicine residency program, a nationally competitive program that has never experienced any difficulty filling, to primary care residents who are now known to be more likely to remain generalists and locate themselves in small towns in the WAMI region than our "traditional" internal medicine residents. Manpower considerations in the rural WAMI region are important again now, as the University of Washington tries to develop a more complete understanding of the decision-making processes that result in career commitments among our medical students (Greer and Carline 1989) and enters into discussion with the state legislatures about medical student entering class "set aside" slots that might be filled by the nominees of small towns without physicians. On a trial basis, subject to examination of such students' subsequent medical school records, residency program choices, and (ultimately) career locations, an experimental program of this nature could be adopted at the University of Washington because it is likely to increase the overall number of candidates for our entering classes, would increase the proportion of our graduates who enter careers in primary care (bringing it closer to our publicly announced target of 50%), and is highly unlikely to erode the "quality" of our enrolled student body. Hypothetically, the University of Washington might even agree to guarantee admissions to these nominees, so long as they meet or exceed explicit thresholds for qualification (pass the Medical College Admissions Test, fulfill our minimum preparatory course requirements, and have an undergraduate grade point average consistent with success in graduate school). The effects on the individual and on the community of a democratic process of nomination and the potential for town-specific incentives (perhaps including defraying costs of education, if the individual returns to practice) might have substantial effects on career decisions. In truth, any such trial program would be likely, in my judgment, to attract ideologically driven, passionate individuals, virtually assuring the University of Washington that these trainees would be at least as likely to succeed as their "over the transom" peers.

Other attributes of individuals entering medical school become salient considerations, in addition to the standard "credentials" reviewed in the admissions process, if the repertoire of roles in the future careers of the medical student alumni/ae are considered. It may be argued, for example, that individuals who are to serve as citizen-advocates for health, participants in the activities of schools, courts, urban housing authorities, and other health-relevant organizations within their community should not have concentrated their "premedical" curriculum on biologic sciences alone. The kind of innate interest in, and social commitment to, the full array of human institutions that would naturally attract physicians to these kinds of societal-mode roles might be more likely to be found among liberal arts majors, who should have a better acquaintance with some of the social history, traditions, and even theoretic constructs that are manifest in these institutions than their science-major peers. Given a sufficient number of these students in medical school, one of the most powerful mechanisms of postgraduate education, the peer–peer interaction, could enhance the education of entire medical school cohorts.

Similar arguments can be made for affirmative action programs on behalf of racial and ethnic minorities, since life experience is the most profound source of appreciation for cultural diversity, and many medical schools do have special relationships to populations in which these minorities are more prevalent than in the general population. The arguments for this kind of affirmative admissions action are complex. The institution may choose to adopt this recruitment and admissions policy on the basis of social justice issues alone, but there is also an educational effectiveness basis for this position. It is unlikely that an African-American studies option, for example, will exist at all in most medical school curricula, and inconceivable that a learning experience of sufficient breadth, depth, and intensity could be made available to produce, by itself, any substantial influence on the attitudes, beliefs, and careers of physicians graduating from that school. The didactic curriculum, enhanced by organized review of the students' experience after working with African-American patients, would have a greater impact. Should a significant proportion of each medical school class *be* African Americans, the medical school educational process might be further enriched by peer–peer interactions drawing on the life experiences of these students for the benefit of all. Clearly, a structure and process would need to be devised that facilitated such peer group education—but read Sara Lawrence Lightfoot's *Balm in Gilead* (1988) and decide whether you thereby learn some things physicians should know about black America. Reflect with Vanessa Northington Gamble (1990) on the gains and losses of medical education. Ask yourself whether you might have been a better physician and educator if a Sara Lawrence's physician-mother Margaret or a Vanessa Gamble had been in your medical school class. Some things really do speak for themselves.

Similar arguments can be stated for recruiting to medical schools the children of families who have lived in poverty, students who have grown up in rural settings, and women. I am convinced that representatives of the latter "medical minority" will enhance our curriculum in, and appreciation for, the relevance of social networks to health, family systems, the physician's roles and transitions, the importance of the construct of "self" to work, communication with others, and healing (Belenky et al. 1986; Dickstein and Nadelson 1986). Acting affirmatively *vis-à-vis* all of these candidate attributes in the admissions process is certainly a major challenge, may require substantial reform in the admissions process itself (Antonovsky 1987), but also clearly constitutes an opportunity for institutional change.

VII. Curricular Opportunities for Change

Several experienced educators have now concluded publicly (Tosteson 1990; Ebert and Ginzberg 1988) that the current content of the medical school curriculum can shrink and still fit the needs of physicians for knowledge of the biomedical sciences. Ebert and Ginzberg even argue that one entire year of the current 4-year curriculum can be dispensed with altogether, permitting a transition into internship after the third year. I contend, however, that physicians require explicit preparation for the broader roles that are legitimately theirs in contemporary society. Disciplinary content not now usually present in the medical curriculum should be introduced and can serve as the knowledge basis for their future competence in these roles, and the faculty should make opportunities available for skill development under tutorial supervision. I argue that new commitments to these cognitive domains and learning experiences should replace the now "unnecessary year" in medical education in the United States.

To produce these new courses and experiences, medical school faculty may first need to divest themselves of the current paradigmatic hierarchical scheme used to assess the relative importances of sciences. The so-called "hard sciences" do not really need to fall in our esteem. Instead, the behavioral and social sciences, including political science, medical sociology, medical anthropology, health economics, and others need to be recognized as "basic" in their own right, serving as the foundation for clinicians' rational understanding and actions in pursuit of their responsibilities. Clinicians also need to learn how to communicate more effectively, verbally and in writing. For all intents and purposes, their "efficacy" as health advocates and physician–citizens will at times be critically dependent on their ability to communicate effectively. These goals for the "new curriculum" may be more readily attainable if strategic decisions are made on a number of matters that medical faculties revisit periodically. These include decisions on how and where learning occurs, what is taught and learned, and who does the teaching.

A number of medical school leaders in the past decade have reexamined the question of how learning occurs (Tosteson 1990; Kaufman et al. 1989). As educators, we seem to have rediscovered the basic principle of adult education (Rogers 1983)—physicians (like other adults) learn best if they can direct the learning experience themselves. Minimizing the hours of didactic, lecture-format, teacher-centered, passive learning and maximizing the number of medical student opportunities to pursue well-defined problems chosen for their heuristic value and relevance to clinical medicine have become the theme of the Harvard "New Pathway," and was always the general procedure of the McMaster and the University of New Mexico curricula in North America, as well as the Newcastle curriculum in Australia. These opportunities for self-directed inquiry seem to have invoked enthusiasm from the students and produced performance on standardized exams at least the equal of traditional approaches. The plausible superiority of this educational approach as a paradigm for the "lifetime learning process" that will follow is clear. This problem-based, learner-centered process may also be less likely to embed the notions of "high science/low science" in medical students, if they find the helpful information for the problems they face as often printed in the journals of public health, health services research, and behavioral medicine as they do in the *New England Journal of Medicine*, *Lancet*, and the *Journal of Clinical Investigation*. Our experience with this kind of inquiry at the University of Washington is encouraging. When medical students are asked to pursue specific case-related problems, even as late in their curriculum as during the third year on clinical clerkships, they rapidly find themselves pursuing such matters as the origins of homelessness, the unavailability of low-income housing, the social constructs for "disability," and the physician's role in arriving at these determinations.

Reviews of the medical curriculum are conducted regularly for all classroom courses. From the perspective of social constructs for physicians' roles, our greatest current need may be for a new curriculum (alluded to above) that can serve as preparation for nonbiomedical roles and varieties of work. In today's world, I believe that all medical schools should offer a well-organized course on physician's responsibilities and social roles, as well as opportunities (at least on an elective basis) for tutored work in such health-relevant helping institutions as the urban housing authority, area agencies on aging, public welfare offices, the courts, the jails, drug abuse detoxification and rehabilitation programs, nursing homes, the public health department, and others. At the University of Washington, one of the most popular courses in the medical school is our second-year course entitled "Medicine, Health, and Society." This course deals with what our medical students refer to as the "big questions" with which physicians grapple. One of its most attractive features, from the students' perspective, are the small-group sessions for the discussion of cases. These cases have involved such nonbiomedical issues as peer pressures among physicians to change their clinical practices to save a financially distressed rural hospital, physicians' personal decisions on the provision (or not) of abortions in the context of divisive community discussions of this issue, and physicians' participation in town council decisions *vis-à-vis* the use of community resources for health services versus other pressing needs. The faculty participating in these sessions act less as "instructors" and more as discussion facilitators and information resources. In practice, the outcomes of these discussions are predictably driven by a student's personal background, family beliefs, constructs of their own work and worth, and views of society. This observation is, of course, the real "lesson" of these discussions and, we hope, part of the basis for future participation by our students in these processes in the communities where they practice.

Decisions on *who* teaches are also important to the evolution of this broader curriculum in medical schools. There are a number of individuals with relevant experience and opinions on the competence of physicians who, I believe, are underrepresented among teaching "faculty." These include such persons as patients, families of patients, administrators of health-related organizations, social service programs staff, malpractice lawyers, law officers, the clergy, nurses, ward clerks, and others. These individuals are more familiar with the "social constructs" for physicians' work than many faculty can be. Where educational occasions provide the opportunity for dialogue between mature physicians and these individuals on matters pertaining to medical need, medical services, and physicians' actions, both agreement *and* disagreement produce student learning. At the University of Washington, such occasions occur regularly in our introduction to clinical medicine course (the freshman and sophomore-year course in which students acquire basic skills), the Medicine, Health, and Society course, family conferences during required courses in internal medicine and family medicine, in the primary care internal medicine and family medicine residents' "psychosocial medicine" seminars, and elsewhere. On these occasions, rapt attention and first-person statements by students and residents revealing their own opinions are commonplace; elsewhere, statements of this kind—evidence of personal exposure and openness to learning—are rare.

Decisions on *where* learning should occur can affect the perceived feasibility and availability of some of the nontraditional experiences referred to above and whether standard rotations (inpatient or outpatient) are sited in community or university-based settings. At this time, many leaders in American medicine are urging the development of additional ambulatory care experiences and the shift of clinical rotations from academic medical centers to their surrounding communities (Greer 1990; Zones and Schroeder 1989; Halperin and Kaufman 1990). The problems with such alternative siting are not insignificant; they include the development of monitoring strategies for the quality of such experience, the availability of faculty effort on a paid or volunteer basis, the economic cost of a decentralized versus a centralized activity, student transportation and safety issues, etc. On balance, the potential for student appreciation of community-based primary care, the presence of an alternative casemix of patient problems, and opportunities for participation in community-based problem-solving activities make alternative siting off the academic medical center campus seem attractive. As electives can be developed that introduce the students to the circumstances of persons living in poverty, those with reduced financial and geographic access, people with work or home-based adverse health risks, and the general role the physician as a member of the community in collaboration with others, all such siting experiments seem likely to be generative and productive, whatever the "medical" content. Small group activities with faculty back at the academic campus to share experiences, reflect together on the meaning of the students' personal reactions, identify topics for further inquiry, and engage in qualitative evaluation of these experiences with peers seem likely to enhance the value of such experiments and to minimize the incidence of serious problems with educational quality. At the University of Washington, student opportunities to see and evaluate specific patients in nursing homes have used this small group mechanism for enhancing and evaluating experiential learning.

VIII. Opportunities for Change through Educational Evaluation

Medical school leadership must ask itself what the available mechanisms are for describing educational process, deciding on the salience of educational outcomes, measuring these outcomes, initiating change in light of apparent successes and deficiencies, and evaluating the effects of change. Some routinely available intelligence about the content and success of the medical curriculum is a prerequisite to managing the curriculum. At the University of Washington the computer database for key word indexing of topics describes the content of the curriculum, a complimentary source of information to course syllabi. Additionally, two student evaluators, recruited prospectively for each course offering and identified to their peers, serve as a "sounding board" and "listening post" for their classmates and submit written qualitative evaluations of the overall course experience, together with suggestions for course/instructor improvement at the conclusion of the course. These and other less extensive student evaluations are taken seriously by the University of Washington faculty, not only because they can be useful for improving the content and pedagogical approaches of our courses, but because they are given considerable weight in the promotional decisions affecting research pathway faculty and are the primary data in the promotional decisions for clinician/teacher pathway faculty. The University of Washington's Department of Medical Education faculty have also developed what we consider to be one of the few validated instruments available for measuring teacher success in clinical settings, both inpatient and outpatient (Irby

1987). This teacher effectiveness instrument has known psychometric properties, captures information on what educators and students consider to be the salient qualities of teacher performance, is submitted by all students and residents with whom the faculty have contact, and generates much of the data from clinical settings for faculty peer feedback as well as retention and promotion decisions. Finally, such postgraduate training programs as our primary care internal medicine and family medicine residencies periodically poll their alumni/ae for retrospective ratings of relevance, adequacy, and quality of their training experiences during residency from their perspective in practice.

Questions about who participates in the evaluation of educational programs are certainly as important as those about content and quality. Where students and faculty are the sole evaluators of the process and its outcomes, professional constructs will be the principal determinants of content and standards. Given the diversity of legitimate physician's roles, I find it entirely plausible to imagine the participation of practice plan managers, clinic and inpatient ward nurses, and ratings from patients in the evaluation the knowledge and skills of students and residents. In the so-called "humanistic skills" domain, the American Board of Internal Medicine (1985), as noted earlier, has in fact initiated such approaches in order to provide feedback to trainees in internal medicine and is exploring analogous procedures for its periodic mandatory recertification process. To evaluate the aggregate accomplishments of a medical school *vis-à-vis* its community organizations and catchment area populations, medical school leadership may have to use routinely collected epidemiologic and utilization information, develop surveillance strategies for critical outcomes ("sentinel events"), elicit evaluative feedback, conduct systematic interviews with representatives of the community, and/or enter into formal health systems/services research with its affiliated organizations (Neufeld 1989). The design of such evaluations, as well as the interpretation of results, should emerge from a dialogue among representatives of the community and the medical school.

IX. Sources of Resistance to Change in Medical Education

Even should many of the prerequisites for managed change in the medical school curriculum be met, the sources of resistance to change in the medical school in the United States are manifold and substantial.

- *Diffusion of power*: Medical schools, acting alone or in their collective organizations, exert limited power. Changes in the medical school curriculum itself of the nature we have been discussing would be subject to the critical review of accrediting organizations, the semiautonomous departments within the school, the affiliated hospitals, professional organizations within the medical community, financing authorities, and others. The financing of postgraduate medical education provides a ready example of this complexity. Suppose the medical school and their affiliated hospital agree that a substantial portion of residency effort and medical student presence should and will shift off-site to a network of teaching clinics. Since Federal support for medical education effort goes to hospitals as an adjustment in allowable charges under Medicare, can these funds be "transferred" in some fashion to the clinic network? Can the affiliated hospital, where there never really was an accounting system that measured the true costs of teaching effort and directed this income to the teachers, do without this income now, when it faces burgeoning deficits? How will its administration replace the patient care effort at their site? Can the medical school's departments forego the hospital's support for the resident stipends? If not, will they simply reduce the number of resident slots in their program, or have they made firm commitments to other organizations for a fixed (at least in the short run) number of resident-months? This may be an especially significant problem in the United States, but these kinds of checks and balances, as well as divided authorities and interests surely exist in the United Kingdom, Australia, and Canada as well, and constitute significant sources of resistance to institutional change.

In fact, one of the least available prerequisites for reform in medical education may be the academic medical center-wide consensus on goals. The separation of responsibilities for undergraduate medical education, residency, and continuing medical education makes it unlikely that such consensus will occur by chance. Differential incentives and constituencies make consensus development difficult even if directly attempted. Medical school retreats are often largely devoted to explicating the rationale for, and inevitability of, different points of view, rather than negotiating or searching for common ground. The faculty, in fact, rarely seem to be the prime movers in institutional change. Instead, major "externalities" such as a change in the financing of medical education by government, or rare and sometimes destructive internal events such as student revolt, serve as the occasion for change because the perception or reality of a significant threat permits the medical school faculty and leadership to "pull together."

The varieties of power in academic medical centers are numerous and, taken together, are also likely to inhibit change. Authority of various kinds (professional, bureaucratic, legal), financial clout, prestige, access to patient populations, relationship to governmental entities—all may serve as special leverage and the basis for relative advantage in disputed issues. New sources of academic medical center complexity in the United States include negotiated contracts with managed care programs (sponsored patient populations with defined benefits served by identified panels of providers), whose administrators serve as "brokers" for enrolled populations. Other "new managers" in the academic medical center who affect educational programs in the clinical years include the staff who establish and run "guest relations" programs (designed to assure the civility of hospital professional and clerical staff to patients and their families), those who develop and feed back information from patient satisfaction surveys, serve as patient ombudspersons, and representatives of unionized hospital employees and residents.

- *Professional inertia*: Conservatism in medicine seems a significant barrier to change, at least in recent history. Examination processes and content emphasize mastery of biomedical material and change slowly. The professional notions of "knowledge base" have certainly not emphasized information vital to physician effectiveness in their "societal-mode" roles. This attention to the narrow technical expertise is, of course, a special responsibility of physicians and must be honored. Should we lavish our attention and energy on the preparation of physicians for their broader roles and produce cadres of well-meaning but technically incompetent physicians with great social consciences, we would surely do harm to our credibility and patients, clearly an abrogation of our social contract. I doubt that anything like this dark scenario could ever occur, even if the accrediting and certifying organizations were to become innovative "at the margins," probably the most "radical" change one could realistically envision. After years of deliberation, for example, the residency review committee for internal medicine recently adopted a recommendation for a minimum of 25% time commitment to ambulatory care experiences during the 3 years of the required residency. Several kinds of experiences, however, qualify as "ambulatory care" time, including service in hospital emergency rooms. The latter experience is usually quite different from the primary care, continuity clinic opportunity that many view as the kind of educational experience most lacking in the education of internists. Even in making this recommendation, the residency review committee may be following secular changes in programs, rather than leading them (Zones and Schroeder 1989). Indeed, some experienced observers of "reform" in medical education suggest that most of the rhetoric for change in academic medical centers has the effect of stultifying, not facilitating change (Bloom 1988).
- *Competition*: Other sources of resistance to change, at least in the United States, include certain characteristics of the competitive "marketplaces" for medical education and medical care services. Schools are clearly in competition with one another for faculty and students. Those who offer nontraditional educational programs or rely on community resources for a substantial fraction of their faculty effort may look unattractive to prospective students, undergraduate premedical advisors, and even their state legislatures, unless they are able to articulate a clear rationale for these kind of approaches, characterize process, and evaluate outcomes in such ways as to provide meaningful information to all the persons who need to be "sold" on these activities. New programs in student recruitment at present are substantially limited by declining undergraduate interest in medical careers (and in primary care medicine in particular) and by the regrettably

small number of minority students in the pool of potential applicants. In the competitive market for medical services, the medical school must provide an attractive, efficient service with reasonable amenities in order to compete for brokered populations and the individual patient. Under these circumstances, student participation may, at times, be viewed as a potential disincentive to prospective patients, rather than an attractive feature of the academic medical center. Further, participation in teaching programs by community physicians may be less likely than ever before—particularly on a voluntary basis—not only because they feel themselves to be under economic pressure to perform in their own practice settings, but also because the medical school may now fairly be viewed by community practitioners as a competitor of theirs in the marketplace.

- *Giving voice to the public*: Finally, I have repeatedly alluded in my comments to the importance of participation by patients, members of the general public served by the medical school's programs, and representatives of affiliated organizations, in our processes to determine needs, appropriateness of services, salience of outcomes, effectiveness of services, social legitimacy of new physicians' roles, and other matters. The embedded problem in all of this, of course, is deciding who speaks for the public (Lukomnik 1987). Where governmentally financed programs are involved, are the representatives of the public the elected representatives, staff of governmental departments or agencies, persons served by the programs of these departments and agencies, someone else, or all of above? If we are asking whether to organize and implement a program of Occupational Medicine, should our advisory group be the medical school's visiting committee, representatives of major industries, representatives of major unions, or staff from the state's Department of Labor and Industries, all of the above, or someone else? In all these matters, vested interests, constituencies, cultural and popular sensitivities, and knowledgeability issues are at work. The proper procedure is elusive, and open dialogue, always difficult to achieve on sensitive matters, is our only recourse.

X. Summary and Conclusions

The structure of my argument in this chapter has been straightforward. I contend, in terms drawn largely from moral philosophy, that the medical school has special responsibilities to the public it serves and needs to examine this charge when developing and implementing its curriculum for the preparation of physicians. The roles and responsibilities these physicians pursue include the technical, biomedical tasks of effective prevention as well as the diagnosis, care, and cure of disease states, but go well beyond the confines of this professional construct to certain other socially legitimate responsibilities of clinicians—case manager, resource rationer, health watcher, physician/citizen health advocate, socially responsible member of professional organizations, and participant in health care organization management who also serves as an advocate of the public's health. Under current circumstances, medical schools may prepare physicians well for their narrow, biomedical responsibilities but inadequately for their expanded roles. The nature of the medical school curriculum, its content, methods, and location, must be subject to change, if medicine is to fulfill public expectations and assume its societal responsibilities. The opportunities and mechanisms for change, at least the kind of change that takes place on an incremental basis, are many, but the prerequisites for such managed change are also many, including the need for well-developed institutional consensus goals for medical education, internal and external information systems, innovative mechanisms for educational program evaluation, public participation in goal setting and evaluation, and garnering the resources to overcome substantial barriers to change. Some of these resources are financial, but the scarcest of all may be nonfinancial—long-lived medical school leadership and a moral authority for change founded on the school's social contract and commitment to continuing dialogue with the population it serves.

The task is substantial; we seek to attune medical schools to their social responsibilities and to return physicians to their native society and culture. We in medicine need not feel that we face this task alone. As Charles Odegaard has recently written (1990) about the persistence of C.P. Snow's two culture problem (the parting of the humanists and scientists) in the modern university, and the adverse consequences of this schism on such fields as engineering, business, and medicine:

The educated citizen who emerges from a university of the present, and certainly of the future, should have some perspective on the world around us, on the world of nature and human beings, and on the human being's responsibility toward the natural environment and participation as a responsible individual in the surrounding social networks. Such a perspective should therefore include an awareness of self and the values which influence one's own conduct as well as knowledge about others with whom one shares participation in this life. Admittedly, this will require a lifetime of effort, but the university should provide learning experiences which help the student get started on these varied tasks.

In medical education, then, as in other fields, what we hope to learn and retain is our place in our society, and the university-based education is merely a good beginning.

Acknowledgments. The following individuals were generous enough to offer constructive criticism of this manuscript in earlier versions: Joseph Chu, Oliver Fein, Harold Goldberg, Nicole Lurie, Charles Odegaard, Michael Whitcomb, and my colleagues on the Planning Committee. This work was supported in part by the Henry J. Kaiser Family Foundation and the Robert Wood Johnson Foundation. The views expressed are those of the author and may not reflect those of the Kaiser or Johnson Foundations, my colleagues, or the University of Washington School of Medicine.

References

Ackerman, B.A. 1980. *Social Justice in the Liberal State*. New Haven: Yale University Press.

Adkins, R.J., Anderson, G.R., Cullen, T.J., Myers, W.W., and Schwarz, M.R. 1987. Geographic and specialty distribution of WAMI program participants and non-participants. *J Med Educ* **62**:810–817.

American Board of Internal Medicine. 1985. *A Guide to Awareness and Evaluation of Humanistic Qualities in the Internist*. Philadelphia: American Board of Internal Medicine.

Antonovsky, A. 1987. Medical student selection at the Ben-Gurion University of the Negev. *Isr J Med Sci* **23**:969–975.

Battista, R.N., and Lawrence, R.S. (Eds.). 1988. *Implementing Preventive Services*. New York: Oxford University Press.

Belenky, M.F., Clinchy, B.M., Goldberger, N.R., and Tarule, J.M. 1986. *Women's Ways of Knowing: The Development of Self, Voice, and Mind*. New York: Basic Books.

Bergman, B.B. 1986. *The "Discovery" of Sudden Infant Death Syndrome: Lessons in the Practice of Political Medicine*. Seattle: University of Washington Press.

Bloom, S.W. 1988. Structure and ideology in medical education: An analysis of resistance to change. *J Health Soc Behav* **29**:294–306.

Bunker, J.P., Gomby, D.S., and Kehrer, B.H. (Eds.). 1989. *Pathways to Health: The Role of Social Factors*. Menlo Park, CA: The Henry J. Kaiser Family Foundation.

Cassell, E.J. 1985. *Talking with Patients, Volume 1: The Theory of Doctor-patient Communication*. Cambridge: The MIT Press.

Committee on Trauma Research, Commission on Life Sciences, National Research Council, the Institute of Medicine. 1985. *Injury in America: A Continuing Public Health Problem*. Washington, D.C.: National Academy Press.

Cullen, M.R., Cherniack, M.G., and Rosenstock, L. 1990. Occupational medicine. *N Engl J Med* **322**:594–604.

Daniels, N. (Ed.). 1985. *Just Health Care: Studies in Philosophy and Health Policy*. Cambridge: Cambridge University Press.

DeVries, M.J. 1981. *The Redemption of the Intangible in Medicine*. London: Institute of Psychosynthesis.

Dickstein, L., and Nadelson, C.C. (Eds.). 1986. *Women Physicians in Leadership Roles*. Washington, D.C.: American Psychiatric Press.

Ebert, R.H., and Ginzberg, E. 1988. The reform of medical education. *Health Affairs* **7**:5–9.

Eisenberg, J.M. 1986. *Doctors' Decisions and the Cost of Medical Care*. Ann Arbor: Health Administration Press Perspectives.

Engel, G.L. 1977. The need for a new medical model: A challenge for biomedicine. *Science* **196**:129–136.

Gamble, V.N. 1990. On becoming a physician: A dream not deferred. In: White, EC (Ed.), *The Black Women's Health Book: Speaking for Ourselves*. Seattle: Seal Press.

Gastel, B., and Rogers, D.E. (Eds.). 1989. *Clinical Education and the Doctor of Tomorrow*. New York: The New York Academy of Medicine.

Geieger, J., Eisenberg, C., Gloyd, S., Quiroga, J., Schlenker, T., Scrimshaw, N., and Devin, J. 1989. A new medical mission to El Salvador. *N Engl J Med* **321**:1136–1140.

Greer, D.S. 1990. Altering the mission of the academic health center: Can medical schools really change? In: *Education of Physicians to Improve Access to Care for the Underserved: Proceedings of the Second HRSA Primary Care Conference, March 21–22, 1990*. Washington D.C.: Health Resources Service Administration, pp. 203–232.

Greer, T., and Carline, J.D. 1989. Specialty choice by medical students: Recent graduate follow-up survey at the University of Washington. *Fam Med* **21**: 127–131.

Halperin, A.K., and Kaufman, A., 1990. Ambulatory medical education: A reconsideration of sites and teachers. *J Gen Int Med* **5**(Supplement):S35–S44.

Iliffe, S., and Haines, A. 1989. Developments in British general practice. *Fam Med* **21**:169–170, 176–6, 229–230.

Inui, T.S. 1988. Though Sydenham fled the plague. *J Gen Int Med* **3**:566–571.

Irby, D., Gilmore, G., and Ramsey, P. 1987. Factors affecting ratings of clinical teachers by medical students and residents. *J Med Educ* **62**:1–7.

Kark, S.L. 1981. *Community-oriented primary health care*. New York: Appleton-Century-Crofts.

Kaufman, A., Mennin, S., Waterman, R., Duban, S., Hansbarger, C., et al. 1989. The New Mexico experiment: Educational innovation and institutional change. *Acad Med* **29**:285–294.

Kellerman, A.L. 1990. Domestic violence and the internist's response: Advocacy or apathy? *J Gen Int Med* **5**:89–90.

Kolata, G. 1990. Wariness is replacing the trust between physician and patient. *New York Times* CXXXIX: February 20.

Koska, MT. 1990. Primary care: Hospitals begin to target community needs. *Hospitals* **5**:24–28.

Lightfoot, S.L. 1988. *Balm in Gilead*. Reading, MA: Addison-Wesley.

Lock, M., and Gordon, D.R. (Eds.). 1988. *Biomedicine Examined*. Dordrecht: Kluwer Academic Publishers.

Ludmerer, K.M. 1985. *Learning to Heal: The Development of American Medical Education*. New York: Basic Books.

Lukomnik, J.E. 1987. Patient and community involvement in different settings. In: Nutting, P.A. (Ed.), *Community-Oriented Primary Care: From Principle to Practice*. Washington, D.C.: Health Resources and Services Administration.

Manning, P.R., and DeBakey, L. 1987. *Medicine: Preserving the Passion*. New York: Springer-Verlag.

Neufeld, V.R. 1989. University partnerships in health systems research. *Bridge* **2**:1–2.

Nutting, P.A. (Ed.). 1987. *Community-Oriented Primary Care: From Principle to Practice*. Washington, D.C.: Health Resources and Services Administration.

Odegaard, C.E. 1986. *Dear Doctor: A Personal Letter to a Physician*. Menlo Park: The Henry J. Kaiser Family Foundation.

Odegaard, C.E. 1990. The structure of the university and goals and values. In: Bjornson, R. and Waldman, M.R. (Eds.), *The University of the Future: Problems and Prospects.* Ohio State University: The Center for Comparative Studies in the Humanities.

Panel on the General Professional Education of the Physician and College Preparation for Medicine. 1984. *Physicians for the Twenty-First Century: The GPEP Report.* Washington, D.C.: Association of American Medical Colleges.

Pendleton, D., Schofield, T., Tate, P., and Havelock, P. 1984. *The Consultation: An Approach to Learning and Teaching.* Oxford: Oxford University Press.

Pickles, W.N. 1972 (reissue). *Epidemiology in Country Practice.* London: The Devonshire Press.

Rogers, C. 1983. *Freedom to Learn for the '80s.* Columbus: Charles E. Merrill.

Sackett, D.L., Haynes, R.B., and Tugwell, P. 1985. *Clinical Epidemiology: A Basic Science for Clinical Medicine.* Boston: Little, Brown.

Schorr, L.B. 1988. *Within Our Reach: Breaking the Cycle of Disadvantage.* New York: Anchor Press.

Schroeder, S.A., Zones, J.S., and Showstack, J.A. 1989. Academic medicine as a public trust. *J Am Med Assoc* **262:**803–812.

Schroeder, S.A., Schuster, B.L., and Gastel, B. (Eds.). 1990. New challenges in resident education. *J Gen Int Med* Supplement to **5**(1):S1–S80.

Seldin, D.W. 1981. The boundaries of medicine. *Trans Assoc Am Physicians* **94:**lxxv-lxxxvi.

Starr, P. 1982. *The Social Transformation of American Medicine.* New York: Basic Books.

Stewart, M., and Roter, D. (Eds.). *Communicating with Medical Patients.* Newbury Park: Sage.

Tosteson, D.C. 1990. New pathways in general medical education. *N Engl J Med* **322:**234–238.

Walton, J.J. 1985. Primary health care in European medical education: A survey. *Med Education* **19:**167–188.

Winkenwerder, W., and Ball, JR. 1988. Transformation of American health care: The role of the medical profession. *N Engl J Med* **318:**317–319.

White, K.L. 1988. *The Task of Medicine.* Menlo Park, CA: The Henry J. Kaiser Family Foundation.

World Conference on Medical Education. 1988. The Edinburgh declaration. *Med Education* **22:**481–482.

Zones, J.S., and Schroeder, S.A. 1989. Evolving residency requirements for ambulatory care training for five medical specialties, 1961 to 1989. *West J Med* **151:**676–678.

Discussion

David Axelrod

Inui has provided an articulate and comprehensive presentation of the responsibilities of the medical school that far transcend some of the current focus on biomedical and biotechnical information. The nurturant role of the medical school is defined in terms of a social contract with the body politic, not unlike the role of medicine described by Virchow in his confrontation with Bismarck.

Rather than suggest that Inui has embarked on a revolutionary confrontation with the current undergraduate medical ethos, I would propose that he is attempting to return us to the precepts of health, if not medicine, contained in the Hippocratic oath. The paradigm is not new, but one that is redefined within the context of a better informed appreciation of the morbidities of our society and a disappointment with the factual revelations on the impact of the technological evolution on the preservation of health, and quality of life, however defined. We have neither exhausted an old paradigm, nor adopted a new one.

The explosion of technological developments of the past 30 years produced an accompanying dynamic within medical schools that focused increasingly on the application of technology rather than on the student–teacher relationship and necessarily the patient–doctor relationship. There was a devolution of essential physician skills and the identification of "quality" for health care with medical interventions. Without definition, without understanding, and without application of the simultaneously burgeoning collection and analysis capabilities, quality rapidly became the inadvertent victim for the promotion of an unparalleled increase in the rate of expenditure for medical care. Academic medical centers adopted new competitive market strategies to capture their share of these revenues and accepted a role for the training of those who would fuel this medical industrial complex. This dynamo

- Produced little in terms of population benefits;
- Increased inequities in the allocation of resources;
- Spawned a new trilogy of concerns for access, cost containment, and a narrowly defined quality
- Blurred the relationships between equity and the macro-view of quality;
- Disillusioned the political and business establishments whose generosity had been virtually unbounded;
- Manifested new entrepreneurial instincts as hallmarks of success in medicine;
- Nurtured a resurgence in guild protectionism among and within the health-related professions;
- Dissipated the remnants of the humanistic traditions in medicine;
- Generated a new dictionary of terms, ambiguously defined, to conceal our failures; and
- Promoted the perversion of a professional educational process.

Small wonder that Inui has suggested a "social contract" to promote corrective actions and a new direction for our zeal. How is that social contract to be defined? Is it to come from an anachronistic paternalism or is it to be defined by those who continue to provide the fuel for our health care engine? Is it to come by revolution or by time-honored incrementalism? How will the social contract address the nonmedical factors in the genesis of health, ill and good? To what extent will the public health problems of homicide, drug abuse, AIDS, and the recrudescence of tuberculosis and sexually transmitted disease be encompassed within the mission of the medical school? How will the allocation of resources be directed to nonmedical interventions through the social contract?

With all of its infirmities, government in each of our respective democracies is likely to develop a prescription for the social contract. The financing of the nurturant function, as well as the preservative, curative, advocative, allocative, and delphic functions, falls within the direct or indirect province of government. Different governmental definitions of ethical and moral responsibilities for universal access to health care are likely to be far more important in the prescription than the focus on academic curricula. It will, however, require

- Attention to the comparatively high level of disaffection with the health care delivery system, particularly in the United States;
- A new level of public accountability and an awareness of distributive injustices in our respective systems;
- A requirement for the integration of medical education at the undergraduate, postgraduate, and graduate levels;
- An awareness of the lack of relationship between consumption of health care resources and health of the population or of the individual;
- An explanation of the rationale for the enormous differences in outcomes and in per capita consumption in different geographic and demographic jurisdictions; and
- A new literacy for humanistic concerns that transcends the implementation of technological innovation.

Those whose "social contracts" are defined in parliamentary systems, rather than in a presidential democracy, are likely to see progress dictated through the majority or ruling party's perception of benevolence in a financially constrained system. That same progress in the United States is more likely to arise from compromise among the virtually limitless special interest groups, all of which have infinite access to a political structure lacking the discipline of party control by an elected leader. The fealty of the elected representative is to his/her own constituencies and not to the elected leader. The distinctions between public demand and public need can become readily confused as each of the special interests attempts to preserve its own share of the allocation through our system of political accessibility and local accountability.

Reform is inevitable, whether it comes through an explicit recognition of the need for a new "social contract," or from our sense of intolerance for the magnitude of the injustices of our current training and organization of the providers of health care. We can either direct the reform through a new infusion of intellect and insight born of our frustrations and disappointments with the population's inevitable mortality or we can abdicate and ascribe our enfeebling to governmental intervention and regulation. The crisis we are so quick to describe will result either in resolution or disaster. How that resolution or disaster evolves depends very much on how we respond to the challenges contained in Inui's analysis.

Sir Christopher Booth

The author makes the case that since medicine is concerned with society at large, medical schools have social responsibilities to the communities in which they live. The case is commendably made for the University of Washington in Seattle, which serves the states of Washington, Alaska, Montana, and Idaho, and has clear responsibilities for providing medical manpower for these predominantly rural areas. It might perhaps be more difficult to make the same case for the many medical schools that exist in urban areas such as New York City, Toronto, Sydney, or London or for those schools and hospitals (for example London's Postgraduate Institutes) that claim a national rather than a local role. Nevertheless, the argument goes much wider than the merely parochial and is generally applicable to medical schools not only in the United States but also in Europe and Australia. In Britain, the argument for increasing the training of physicians in the social and behavioral sciences was largely won with the publication of the 1968 Report of the Royal Commission on Medical Education, chaired by Lord Todd (Royal Commission 1968). Since then, pioneering medical schools, particularly McMaster in Canada, have successfully transformed their educational programs from the traditional bias toward biomedical science that so dominates the medical educational scene in the United States and in many universities in Britain. If one had any criticism of Inui's thesis, it would be that there is a faint undercurrent of unnecessary apology to the scientific grandees who so firmly control American medical schools and who hail their accomplishments as "bastions of biomedical science."

The argument that physicians should have greater exposure to ambulatory care, primary care, and the public health problems of their communities is compellingly presented. Yet at the end of the day, financial concerns drive health care systems. If the funding of care is predominantly left to the private sector, then those seeking to practice medicine and earn their living at it will inevitably seek to learn those practices that ensure that a gainful living may be made. If medical schools are to remain financially viable, they too have to seek their financial salvation from those areas of health care that can pay. Inui argues, quite rightly, that intending physicians should know more of the problems of underprivileged ethnic minorities, the mentally disabled, and the physically handicapped. Yet if these groups remain uninsured, how can medical schools effectively provide such educational opportunities without extra financial support? Is the answer to support the proposals for a national system of insurance recently put forward by the American College of Physicians?

There is clearly a need for a greater concern with public health matters in medical schools. Yet one has to question whether the national trend towards creating, within universities, Schools of Public Health that are separate from the medical schools has not inhibited the development of educational facilities for medical students. For too many, public health has been a postgraduate activity.

Finally, there is the question of research. The success of many medical schools has been in research in the biomedical sciences. The requirement for innovative research in the areas of social concern identified by Inui is no less important.

Reference

Royal Commission on Medical Education, 1965–68. 1968. *Report*. Cmnd. 3569. London: Her Majesty's Stationery Office.

Ian R. McWhinney

I agree totally with Inui's two main statements: that the medical school has a social responsibility to the population it serves and that its central responsibility is for the education of physicians. I wish, however, to express my skepticism that these responsibilities can be met by changes in the formal curriculum, by the attaining of "competencies," and by the provision of "intelligence."

I make a distinction between the formal curriculum, the foreground of education—the written objectives, courses, group teaching, laboratory work—and the background or context: the environment of learning and the mind-set of teachers. The background or informal curriculum is a far more powerful influence on students than the formal curriculum to which we tend to give most of our attention. Marshall McCluhan's insight—one he derived from H.A. Innis (1972)—is summed up in the aphorism "the medium is the message." If students have their clinical training mainly in hospitals, especially tertiary care hospitals, they will get the message: "this is what disease is, and this method for investigating it is **the** method of medicine." If they never care for a patient at home, the message will be "the home is no place for a physician." If they are taught mainly by specialists, they will get the message: "this is where authority, prestige, and power lie." If they are never taught by a nurse or social worker, the message will be: "nurses and social workers have nothing to teach me." On the cognitive level, the environment has a potentially biasing effect on the learning of clinical method. The predictive value of symptoms, signs, and tests varies with the prevalence of the target disorder in the population of the clinic or practice (Sackett et al. 1985). The sensitivity of tests varies with the stage of the target disorder (McWhinney 1989). The range of attributes used to define a category (disease) is strongly influenced by the range of attributes available during training (Bruner et al. 1956). This has important implications for early diagnosis and secondary prevention (McWhinney 1989). If, therefore, students are trained mainly in a hospital setting, they will acquire diagnostic habits that are inappropriate for primary care. I will return to this issue after some comments about different types of population.

I think it is important to identify the different levels of population that are germane to our subject. All clinicians relate to families as well as to individual patients. Meeting the needs of families can be taught in any clinical setting, provided the teacher is a model of good family care. Often this is not the case. I find that talking to families is often delegated to unsupervised house staff. Reform on this level has to start in the hearts and minds of the teachers.

The next level is the population of a practice for which a primary physician provides continuing care. This may be synonymous with a neighborhood, although in North America urban practices have tended to become dispersed. This requires competence in identifying health risks in individuals, in thinking of the whole practice as a population at risk, and in identifying health risks in a neighborhood. Prior to competence must come the appropriate mind-set and this, in my experience, is rare—at least for the latter two competencies. The next level is the large population of the city, country, or region. From this level, the clinician acquires a background awareness of the larger context within which he/she practices. Each of these levels requires different mind-sets, information, and skills.

We must not, however, make too much of a distinction between clinical and population competency. For the great majority of physicians, their "population competency" will be applied in clinical practice: hence the need for a reformed, patient-centered clinical method that views patients in their social context as a matter of course (McWhinney 1986).

Let me now return to my original point. In attending mainly to the formal curriculum and to health information, I fear that we are merely adding to the abstractions that already dominate medical education instead of providing the appropriate learning environment for students, and changing the hearts and minds of those who teach them.

A.N. Whitehead (1926) criticized professional education for its reliance on abstractions rather than concrete experience. "It holds if you apply it to a nation, a city, a district, an institution, a family, or even to an individual. There is a development of particular abstractions and a contraction of concrete appreciation." According to Whitehead, this diet of abstractions has produced a "celibacy of the intellect" that he compares with the celibacy of the medieval learned class. Information alone will not change people. The article by Kerr White et al. (1961), with its overwhelming message, was published 30 years ago. Yet medical students and residents are still taught mainly by specialists and mainly in tertiary care hospitals. Sophisticated intelligence was not needed to see that the Love Canal in Niagara Falls was an environmental and public health disaster. The local physicians did not see it because they were not there in the homes of the people and in the neighborhood. They were in the hospitals with their backs to the community. The conditions were exposed in the end by a journalist (Brown 1979).

The reform of medical education requires a redefinition of the medical school (McWhinney 1980). Instead of a place, a campus, a group of buildings, it should be an organization that is immanent in the whole health care system. It should be as much a presence in the rural hospital, the nursing home, the public health unit, and the inner city or rural practice, as it is in the tertiary care hospital and the laboratory. It follows also that those who teach should represent the whole profession in some proportion to their numbers, as well as our sister health professions from whom we have so much to learn.

If the medical school is to be immanent in the health care system, it follows that the school should not own any one part of it, or provide any service directly. The school can then provide learning environments by entering into agreements with institutions of many different kinds. My own school—the University of Western Ontario—is an example of this (McWhinney 1980). Most of the competencies we are discussing can be learned only in the primary care and community setting. We need, therefore, a major shift in the center of gravity of medical education from tertiary to primary care, and from teaching by specialists to teaching by generalists (McWhinney 1980). The great turning points in medicine have been associated with revolutionary changes in the environment in which medicine is practiced: the birth of modern medicine after the French Revolution (Foucault 1975) and the Flexner (1910) reforms earlier in our century. The change we need now will, I believe, be of the same magnitude. As Inui implies, the process will be difficult and painful, and it will necessarily involve a change in the power structure of medical education.

References

Brown, M.H. 1979. Love canal and the poisoning of America. *Atlantic Monthly* December.

Bruner, J.S., Goodnow J.J., and Austin C.A. 1972. *A Study of Thinking*. New York: Wiley.

Flexner, A. 1910. *Medical Education in the United States and Canada*. A Report to the Carnegie Foundation for the Advancement of Teaching. New York.

Foucault, M. 1975. *The Birth of the Clinic: An Archaeology of Medical Perception*. New York: Vintage Books.

Innis, H.A. 1972. *The Empire and Communications*. Toronto: University of Toronto Press.

McWhinney, I.R. 1980. The reform of medical education: A Canadian model. *Med Education* **14**:189–195.

McWhinney, I.R. 1986. Are we on the brink of a transformation of clinical method. *Can Med Assoc J* **135**:873–878.

McWhinney, I.R. 1989. *A Textbook of Family Medicine*. New York: Oxford University Press.
Sackett, D.L., Haynes, R.B., and Tugwell, P. 1985. *Clinical Epidemiology: A Basic Science for Clinical Medicine*. Boston: Little, Brown.
White, K.L., Williams, T.F., and Greenberg, B.G. 1961. The ecology of medical care. *N Engl J Med* **265**:885–892.
Whitehead, A.N. 1926. *Science and the Modern World*. Cambridge: Cambridge University Press.

General Discussion

There was unanimous agreement that despite obstacles and problems, the concept of the social contract between medical schools and the population was valid. Organized efforts should now be made not only to "graft the population-based paradigm" onto the educational environment for physicians and other health professionals but to expand medicine's fundamental perspectives and develop specific mission statements. Consideration of the institutional mission should be based on continuing dialogue that actively engages the faculty and in appropriate ways the "community." As important are faculty and institutional "role-modeling"—probably the most important pedagogical instruments available to influence attitudes and behavior. Teaching and learning need to be based on information about the population leavened by experience within the community.

The political basis of societal actions needs to be understood at a deeper level than is now generally the case for medicine. The nature of the health care system is as critical a determinant of physician behavior as the educational environment. Medical faculty can play a role in changing both. To these ends a broadened epistemology of medicine beyond that currently embraced is needed. It requires deeper, more sophisticated understanding of and experience with politics, history, cultural anthropology, ethics, and the law. There is an urgent need to "demedicalize" health, on the one hand, and, on the other, to distinguish between public "need" and public "demand." To further these goals, medicine should help the other health professions to incorporate the population perspective, and to build closer links with the social and behavioral sciences.

3
Measuring the Burden of Illness in General Populations

MICHAEL G. MARMOT and ANTHONY B. ZWI

I. Introduction

This chapter has two themes: *medical schools have traditionally failed to devote attention to the determinants of health* and *medical students are taught on an unrepresentative sample of patients and health conditions.* The availability of population-based data may assist medical schools to understand and appreciate the distribution of health, disease, and death, as well as their determinants, in the population they serve. Awareness of these patterns should influence medical education, clinical practice, and research, thus making them more responsive to public health priorities.

It has been proposed that medical schools should establish a "Health Intelligence Unit" to collate, analyze, and interpret statistics relevant to health and health services (White 1988). This could be in partnership with a local health department or authority. A range of data should be collected by such a unit: we draw on available information from the United Kingdom, United States, and Canada, to illustrate those available.

Three principles should inform the use of such data:

- They need to be *population based* rather than counts of cases: a denominator as well as numerator is required;
- Their *form depends on the questions being clearly defined:* are we looking at care or cure, prevention or treatment, causes or mechanisms? and
- *Heterogeneities and inequalities within and between populations help identify issues* requiring explanations, interventions, and further research.

We argue that *every medical school and its faculty should be thoroughly familiar with the distribution of health problems in general populations, including those living in the institution's "catchment" or service area.*

Three general points should be borne in mind about the data assembled:

- Data are powerful. If they were not so, politicians would not try to suppress or distort them.
- Data, like science itself, are not value neutral. The data collected relate to the questions posed.

- Data do not make decisions; people do. We argue that the medical curriculum should be influenced by the data on health and social problems in the communities or populations served by the medical school. There will not, however, be a straightforward correspondence between the magnitude of problems and the space devoted to them in the curriculum.

II.　Appropriate Medical Education

Medical education needs reshaping. Health services have altered. New structures and forms of organization are in existence or are proposed; there is greater recognition of the role of primary care and care in the community; there is heightened awareness of limited resources; there are fewer hospital beds available and lengths of stay have shortened; and costs are of great concern. Populations too have varied over time and are socially and ethnically diverse; life expectancy is greater; chronic diseases are more common; and populations are aging. Changed too are some of our perceptions of health: there is greater recognition of the variety of influences on health and of the importance of behavior and social conditions; there is concern about the quality and not only the quantity of life. Despite these many fundamental changes, medical education generally takes place in the laboratory or at the bedside of sick individuals in tertiary care institutions, oblivious to many of the debates raging around health in our society.

Medical students must have an understanding of biology. The challenge and excitement of molecular genetics assure it a prominent place in the curriculum, but this should not be at the expense of other priorities. Teaching and research in a medical school rarely reflect the burden of illness in the general population. Rather, they tend to echo the clinical and research interests of the faculty and the pattern of patients admitted to teaching hospitals.

A model of the range of influences on health status is shown in Figure 3.1 (Evans and Stoddart 1990). A comprehensive analysis of health and illness necessitates consideration of the social, physical, and genetic environment, as well as of the host response (especially behavior) and the health care system. The political environment influences the pattern and distribution of health care, as well as having a more direct influence on health status.

The need for medical schools to be at the frontiers of innovation in technical and molecular medicine has to be balanced against the necessity to train medical students appropriately and for the medical school itself to take the lead in shaping services oriented to the needs of the community. Medical education must reflect an awareness of

- The distribution of health, disease, disability, and death in the population;
- The causes of disease that reside in the economy, the physical, occupational, social, and cultural environments, as well as in the genetic make-up of individuals, and in their behavior; and

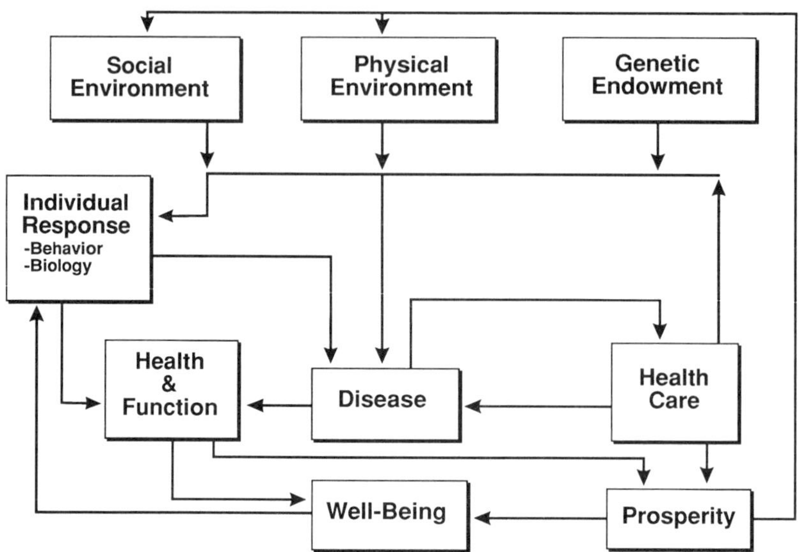

FIGURE 3.1. Model of relationship between health and its determininants (Evans and Stoddart 1990).

- Health conditions presenting (or not presenting) at different levels of the health services operating in the community.

An understanding of the composition of the community by age, sex, ethnic group, employment status, social class, and other factors will be crucial to exploring the population distribution of causes of health states and the services needed to deal with them. Without this awareness, the thrust of teaching, research, and service undertaken by the medical school may be misdirected, neglecting important health problems. Three approaches warrant emphasis:

Medical Schools Should Consider the Determinants of Health

Medical schools devote little attention to the determinants of health in society. The relationship to health of income, employment, social class, housing, water supply, sanitation, or the health care system itself receive cursory, if any, consideration. Traditionally, clinicians focus on treatment of disease. Broadening the focus of medical attention to the health problems of the population, as in Figure 3.1, should influence the subsequent practice of medicine. Neglecting the determinants of health confines medicine to the important but limited role of patching up and treating the ill. Medicine should participate in addressing the causes of ill-health that reside in individual behaviors and in the community and its social and political structure.

Education Should Reflect the Distribution of Health in Society

In their preclinical work, medical students are exposed to a very limited extent, through study of the social sciences, to understanding their future patients in their social context. At the clinical level, students spend the majority of their time in tertiary referral hospitals studying health problems requiring care and treatment at a superspecialty level. The limited attention to ambulatory care revolves around patients presenting to hospital clinics. Little attention is given to primary care and even less to considering the determinants of ill-health in the community.

It may be argued that the role of the medical school is to develop an undifferentiated doctor who has the knowledge, skills, and attitudes required to go into any branch of medicine for postgraduate training. It follows, therefore, that specialist care should not be overemphasized at the undergraduate level at the expense of greater emphasis on health in the community. Students should gain experience of treating people in a range of settings and should be competent to deal with health problems affecting the majority of people. They should understand the proportion of the population and the nature of the problems that present at different levels of the health service.

Even where students indicate a preference for working in primary care, medical education generally fails to provide relevant experience. An enquiry into career choices of recent graduates from five United Kingdom medical schools showed that the largest single group, nearly 40%, intended pursuing a career in general practice (University Hospitals Association 1989). A minority of students plan to pursue careers resembling those of the majority of their teachers, yet the education of medical students tends to follow their teachers' clinical activities and research interests.

Establishing a Health Information and Analysis Unit

Understanding the range and distribution of health and ill-health in the community is clearly important. Kerr White (1988) suggests the establishment of "Health Intelligence and Analysis Units" at medical schools may be useful in this regard. These would have the task of monitoring, among other things, the health status of the population served, changes in its status, the distribution of health problems and associated disability, new interventions and technologies, and assessing the value of care provided. An experimental unit of this sort has been set up at McMaster University as described in Chapter 4. Neufeld has described a mechanism for utilizing information on

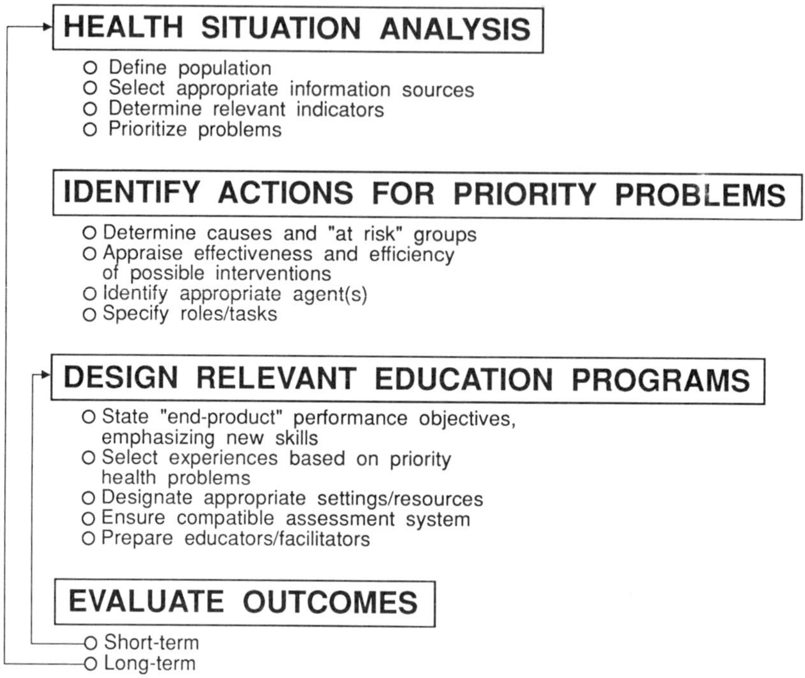

┌─────────────────────────────────────┐
│ **HEALTH SITUATION ANALYSIS** │
└─────────────────────────────────────┘
- Define population
- Select appropriate information sources
- Determine relevant indicators
- Prioritize problems

┌─────────────────────────────────────┐
│ **IDENTIFY ACTIONS FOR PRIORITY PROBLEMS** │
└─────────────────────────────────────┘
- Determine causes and "at risk" groups
- Appraise effectiveness and efficiency
  of possible interventions
- Identify appropriate agent(s)
- Specify roles/tasks

┌─────────────────────────────────────┐
│ **DESIGN RELEVANT EDUCATION PROGRAMS** │
└─────────────────────────────────────┘
- State "end-product" performance objectives,
  emphasizing new skills
- Select experiences based on priority
  health problems
- Designate appropriate settings/resources
- Ensure compatible assessment system
- Prepare educators/facilitators

┌─────────────────────────────────────┐
│ **EVALUATE OUTCOMES** │
└─────────────────────────────────────┘
- Short-term
- Long-term

FIGURE 3.2. Priority health problems model. *Source:* Network of Community-Oriented Health Sciences Education (1989).

health in the community for medical education (Fig. 3.2); this is described below (p. 101–102).

III. Data Collection Must Be Population Based

Data on individual cases are obtained during clinical interview and examination. To assess the health status of a community, epidemiological methods need to be employed. These relate counts of events or people to a population denominator and allow the calculation of rates. Rates enable data to be compared across different populations or within a population between sexes or ages. Focusing on the numerator alone (counts) would lead to erroneous conclusions about the relative burden of illness in a section of the community.

International, national, intranational, or local populations may be relevant. A comprehensive set of information (Table 3.1) could be specified as a minimum standard data set to be collected by all schools. Many of these data are routinely published (Table 3.2). Others may appear in the medical

TABLE 3.1. Data on the health of the community.

Perceptions by community
  Perception of state of health
  Views on appropriateness of services
  Attitudes to health promotion, screening, etc.

Physical environment
  Occupational hazards
  Housing conditions
  Water supply and sanitation
  Radiation, etc.

Behaviors
  Smoking
  Alcohol
  Drug misuse
  Exercise
  Diet
  Stress
  Sex, etc.

Social and demographic
  Population size by
    Age and sex
    Ethnic, religious, and language group
    Income, employment, and social class, etc.
  Population projections

State of health
  Morbidity
  Disability
  Mortality
    Neonatal, perinatal, postnatal
    Infant and childhood
    Crude
    Age, sex, and cause-specific
  Incidence and prevalence
  Attack rates
  Survival rates
  Notification rates
  Disease registers
  Potential years of life lost by cause
  Fertility, low birthweight, stillbirth, abortion rates, etc.

Genetic
  Genetic diseases
  HLA types etc.

Health services
  Utilization, e.g., hospital bed use or general practice consultations
  Access, e.g., waiting times, consultations by social class
  Equity, e.g., social class differences in health care given same condition
  Cost and affordability, to individuals and society
  Considerations of effectiveness and efficiency, including readmission rates
  Prescribing rates
  Procedures undertaken
  Levels of staffing

TABLE 3.1. *Continued.*

Societal costs
  Health as proportion of GDP, GNP
  Sickness absence
  Days of work lost
  Value of care provided by families, etc.
  Health services
  Insurance costs to individuals and employers

or social sciences literature. The need for detail may necessitate specific study and the collection of data at local level. In the USA, much data are routinely presented by the National Center for Health Statistics (Woteki et al. 1988). In the United Kingdom, district and regional health authorities have recently been required to produce an Annual Health Report examining the state of health of the community served by the authority; a common data set to be used for this purpose is made available on floppy disk by the Department of Health to the organizations concerned. Such data would be extremely valuable to the medical schools operating within those geographic boundaries.

An example of locally available data is the 1989 Annual Health Report from the Bloomsbury Health Authority, the district in which the authors' medical school is based. This describes the composition of the population, birth, death, perinatal and low-birthweight rates, standardized mortality ratios, infectious diseases rates, and details of service utilization and cost. Using Bloomsbury data for deaths in 1987, for example, reveals three conditions for which the standardized mortality ratio in the district is substantially higher than the national average: cancer of the breast, accidents and injuries, and tuberculosis (Bloomsbury Health Authority 1989). This highlights the need for further research both into the causes of these conditions and into the accessibility and effectiveness of services.

Local health surveys will be required to gather information on self-perceived health (which predicts subsequent mortality), use of health services, and use of screening services and behaviors. This is essential to understanding the community in which the medical school is based.

IV. Different Forms of Information Convey Different Messages

Different forms of information provide different insights into health and health services. Data useful for health planning, evaluation of health services, assessing changes over time, identifying inequalities, and developing public health approaches to reducing causes of ill-health will vary. Data on perceptions of health, behaviors and life-style, disability, morbidity, and mortality are necessary.

TABLE 3.2. Sources of information in the United Kingdom, Canada, and United States.

United Kingdom
  Morbidity Statistics from General Practice
  Hospital In-patient Enquiry
  Hospital Activity Analysis—Hospital Episode System
  General Household Survey
  Social Trends—annual reports
  Registrar General's Decennial Supplement on Occupational Mortality
  OPCS Longitudinal study
  Mortality statistics, including infant mortality
  Abortion, cancer registration, congenital malformations
  Health service indicators
  District and regional annual health reports
  Social Security Statistics
  OPCS Survey of disability

Canada
  Labor Force Survey
  Canada Health Survey and Canada Health Promotion Survey
  Canada Fitness Survey
  Ontario Health Promotion Survey
  Sources of routine statistics such as Chronic diseases in Canada, etc.

United States
  National Vital Statistics System
  National Health Interview Survey
  National Health Examination Survey
  National Survey of Family Growth
  National Health and Nutrition Examination Survey
  National Hospital Discharge Survey
  National Nursing Home Survey
  National Master Facility Inventory
  National Ambulatory Medical Care Survey
  National Occupational Hazard Survey
  National Occupational Exposure Survey
  National Survey on Drinking
  National Household Survey on Drug Abuse

Other
  Local surveys
  Censuses
  Commissions of enquiry
  Registers of disease
  Infectious disease surveillance
  Abortion surveillance
  Immunization surveillance
  Workmens compensation data
  Voluntary organizations
  Private sector health and welfare services

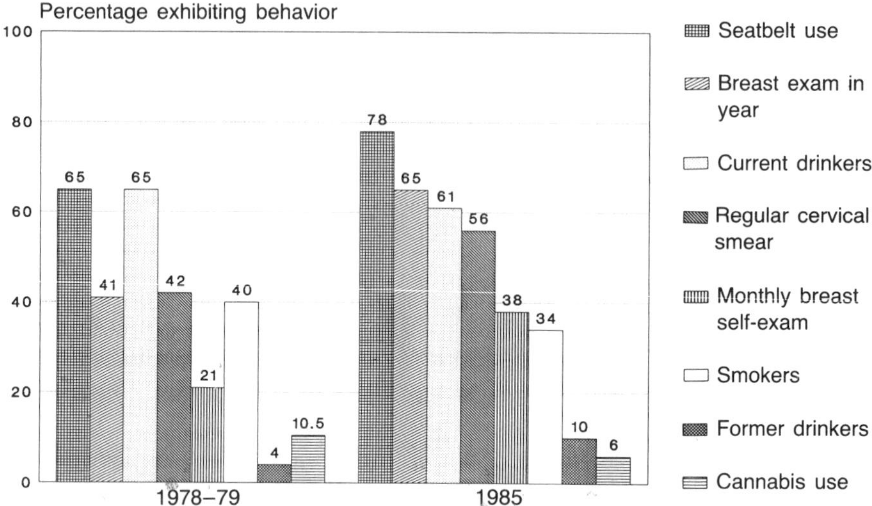

FIGURE 3.3. Improvements in preventive practices, people aged 15+, Canada 1978/ 1979–1985. *Source:* Canada Health Promotion Survey (1985) and Canada Health Survey (1978/1979).

Perceptions of the Community

Attitudes and perceptions of the community may influence the utilization of services, behavioral change in response to health education, and compliance with medical treatment. Routine surveys used to collect such information include the United States National Health Interview Survey and the General Household Survey in the United Kingdom.

Figure 3.3 presents data from the Canada Health Survey and Canadian Health Promotion Survey (Rootman et al. 1988). Almost all the health behaviors examined showed positive changes from 1978/1979 to 1985. For example, while 65% of people generally wore seatbelts in 1978–1979, 78% did so in 1985; 41% of women had had a breast examination in the previous year in 1978–1979; this had increased to 65% by 1985.

Monitoring of preventive practices is essential to determining whether health promotion messages are reaching the population. More specific data are required to see if all sections of the community are heeding messages; if not it may be that the educational material is culturally inappropriate or that it fails to take account of the objective difficulties in making the changes advocated.

The Health and Lifestyles Survey (Blaxter 1990) examined the opinions and attitudes to health and health services of a sample of the population of England, Wales, and Scotland. Such a survey is invaluable to medical education—it indicates the links between social position and health-related attitudes and behaviors. The survey showed that lower income groups perceived their health as being worse; the most common illness symptoms were those of colds or flu, headaches, "bad back," "trouble with periods," and indigestion. In general, health was considered to be more than the absence of disease: older people considered functioning to be important while women included more psychological factors in their definition of health. The survey found that determinants of health related more closely to specific local conditions than geographic location alone. The protective effect of good health behavior was most evident in those living in favorable environments while it was less apparent in those exposed to poor living and environmental conditions (Blaxter 1990).

The medical curriculum should include a component on health promotion (Gillies and Elwood 1989). The aim of such a course would include the ability to identify personal, cultural, and sociodemographic factors (e.g. age, sex, social class, education, marital status, and economic status) that influence the perception and experience of health and illness, understanding the concepts of health education and health promotion and appreciating community and individual-based approaches.

Life-style

A wide variety of life-style factors affect health. Many, such as alcohol consumption, tobacco use, and sexual behavior, are described elsewhere in this chapter. Diet affects a range of health conditions including cancer, heart disease, and conditions affecting the gastrointestinal tract. Information on dietary habits is available from a number of sources in the United States, including the National Health Interview Survey (Adams and Hardy 1989) and the National Health and Nutrition Examination Survey.

Such surveys have demonstrated, for example, that 20% of whites, 26% of Hispanics, and 35% of blacks are more than 20% above their recommended weight (Dawson 1988). Black women were, however, less likely to perceive themselves as overweight—this has implications for diet and nutrition-related programs.

In the United Kingdom, a recent survey of adult nutrition has been completed. This revealed differences in food consumption between men and women (men consuming greater quantities, less wholemeal bread, more fat, less fruit, more meat, and more fried potato chips). Obesity, defined as a body mass index over 30, was present in 12% of women and 8% of men, compared with 8% and 6%, respectively, in 1980. Only 12% of men and 15% of women had fat intake that met the Committee on Medical Aspects of Food Policy (COMA) target of 35% or less of food energy from fat. Details of cholesterol, vitamin, and mineral consumption were assayed in a carefully conducted study. Twenty-one percent of men and 35% of women were classified as nondrinkers. Energy intake was lower for unemployed than other men. Lower social class people were found to be shorter than others. Unemployed men who consumed alcohol did so more than employed men who consumed alcohol (Office of Population Censuses and Surveys 1990). Knowledge of dietary and other life-style factors, such as exercise and stress, provides a basis for educational and health promotion interventions and may provide valuable insights into causes and mechanisms of disease, offering opportunities for research and necessary background for clinical interventions.

Disability

The study of disability features rarely in medical education despite the fact that disability poses a significant health burden within communities. The Health and Activity Limitation Survey was conducted in Canada in 1986 and 1987. It gathered comprehensive data on the prevalence of mental and physical disabilities among Canadians of all ages. It used the standard definition of disability as "any restriction or lack resulting from an impairment of ability to perform an activity in the manner or within the range considered normal for a human being" and used questions on activities of daily living to assess this (Jordan-Simpson and Dowler 1990). Disability was present in 1.7 million women (14%) and 13% of men. Impaired mobility and impaired agility were most often cited. Disabilities increased in severity with age and were more common in women than men. The level of institutionalization in women was also higher—possibly reflecting longer life expectancy or the lack of household support systems at home. These and other insights may provide useful information about the community that is served by a medical school.

In the United Kingdom, the Office of Population Censuses and Surveys (Martin et al. 1988) conducted four surveys of disability from 1985 to 1988, covering adults or children in private households or communal establishments. About 14% of adults in private homes had some form of disability. The rate rose with age, accelerating after 50 and rising very steeply after 70. The north of the country had the highest rates.

Longitudinal studies may provide unique and salient information about trends over time, not only in terms of death and disease, but also in terms of disability, exposures, perceptions, and the relative influence of environment, genetic, and health service factors. The merits of such studies have been described by Wadsworth and Rodgers (1987); medical schools would do well to monitor the output from such surveys and use them to enhance their understanding of the aging process and the contribution of early life influences on subsequent health. A number of such national surveys exist in the United Kingdom and provide unique insights into these processes. The earliest of these is the Medical Research Council Survey of Health and Development (Wadsworth 1987).

TABLE 3.3. Death rates per million population for England and Wales by sex and cause 1987.

ICD chapter	Males	Rank	Females	Rank
All causes	10654		10304	
Circulatory system	5075	1	4940	1
Neoplasms	2900	2	2574	2
Respiratory system	1096	3	956	3
Injury and poisoning	436	4	253	6
Digestive system	283	5	368	4
Nervous system and sense organs	199	6	208	7
Endocrine, nutritional, metabolic, and immunity	161	7	203	8
Mental disorders	148	8	283	5
Genitourinary system	125	9	148	9
Symptoms, signs, ill-defined conditions	57	10	81	11
Infectious and parasitic	47	11	43	13
Musculoskeletal and connective tissue	45	12	139	10
Congenital anomalies	38	13	33	14
Blood and blood-forming organs	33	14	50	12
Skin and subcutaneous tissues	6	15	19	15
Certain conditions originating in perinatal period	5	16	3	16
Pregnancy, childbirth, and puerperium			2	17

Source: Office of Population Censuses and Surveys (1989).

Expectation of Life: Risk of Death

Life expectancy is higher in women than men in the United States, Canada, and the United Kingdom and is approaching 80 in all of them. In the United Kingdom, this hides differences that arise on closer examination: life expectancy is lower for lower social classes, those living in the north of the country, and members of ethnic groups.

The major causes of death in England and Wales for males and females in 1987 are diseases of the circulatory system, neoplasms, and respiratory diseases (Table 3.3). Collectively, these three disease groups account for over 85% of all deaths in males and 82% in women. The fourth biggest killer in men are injuries and poisoning; in women it is diseases of the digestive system. Mental disorders rank fifth in women and show double the male rate. Death rates are higher in men than women for each of the top four causes.

In the United States the pattern is slightly different (Fig. 3.4). The four main causes of death among whites and blacks are heart disease, cancer, "accidents and adverse effects," and cerebrovascular disease. Deaths from HIV disease are included in Figure 3.4 to illustrate the emerging importance of this major public health problem. HIV disease, unknown before the 1980s, was the fifteenth leading cause of death in the United States in 1987 and was ranked tenth for the black population. In 1990 it is one of the leading causes of death in young adults. Time trends provide additional insights:

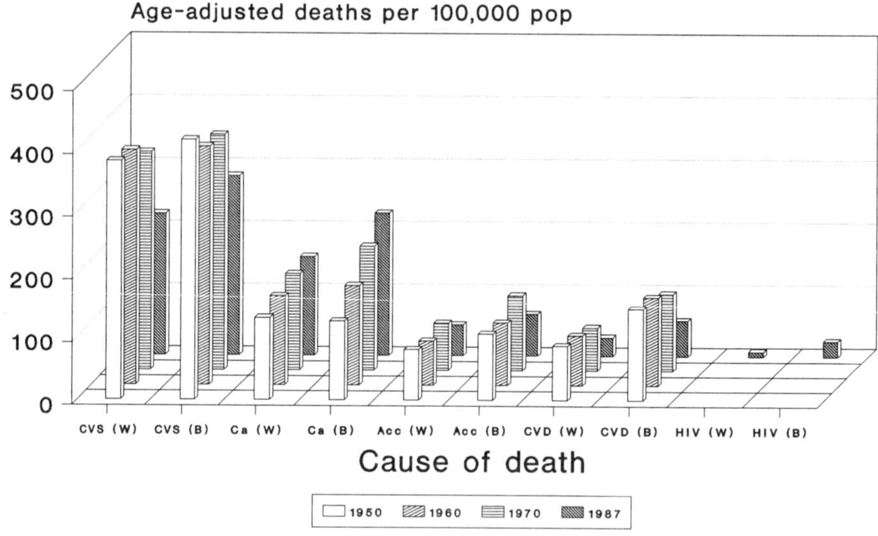

FIGURE 3.4. Most important causes of death for black (B) and white (W) Americans (1987). Deaths from cardiovascular (CVS); cancer (Ca); accidents and adverse effects (Acc); cerebrovascular (CVD); and HIV disease (HIV). *Source:* United States Department of Health and Human Services (1989).

heart disease and cerebrovascular disease rates show marked declines, particularly since 1970, whereas age-adjusted death rates from cancer have increased. Marked disparities in mortality between blacks and whites are revealed for all causes shown; HIV disease, for example, disproportionately affects black and Hispanic people.

Impact of Disease at Different Ages

- *Age-specific rates:* Rates for the whole population do not show the burden of conditions at particular stages of life. Table 3.4 shows the three leading causes of death for males at each age in England and Wales in 1987. Sudden infant death syndrome is the leading cause of death in those under a year of age, but injury and poisoning are the foremost cause of death among those between 1 and 35 years and remain among the top three to age 55. Heart disease, cancer, and respiratory disease are the most important killers over all ages, but assume most significance from the age of 35 onward. The pattern differs for women: cerebrovascular disease is more important at all ages above 25 years than respiratory disease. A focus on a particular age group may be most revealing. In the United States, the homicide rate among blacks aged 15–24 was 85.6 per 100,000—seven times the rate for whites (United States Department of Health and Human

TABLE 3.4. Top three causes of death (per million population) in males and females in England and Wales, 1987.

Age group	First		Second		Third	
Under 1	Sudden infant death	2551	Congenital anomalies	786	Respiratory disease	565
1–4	Injuries and poisoning	121	Congenital anomalies	93	Nervous system disease	50
5–14	Injuries and poisoning	90	Malignant neoplasms	39	Nervous system disease	23
15–24	Injuries and poisoning	526	Malignant neoplasms	68	Nervous system disease	20
25–34	Injuries and poisoning	462	Malignant neoplasms	129	Heart disease	68
35–44	Heart disease	455	Injuries and poisoning	410	Malignant neoplasms	388
45–54	Heart disease	2094	Malignant neoplasms	1498	Injuries and poisoning	434
55–64	Heart disease	6657	Malignant neoplasms	5347	Respiratory disease	973
65–74	Heart disease	15739	Malignant neoplasms	12741	Respiratory disease	3876
75–84	Heart disease	32136	Malignant neoplasms	23325	Respiratory disease	12511
85+	Heart disease	57905	Respiratory disease	36811	Malignant neoplasms	31284
All ages	Heart disease	3759	Malignant neoplasms	2871	Respiratory disease	1096

Source: Office of Population Censuses and Surveys (1989).

Services 1990). For black males aged 15–19, homicide has been the leading cause of death since 1968.

- *Years of potential life lost (YPLL):* One measure of the relative importance of different conditions is the YPLL; this measures the impact of various diseases and lethal forces on society, emphasizing the particular loss from youthful or early deaths (Last 1988). Table 3.5 illustrates these data for the United Kingdom, for both sexes, for years of working life (age 15–65) lost. Besides ischemic heart disease, motor vehicle accidents and suicide are the major causes of premature death in males, while in females breast cancer and cervical cancer are the first and second (with ischemic heart disease) most important causes of death. The ranking of causes is different from the all-age mortality rates in Table 3.3. Despite relatively few numbers of deaths in motor vehicle accidents per year (3319 in males in 1987) compared with 86,978 for ischemic heart disease, they contribute a large number of YPLL because of the younger age at which they exert their effect. The average age at death was 38 and 71.3 years for motor vehicle accidents and ischemic heart disease respectively.

It is worth noting that the ranking of causes changes depending on the

TABLE 3.5. Major causes of years of life lost between ages 15 and 65 for England and Wales (1987).

Rank		Thousands of years of life lost	Years of life lost per 10,000 population
	Males		
1	Ischemic heart disease	181	85
2	Motor vehicle accidents	95	45
3	Suicide	57	27
4	Neoplasm of digestive organs and peritoneum	44	23
5	Neoplasm of trachea, bronchus, and lung	42	20
6	Sudden infant death syndrome	41	19
7	Cerebrovascular disease	30	14
8	Other heart disease and hypertension	25	12
9	Leukemia	16	8
10	Other diseases of the respiratory system	14	6
	Bronchitis, emphysema, and asthma	14	6
	Females		
1	Neoplasm of female breast	60	29
2	Ischemic heart disease	40	19
2	Neoplasms of genitourinary organs	39	19
4	Neoplasm of digestive organs and peritoneum	30	14
5	Sudden infant death syndrome	28	13
5	Motor vehicle accidents	28	13
7	Cerebrovascular disease	27	13
8	Neoplasms of trachea, bronchus, and lung	21	10
9	Suicide	17	8
10	Other heart disease and hypertension	15	7

Source: Office of Population Censuses and Surveys (1989).

age band examined (Blane et al. 1990). YPLL to age 65 emphasizes those causes of death that strike young people in particular, but fails, however, to consider the impact of any disease causing death after the age of 65. Canada, for example, uses age 25–74 for these calculations (Fig. 3.5). Most conditions affect men more than women, with the exception of breast cancer, which is the second highest cause of potential years of life lost in Canadian women aged 25–74.

YPLL may reveal the changing pattern of mortality for particular conditions. Breslow and Cumberland (1988) show that in the United States, there were 300,000 fewer YPLL before age 65 from cancer in 1980 than would have been the case if 1950 age-specific cancer rates still applied. Nevertheless, cancer still accounted for 1.8 million lost years of potential life before age 65 in 1980 and cancer mortality rates were rising. This "saving" of YPLL in the face of increasing mortality rates from cancer reflects a drop in cancer mortality rates (predominantly from lung cancer)

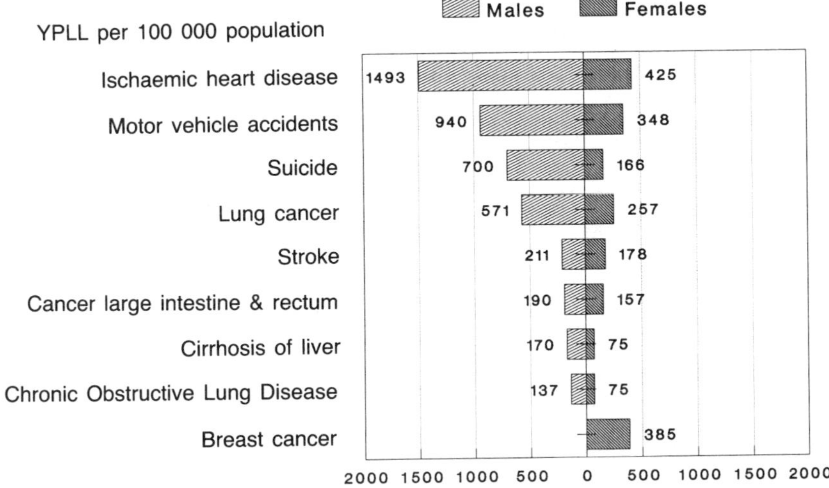

FIGURE 3.5. Years potential of life lost—Canada, ages 25–74 years (1985). *Source: Chronic Disease in Canada* (June 1987).

at younger ages, and an increase at older ages. These deaths at older ages contribute little, or nothing, if over 65, to the YPLL.

The use of YPLL reveals conditions that cause considerable mortality at early ages and that would otherwise receive little attention. Accidents and injuries are clearly most important in this respect and should arguably receive greater priority in medical education and research.

Preventable Deaths

Much disease and death are preventable. McKeown (1976) argued that the main reasons for the downward trend in mortality over the generations have been, in order of importance, rising standards of living (including dietary change), developments in hygiene and the control of the physical environment, limitations of population growth, and the introduction of preventive and therapeutic medical measures, including immunization, antibiotics, screening, and changes in behavior.

- *Deaths avoidable by medical care:* A relatively small proportion of deaths in industrialized countries result from inadequate access to good health care. In England in 1987, 13,794 of 531,150 (2.6%) were considered "medically preventable." These included deaths from cervical cancer, Hodgkin's disease, respiratory diseases in children, asthma in the under 45's, tuberculosis in those under 65, hypertension and stroke before 65, perinatal deaths, and those from chronic rheumatic heart disease. Compared with 1980, most of these are showing declines, except for tuberculosis (Department of Health 1989).

The moves toward improving clinical practice through medical audit in the United Kingdom will help identify inappropriate practices that should be modified to avoid unnecessary deaths. Table 3.6 indicates "avoidable" mortality from tuberculosis in the 16 districts of the North East Thames region of the United Kingdom in people aged 5–64 over 1983 to 1988. The figure indicates how the standardized mortality ratio (SMR) for tuberculosis in each of the 16 districts rate relative to distribution of SMRs in the 190 United Kingdom health districts. It illustrates graphically which districts have the worst experience of tuberculosis mortality; this could result from increased incidence and prevalence or from poorer health services. In this case, part of the explanation may be that a number of the districts cover deprived communities with high ethnic populations. Also, four of the six worst districts have teaching hospitals and therefore may be dealing with the most severe cases.

"Avoidable" suggests they need not have happened. Knowledge of these problems and improved approaches to treatment will reduce the risk of these unnecessary deaths. Focusing on them will help identify practical skills that medical students should acquire, such as recognizing the section of the community most affected by such conditions, improved ability to establish the diagnosis, knowledge of the referral chain, and improving access to treatment early in the course of illness.

- *Preventable by changing exposures:* The traditional understanding of "cause of death" is the disease that terminated life. Presenting ill-health, disease, and death in a way that emphasizes their social or behavioral origin can be very powerful, revealing priorities for prevention. Poverty, employment, smoking, alcohol consumption, stress, diet, exercise, infection, drug misuse, and sexual behavior all have profound influences on health and disease states in our societies; changing risky behaviors will do an enormous amount for the promotion of health (although the influence of societal structures on behaviors should not be neglected).

There is value, therefore, in presenting health, disease, and death data by "true cause" rather than by disease. Alcohol or tobacco-related conditions, for example, account for vast damage to health. Smoking has its main influence through premature deaths from cancer, coronary heart disease, and chronic obstructive lung disease, but many other disorders such as deaths from fires, peptic ulcer disease, strokes, atherosclerosis, and other heart disease should also be taken into account when assessing the impact of tobacco on raising death rates.

Semenciw (1987) estimated that more than 362,000 deaths among Canadian males and nearly 208,000 in females, between 1960 and 1984, were attributable to smoking. In the period 1980–1984, an average of 22% of the 16,553 deaths annually in men and 19% of the 9,913 in women aged 35–84 occurred each year due to smoking. Deaths from cancer of the lung and chronic respiratory disease have increased more than any other conditions in Canadian women from 1966 to 1986 (Arraiz and Wong 1990).

TABLE 3.6. Location of 16 districts in northeast Thames region, by centile of SMR relative to all English health districts, for "avoidable" mortality[a] from tuberculosis.

| | Position relative to other English health districts by centile | | | | | | | | | |
District	1–10 (lowest SMR)	11–20	21–30	31–40	41–50	51–60	61–70	71–80	81–90	91–100 (highest SMR)
Northeast Essex	X									
Southend			X							
Enfield				X						
Barking, Havering, and Brentwood				X						
Mid Essex						X				
Basildon							X			
Redbridge							X			
West Essex								X		
Waltham Forest								X		
Islington									X	
Newham										X
Haringey										X
Hampstead										X
City and Hackney										X
Bloomsbury										X
Tower Hamlets										X

[a]Standardized mortality ratio for tuberculosis, for ages 5–64 years for years 1983–1988.
Source: Department of Health, Health Services Indicators Package (1990).

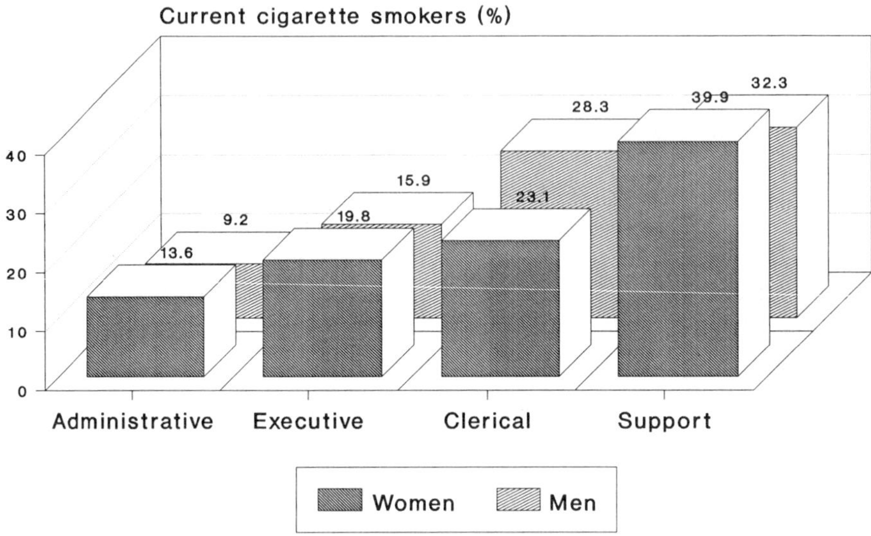

FIGURE 3.6. Prevalence of smoking: men and women civil servants—Whitehall II 1986–1988 (Marmot et al. 1991).

In the United States with its larger population, 390,000 deaths, nearly one-fifth of all deaths in 1985, were attributable to smoking (Warner 1989). More specifically, 30% of cancer deaths, 21% of coronary heart disease deaths, 18% of stroke deaths, and over 82% of chronic obstructive pulmonary disease deaths were due to smoking.

The decline in smoking in the United Kingdom has been greater among men than women and more in high than low social classes. Figure 3.6 demonstrates the smoking behavior of men and women in the Whitehall II study, a study of 10,314 civil servants working in and around Whitehall, London in 1986 to 1988 (Marmot et al. 1991). In nearly all civil servant grades, the prevalence of smoking among women was greater than among men. Already lung cancer is the most important cause of cancer mortality in women in Scotland; this is likely to be the case in England and Wales too as lung cancer deaths approach those from breast cancer (Smith and Jacobson 1988). In the United States the declining rate of smoking in men under the age of 50 has already been manifest in reduced rates of lung cancer in these age groups (Breslow and Cumberland 1988). Thus trends in behaviors now or in the past will have effects on disease rates in the future.

Alcohol has marked impacts on morbidity and mortality. Table 3.7 shows the large number of deaths that were directly or indirectly attributable to alcohol in the United States in 1987 (Shultz et al. 1990). Alcohol exerted its influence through direct toxicity (for example, alcoholic psychoses, alcoholic cardiomyopathy, and alcoholic cirrhosis of the liver), or as a contributory cause through certain cancers (such as cancer of the lip or stom-

TABLE 3.7. Major causes of alcohol-related mortality in the United States, 1987.

Diagnosis	Percentage of deaths by diagnosis due to alcohol (%)	Age (years)	Males		Females	
			Number of deaths	Alcohol-related deaths	Number of deaths	Alcohol-related deaths
Cancer of the esophagus	75	35+	6705	5029	2365	1774
Cerebrovascular disease	7	35+	58302	3790	90068	5854
Alcoholic cirrhosis of the liver	100	15+	5517	5517	1991	1991
Motor vehicle accidents	42	0+	33904	14240	14386	6042
Accidental falls	35	15+	6091	2132	5485	1920
Suicide	28	15+	24073	6740	6472	1812
Homicide	46	15+	15007	6903	4792	2204
All causes				70168		34927

Source: Shultz et al. (1990).

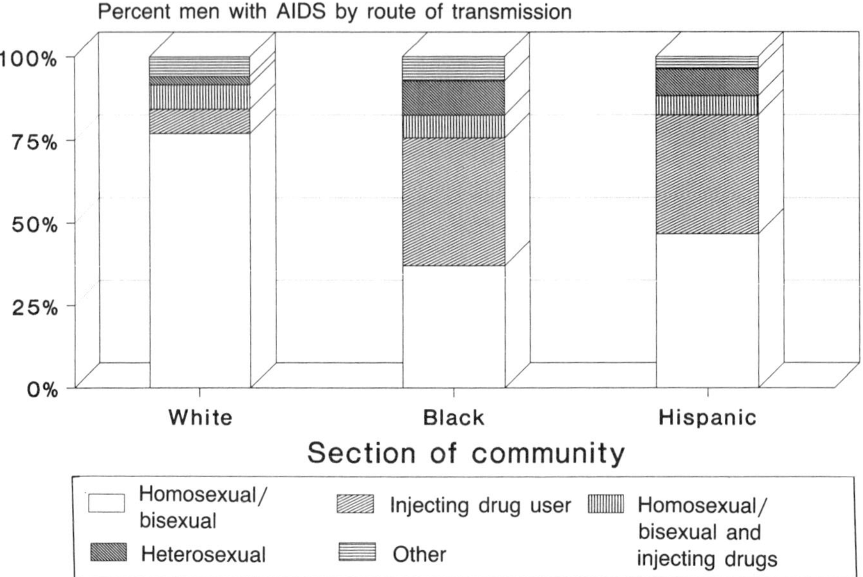

FIGURE 3.7. Transmission of HIV in U.S. men up to 1989. *Source:* United States Department of Health and Human Services (1990).

ach), other diseases (such as diabetes mellitus and pneumonia), accidents and violence—together accounting for over 105,000 deaths in the United States, 4.9% of total mortality (Shultz et al. 1990). This was an increase from 4.5% of deaths in 1985. Besides deaths, the impact on non-fatal injuries, disability, and deteriorating quality of life should not be underestimated.

Sexual and drug-taking conduct have major influences on sexually transmitted diseases and HIV infection. Figures on AIDS transmission highlight the differing modes in various communities in the United States. Among white men, the main mode of transmission is between men who have sex with men, accounting for over three quarters of cases reported up to 1989 (Fig. 3.7) whereas in Black and Hispanic men with AIDS, intravenous drug use is responsible for nearly 40% of cases (National Center for Health Statistics 1990). Identifying risk behaviors in different communities will play some part in developing appropriate educational, service development, and other intervention strategies. Care should be taken in using such data to avoid stereotyping and stigmatizing members of the community and to recognize the social and economic determinants of risky behaviors.

Use and Planning of Services

Epidemiology has a role both in health planning (for example, measurement of determinants of health, sickness and social performance, and the prevention of disease) and health care planning (Knox 1979). Different activities may be recognized as part of the health care planning function: measuring need and demands, assessing the deployment and future need for resources, monitoring current and future provision of services, setting standards and targets for the provision of appropriate services, implementing programs, and evaluating initiatives.

- *Measuring need:* The data required for assessing needs depend on how and who defines "need." The concept is also linked to the possibility for effective action—in the absence of an appropriate intervention, "need" is less (Knox 1979, 48). For preventive purposes, assessment of "risk" for particular groups may help determine the level of need.

  Data on the use of health services may provide some information, but by no means a comprehensive assessment, of health needs. Variation in use of health services is strongly related to income, ability to pay, and the nature of the health service. A recent report indicated that nearly 37 million people (15% of the total civilian noninstitutionalized population in 1987) in the United States are covered by neither private health insurance nor by public programs (Short et al. 1989); those without adequate cover were mostly young adults, blacks, Hispanics, the unmarried, and families without a working adult. Thus, measurement of health service use by such groups will not generate an accurate idea of the distribution of health problems in these communities, nor of their "needs." Even in the presence of a national health service there are wide disparities in health and service utilization (Townsend and Davidson 1988; Radical Statistics Health Group 1987; Whitehead 1988; Smith and Jacobson 1988; Davey Smith et al. 1990), limiting the value of utilization data as a source for the measurement of needs. Consultation with general practitioners is related to a range of social and economic attributes; single people tend to consult less than those married, widowed, or divorced; those renting or living in council (public) housing consult more than those owning their homes (this differential was especially great for serious illnesses); people seeking work were more likely than those in employment to consult for serious illness; lower social class people were more likely to consult their general practitioners with the gradient being highest for serious illnesses (McCormick et al. 1990). There is worse health in lower social classes despite higher rates of consultation.

- *Load on different types of service:* Different pictures of the health problems of the population are provided by data from different components of the health service. This has previously been well-illustrated by Black and Pole (1975) and also by McCarthy (1982). Although medical students spend the majority of their clinical training in tertiary care hospitals, 98% of all episodes of illness resulting in medical consultation are managed within the general practice setting (Goldacre and Vessey 1987).

  The distribution of consultations between primary care, hospital, and tertiary care services provides insight into the load placed on different levels of health service by a variety of conditions. These are summarized for

TABLE 3.8. Mortality, morbidity, and service use for selected conditions in England and Wales.

	Ischemic heart disease		Stroke		Cancer		Hypertension	
	Males	Females	Males	Females	Males	Females	Males	Females
Mortality (1987)								
Mortality, all ages (number)	86978	68257	26051	43399	74325	68126	1637	2123
Age-specific death rates/10,000 people (all ages)	35.10	26.30	10.57	16.73	30.19	26.37	0.66	0.81
Mortality rate for age 55–64 rate/ 10,000 people	60.90	18.96	9.04	6.64	53.48	42.81	1.00	0.59
Morbidity (1981–1982)								
Episodes/10,000 people at risk (age 45–64)	1.13	0.47	0.44	0.27	—	0.44	7.95	9.50
Consultations/ 10,000 people at risk (age 45–64)	397	129	158	78	178	52	2673	3161
Hospital discharges and deaths/10,000 population England (all ages)	52.5	27.6	23.7	26.6	89.7	81.4	2.7	2.7

Sources: Royal College of General Practitioners and Office of Population Censuses and Surveys (1986). Office of Population Censuses and Surveys (1986). Office of Population Censuses and Surveys (1989). Department of Health (1989). The categories presented are chronic ischemic heart disease (CC183), other cerebrovascular disease (CC196), neoplasms of the larynx, trachea, bronchus, and lung (CC041), and uncomplicated hypertension, primary or secondary (CC194).

four conditions in Table 3.8, which describes the mortality and morbidity associated with ischemic heart disease, stroke, cancer, and hypertension. It reveals marked differences in utilization of different services for specific conditions. For example, although hypertension accounts for high levels of morbidity and many consultations with general practitioners, it leads to little mortality or hospital bed use. Cancer, on the other hand, accounts for few general practice consultations but large numbers of deaths and hospital use. Goldacre and Vessey (1987) calculated that of 2500 general practice consultations, 461 (18.4%) would be for acute nasopharyngitis, pharyngitis, or tonsillitis, 181 (7.2%) for anxiety or depressive neurosis, 148 (6%) for acute bronchitis or bronchiolitis, and 2.9% for otitis media. Acute myocardial infarction accounted for only 0.4% of consultations; lung cancer for 0.08%.

The rank order for general practice consultations in England and Wales

TABLE 3.9. Consultation rates in general practice per 1000 people at risk in the United Kingdom, 1981–1982.

Diagnostic code	Males	Females
Osteoporosis	0.2	1.8
Malignant respiratory neoplasms	8.8	2.4
Chronic abuse of alcohol	6.7	3.1
Schizophrenia	6.5	7.1
Acute myocardial infarction	20.6	9.4
Malignant neoplasm of breast	0.1	9.7
Iron deficiency anemia	3.5	16.0
Constipation	9.7	16.4
Dizziness, giddiness	10.2	18.8
Diabetes mellitus	25.4	26.7
Excessive menstruation	—	30.7
Cough	29.6	32.5
Obesity	9.2	38.8
Conjunctivitis	30.8	41.4
Back pain	46.8	48.1
Abdominal pain	33.5	56.9
Acute bronchitis/bronchiolitis	99.1	95.6
Depressive disorder	35.2	105.7
Upper respiratory infection, acute nonfebrile	112.8	134.1
Uncomplicated hypertension	109.1	150.4
Advice on contraception	2.9	199.0

Source: Royal College of General Practitioners and Office of Population Censuses and Surveys. (1986).

is different to that of deaths. The four major reasons for men consulting a general practitioner are respiratory disease, circulatory disorders, musculoskeletal and connective tissue disease, and nervous system disorders, whereas for women they were respiratory, musculoskeletal, "ill-defined," and circulatory disorders. A selection of problems presenting to general practitioners, as well as their rates of consultation in the United Kingdom is presented in Table 3.9.

The International Classification of Primary Care attempts to take account of the variety of presentations in the primary care setting and includes a description of problems by organ system involvement, mental and social problems, and patient complaint (Bentsen 1986; Lamberts and Wood 1987). Primary care presentations are monitored in the United Kingdom through the General Practice Morbidity Survey. In the United States, the National Ambulatory Medical Care Survey (National Center for Health Statistics 1987 and 1990) and the Ambulatory Sentinel Practice Network provide valuable information on the surveillance of health problems presenting at primary care sites as well as the service responses (Green et al. 1984).

An iceberg effect is present with the vast majority of people with a given condition consulting primary care physicians, a smaller number being seen

TABLE 3.10. Causes of daily hospital bed use in England, 1985.

ICD chapter	Beds used daily	Rank
All causes	145622	
Circulatory system	31423	1
Symptoms, signs, and ill-defined conditions	15948	2
Neoplasms	14344	3
Respiratory system	14038	4
Injury and poisoning	13689	5
Nervous system and sense organs	10802	6
Musculoskeletal and connective tissue	10231	7
Digestive system	9878	8
Genitourinary system	6850	9
Mental disorders	5294	10
Endocrine, nutritional, metabolic, and immunity	3387	11
Skin and subcutaneous tissues	2791	12
Certain conditions originating in perinatal period	1709	13
Infectious and parasitic	1560	14
Congenital anomalies	1440	15
Blood and blood-forming organs	1270	16
Pregnancy, childbirth, and puerperium	968	17

Source: Office of Population Censuses and Surveys (1987).

at district hospitals, and still fewer (with more complicated presentations) being seen at tertiary care institutions. Therefore, analysis of the distribution of patients seen at tertiary hospitals diverges quite substantially from the pattern in the primary care setting.

Hospital bed use provides information on the small percentage of illnesses that require emergency care, surgery, or continuous inpatient assessment. Community-based studies of fatal myocardial infarction show that the majority of deaths occur outside hospital and that 40–50% of deaths occur within an hour of the onset of the acute attack. These findings indicate that the outcome of heart attack is far worse than that found in examining hospitalized patients; estimation of risk factors would also be erroneous if it focused only on the selected group of patients who reach hospital.

Cerebrovascular disease and other circulatory disorders, signs, symptoms, and "ill-defined" conditions, neoplasms, and respiratory disorders accounted for nearly 45% of hospital bed-use in males in 1985; in females cerebrovascular disease was responsible for 14.4% of National Health Service (NHS) hospital bed use (Table 3.10).

Table 3.11 describes spells of hospital admission, indicating the importance of diseases of the digestive system, and in women, conditions related to childbirth, pregnancy, and the puerperium, and diseases of the female genital organs and breast. There are some limitations to such data, however; they indicate episodes or spells of illness, rather than individuals, and therefore may count, more than once, people who are admitted on a number of

TABLE 3.11. Hospital admission spells in the United Kingdom,[a] 1985.

Males			Females		
Diagnosis	Spells per 10,000 population	Rank	Diagnosis	Spells per 10,000 population	Rank
All causes	1032.1		All causes	1114.5	
Signs, symptoms, and ill-defined conditions	141.4	1	Signs, symptoms, and ill-defined conditions	149.1	1
Diseases of the digestive system	116.6	2	Complications of pregnancy, childbirth, and puerperium	142.6	2
Diseases of the respiratory system	111.5	3	Diseases of female genital organs including breast	115.6	3
All neoplasms	99.7	4	All neoplasms	109.9	4
Other injuries and reactions	86.9	5	Diseases of the digestive system	99.8	5
Heart disease	84.7	6	Diseases of the respiratory system	84.9	6
Diseases of the musculoskeletal and connective tissues	54.2	7	Diseases of the musculoskeletal and connective tissues	64.6	7
Cerebrovascular disease and other diseases of the circulatory system	51.3	8	Other injuries and reactions	60.4	8
Fractures, dislocations, sprains, and strains	43.9	9	Heart disease	59.6	9
Diseases of the male genital organs	37.2	10	Cerebrovascular disease and other diseases of the circulatory system	53.0	10

Source: Office of Population Censuses and Surveys (1987).
[a]Psychiatric and maternity bed use are excluded.

occasions for the same condition. They also provide no data on people seeking hospital care outside of the NHS—in some regions, and for certain conditions, use of private hospital beds may be significant. Spells of hospital admission provide some idea of the number of hospitalizations due to a particular cause; this needs to be differentiated from bed days, which indicates the length of time in hospital associated with defined causes.

Length of stay indicates the average duration of hospital stays associated with the main categories of disease (Table 3.12). This provides some idea of the load placed on the hospital service. Mental disorders account for the

TABLE 3.12. Mean duration of hospital stay in England, 1985.

ICD chapter	Average days	Rank
All causes	10.7	
Mental disorders	44.9	1
Circulatory system	19.6	2
Endocrine, nutritional, metabolic, and immunity	15.6	3
Nervous system and sense organs	13.3	4
Musculoskeletal and connective tissue	13.3	4
Skin and subcutaneous tissue	12.3	6
Respiratory system	11.1	7
Certain conditions originating in the perinatal period	10.8	8
Neoplasms	10.6	9
Blood and blood-forming organs	10.1	10
Injury and poisoning	9.2	11
Symptoms, signs, and ill-defined conditions	8.5	12
Congenital anomalies	7.5	13
Infectious and parasitic	7.4	14
Digestive system	7.1	15
Genitourinary system	5.3	16
Pregnancy, childbirth, and puerperium	2.4	17

Source: Office of Population Censuses and Surveys (1987).

longest hospital stays, with an average of one and a half months; this is followed by circulatory system disorders (less than 20 days stay on average). Digestive system disorders, although accounting for frequent admissions, tend to involve short stays that average 7.1 days.

The conditions which account for the longest average hospital stays (Table 3.13) include a range of conditions, such as cerebral atherosclerosis and infantile cerebral palsy, which account for average stays of 220 and 60 days, respectively. They may prevent hospital beds being used for other conditions and place a considerable strain on existing services. Thus each data source provides a particular type of information, which may collectively be used

TABLE 3.13. Leading causes of long hospital stays in England.

Condition	Average days in hospital
Cerebral atherosclerosis	219.7
Senility without psychosis	84.6
Atherosclerosis	76.2
Infantile cerebral palsy	60.4
Acute but ill-defined cerebrovascular disease	52.7
Parkinson's disease	50.9
Cerebrovascular disease	48.8
Fractured femur (not head)	40.0

Source: Office of Population Censuses and Surveys (1987).

TABLE 3.14. Burden of cardiovascular disease on hospitals and disability in the United States, 1980.

	Hypertension alone	Cardiovascular disease with hypertension	Cardiovascular disease alone	Cardiovascular disease with complications
Ambulatory visits (% of all visits)	11.9	4.3	7.2	8.0
Hospital admissions (% of all)	8.3	6.9	11.6	9.1
Hospital days (% of all)	6.4	9.2	14.4	12.9
Bed-disability days (% of all)	9.1	6.2	10.4	10.1
Work-loss days (% of all)	8.1	2.6	3.9	2.5
Restricted-activity days (%)	11.0	6.2	9.9	8.5

Source: Harlan et al. (1989).

for determining priorities and understanding what problems present to which levels of the health service.

Data from the United States illustrate the burden of cardiovascular disorders on different health service indicators. Cardiovascular disease, affecting 17% of the population, accounted for over 30% of all ambulatory visits and over 35% of all hospital admissions in the United States in 1980 (Harlan et al. 1989). This demonstrates a reverse iceberg effect—a condition appearing to be particularly common at tertiary level is less common in the primary care and general community setting. Hypertension (without complications) accounts for 11.9% of ambulatory visits, 8.3% of hospital visits, and 6.4% of hospital days (Table 3.14). This is in marked contrast to cardiovascular disease with complicating conditions which accounted for 8% of ambulatory visits, 9.1% of hospital admissions and 12.9% of hospital days. Hypertension is treated mostly in the primary care setting, while cardiovascular disease with complications requires hospital care.

Accidents and injuries are a major cause of death and morbidity in the United Kingdom (see Tables 3.3, 3.4, and 3.5), resulting in more than 500,000 hospital admissions per year (8% of all admissions) and about seven million attendances at accident and emergency services (45% of all attendances!) per year (National Association of Health Authorities/Royal Society for the Prevention of Accidents 1990). A recent study of YPLL by social class in the United Kingdom (Blane et al. 1990) demonstrated the increasing importance of injuries and violence as a contributor to widening social class differences in premature mortality from 1971 to 1981.

The thrust of this contribution is that the health problems of the population should have a substantial impact on determining the priorities of the medical school in education and the provision of care. This is not to say that because conditions occur commonly they necessarily take highest priority (they may cause little discomfort, disability, death, or resource utilization), but that medical schools, their faculty and students, should be aware of these conditions, their causes and scope for prevention and treatment.

It is beyond the scope of this chapter to consider the approaches to measuring the effectiveness and efficiency of care, although these should clearly play a major part in determining priorities.

Cost of Services and Costs to the Community

Consideration of the cost of services is necessary for determining priorities, evaluating efficiency of services, and because resources are always finite and need to be deployed where maximum gain can be achieved. This should be an essential part of medical education. Costs to society, to the health services, to insurers, to the individuals themselves, and to their careers should all be considered. It would be undesirable to shift the financial burden of caring from the health services to individuals and their families.

Harlan et al. (1990) draw attention to the limited research focus on injury and poisoning despite the fact that they accounted for about 12% ($16.7 billion) of the total direct medical costs of $136 billion and were second only to circulatory disease which cost over $20 billion in 1980 (Fig. 3.8). The total work-loss attributable to injuries in the United States was nearly 250,000 person years, representing 14% of all work-loss days attributable

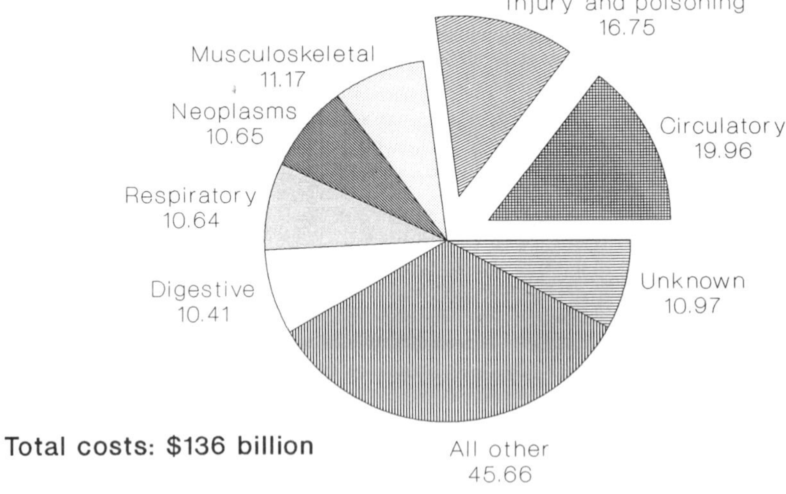

FIGURE 3.8. Direct medical costs (US$ billion) 1980 for noninstitutionalised population. *Source:* Harlan et al. (1990).

to illness. The potential years of preretirement work life lost as a result of premature mortality from intentional and unintentional injuries was over four million years in the United States in 1982 (Harlan et al. 1990)—roughly twice the years of potential work life lost from either neoplasms or heart disease.

In the United Kingdom, annual treatment costs for accidents and injuries alone are estimated to be a billion pounds—nearly 5% of the total National Health Service budget. The additional costs of follow-up and rehabilitation have yet to be calculated (National Association of Health Authorities/Royal Society for the Prevention of Accidents 1990). The same study indicated that further costs are incurred as a result of avoidable health service utilization, causing delays to other services. For example, it has been estimated that the health service burden of one compound fracture of the tibia and fibula in an elderly woman following a fall may defer six hip operations; one serious head injury in a young cyclist defers 10 hernia operations.

The impact of conditions on work-loss, bed-disability, and restricted activity also warrants attention. Table 3.15 describes the leading causes of certified sickness absence in the United Kingdom in 1987–1988 by sex. Musculoskeletal disease assumes far greater importance when considering disability and health service use than if one merely considered deaths. These data provide some indication of the economic impact of these disorders, although it should be noted that the figures are derived from *certified* absences and a quite different distribution may be present in uncertified absences which are of shorter duration.

TABLE 3.15. Millions of days certified incapacity due to sickness in 1987/1988 by sex.

ICD chapter	Males	Rank	Females	Rank
All diseases and conditions	284.6		96.9	
Circulatory system	73.6	1	10.1	3
Musculoskeletal and connective tissue	63.7	2	27.5	1
Mental disorders	39.3	3	23.1	2
Respiratory system	28.1	4	4.6	6
Nervous system and sense organs	22.2	5	7.7	4
Accidents, injuries, and poisoning	18.6	6	4.6	6
Symptoms, signs, and ill-defined conditions	10.8	7	5.2	5
Digestive system	9.2	8	2.3	10
Endocrine, nutritional, metabolic, and immunity	7.2	9	2.2	11
Neoplasms	3.7	10	1.2	12
Genitourinary system	2.9	11	2.6	9
Infectious and parasitic	2.3	12	0.9	13
Skin and subcutaneous tissue	2.0	13	0.7	14
Congenital anomalies	0.6	14	0.6	15
Blood and blood-forming organs	0.4	15	0.3	16
Pregnancy, childbirth, and puerperium	0	16	3.3	8

Source: Department of Health (1989).

Estimated costs should also include hidden costs such as those incurred by families in looking after sick relatives or the money and time spent on gaining access to the health service. The impact of an ill family member will be felt by other members of the household, some of whom (usually women) may have to give up some of their own employment or activities outside the home. Although the opportunity costs of this should be taken into account in calculating the cost of an illness, this is rarely done.

The Limitations of Data

Data should never be uncritically accepted. There are invariably limitations and weaknesses which need to be taken into account in assessing their value. Knox (1979), for example, draws attention to some of those which result from the information-ascertainment techniques employed. Screening programs lead to an *apparent increase* in incidence, notification of a disease outbreak will lead to *additional* cases being identified where they previously would not, changes in diagnostic patterns and classifications may impact on reported incidence and prevalence rates, and improving access to certain facilities will change the distribution of health problems within the service.

Health service utilization and the rate of medical procedures vary substantially among countries as well as among small areas within a country (McPherson et al. 1982; Wennberg 1988). This makes it difficult to estimate incidence and prevalence of health problems on the basis of surgical and other interventions undertaken.

Other limitations abound. Data from general practice consultations exclude those who go straight to accident and emergency departments in hospitals and give an erroneous impression of needs; rates of National Health Service (NHS) bed use fail to consider private sector hospital utilization and therefore underestimate the need for hospital care. In the United States, the National Ambulatory Medical Care Survey provides details of office-based consultations, but until 1990 excluded those taking place in hospital emergency rooms. Furthermore, estimates may be based on small numbers or samples may be systematically different from the truth, resulting in bias. The validity of measurements on which study results are based should at all times be examined. More profoundly, many measures of the NHS revolve around health service activity and not the original objectives of making care more available (Knox 1987).

All of these need to be considered in assessing the value of collated information. Medical students need to be imbued with a critical approach to data derived from clinical, epidemiological, or routine study. Experience of handling and examining data relevant to the health of the community served by the medical school will play some part in generating these skills.

V. Heterogeneity in Society Raises Questions

Ethnicity, race, culture, sex, and age all impact on health, health service utilization, behaviors, needs, and the articulation of demands. Figure 3.9 shows variation in the prevalence of risk factors for heart disease in Canadians aged 20 to 69 (Miller and Wigle 1986). Cigarette smoking, obesity, and physical inactivity vary by sex and level of education, with rates of smoking being higher in males, and physical inactivity and obesity higher in females. For almost all adverse risk factors, including diastolic blood pressure, alcohol consumption, cholesterol level, and overweight (not shown in the figure) there are similar patterns and fewer healthy behaviors apparent in those with lesser education (Miller and Wigle 1986). Any attempt to control heart disease must recognize these variations and target interventions appropriately; different methods may need to be employed to reach different groups. Medical students should learn this as a matter of course: rates of health and disease vary in the population; the intervention and approaches adopted need to vary as a result.

Age and Sex

Age and sex are fundamental descriptors of health in the community. Use of services, risk behavior, mortality, morbidity, perceptions of health problems, and attitudes to the conditions vary with age and sex. Figure 3.10 shows the incidence of new cases of coronary heart disease

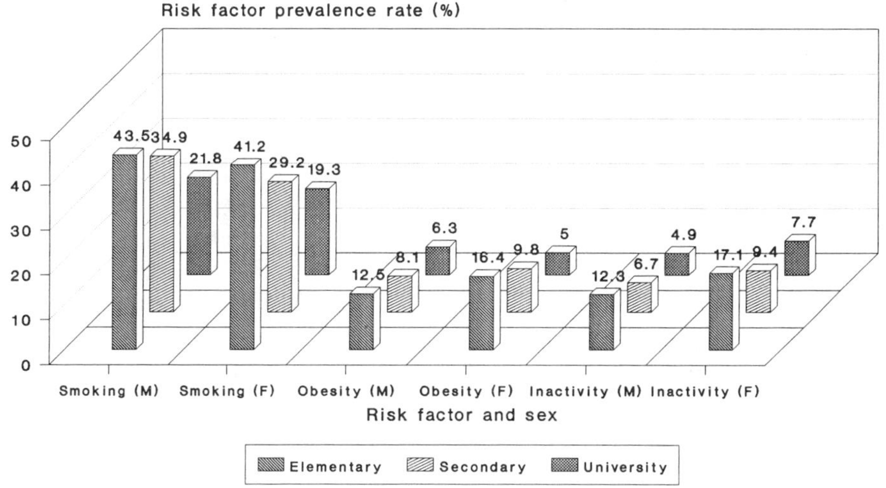

FIGURE 3.9. Prevalence of risk factors for cardiovascular disease among Canadians by educational group. *Source:* Miller and Wigle (1986).

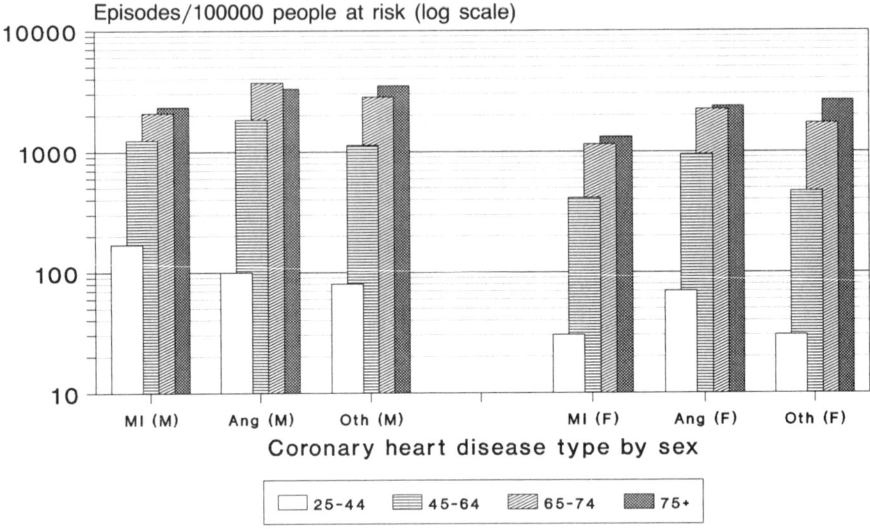

FIGURE 3.10. Incidence of coronary heart disease by sex and age group (1981–1982), England and Wales. MI, myocardial infarction; Ang, angina; Oth, other. *Source: Royal College of General Practitioners (1986).*

in a defined time period, by sex and age in England and Wales in 1981–1982. Based on general practice consultation rates it demonstrates clear age and sex variations of consultations for all forms of coronary heart disease. Those aged 45–64 have 10 times higher rates of consultation than those aged 25–44; this doubles again for those over 65. Women have substantially lower rates of consultation for coronary heart disease at all ages. The consultation rate for these three forms of coronary heart disease together varied from 0.55 consultations annually per 1000 male population aged 25–44 to 5.14 consultations annually per 1000 male population aged 75 years and above.

Priority health problems vary with age; so do behaviors and perceptions. Engendering an understanding of these in medical students can be achieved by presenting students with problems faced by different age cohorts and having them learn about their state of health, beliefs, and social conditions.

Social Class

Social class differences are apparent for use and access of services, health status, health behaviors, and the distribution of determinants of health. A variety of measures of social class have been employed: income, occupation, education level, and housing tenure. Whichever is used, major differences are apparent.

The Black Report and The Health Divide (Townsend and Davidson 1988; Whitehead 1988) collate the substantial data indicating class inequalities in

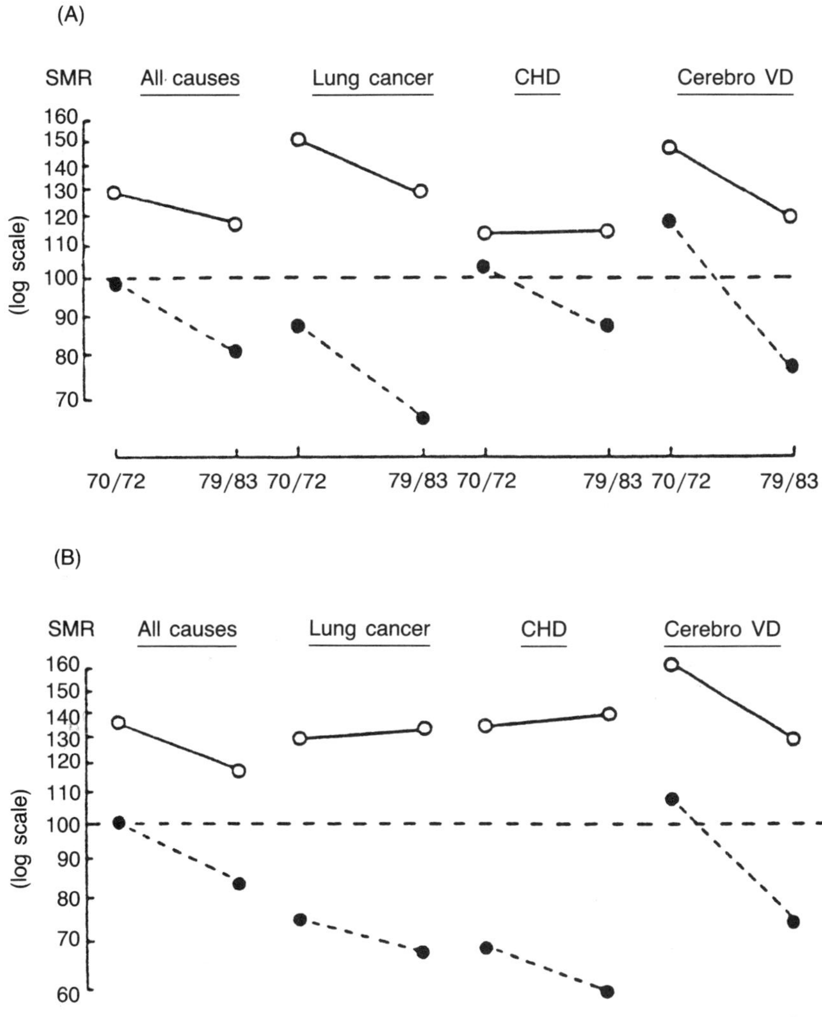

FIGURE 3.11. Standardized mortality ratios for select causes of death in the United Kingdom 1970–1972 and 1979–1983 for manual (open dots) and manual (solid dots) groups. (A) Men aged 20–64: (B) Married women aged 20–54 classified by husbands occupation. *Source:* Marmot and McDowall (1986).

health and health care in the United Kingdom. Mortality data are among the most readily accessible. Marmot and McDowall (1986) showed widening social class inequalities in mortality between 1970–1972 and 1979–1983 (Fig. 3.11); a recent review by Davey Smith et al. (1990) drives home this point with up-to-date information.

In 1981, men in the manual worker classes had death rates 45% higher than men in the nonmanual classes while women had rates 43% higher; the excess mortality associated with being in the manual worker classes was greater than the total number of deaths from stroke, infectious disease, accidents, lung cancer, and other respiratory diseases combined and if manual workers had the same mortality experience as nonmanual workers, there would have been 42,000 *fewer* deaths in 1981 among those aged 16–74 (Smith and Jacobson 1988).

Although mortality is only one measure of the health of a community, it may provide important indications of other inequalities. An editorial in the Lancet stated:

a whole conglomerate of undesirable exposures is concentrated among those, who, being less socially privileged, tend to have worse education, less money, worse housing, less access to medical care—in many kinds of ways less personal and material resources for health. Society's inequitable distribution of those resources, and their effects on health and survival, seem to be remarkably well measured by social class differentials in mortality. (Editorial 1986)

Receptiveness to educational messages also varies by social class and level of education. In the United States, the age-adjusted prevalence of current smoking among men 25 years and over declined by 40% from 1974 to 1987 in those with college education, while the decline in those with fewer than 12 years of education was only 13% (United States Department of Health and Human Services 1991).

In the United Kingdom, smoking prevalence declined over time in male civil servants of all grades in London. It was, however, greatest in those of higher status, where the rates decreased by well over 50% (Fig. 3.12). In the others, the declines were less marked, although still considerable. Despite the decline in smoking rates, the social gradient persists (Marmot et al. 1991).

More attention needs to be devoted to reducing smoking rates in working class people. It is apparent that the messages that have succeeded in changing the habits of the middle classes may need to be different for the working classes, or, more fundamentally, that structural conditions need to be changed to enable health promotion messages to achieve their objectives.

Doctors are taught to speak with and treat individuals. This is highly appropriate to the clinical care setting. However, social class and ethnic differences in a wide range of health-related indices suggest that failure to recognize that health status and behavior are influenced by social and political circumstances will virtually ensure that interventions by the medical profession, other than providing care, will be extremely limited.

Race and Ethnicity

Race and ethnicity are major influences on health. For example, Figure 3.13 shows that the excess in mortality for blacks is much greater in Harlem, New York than it is nationally (McCord and Freeman 1990). Standardized

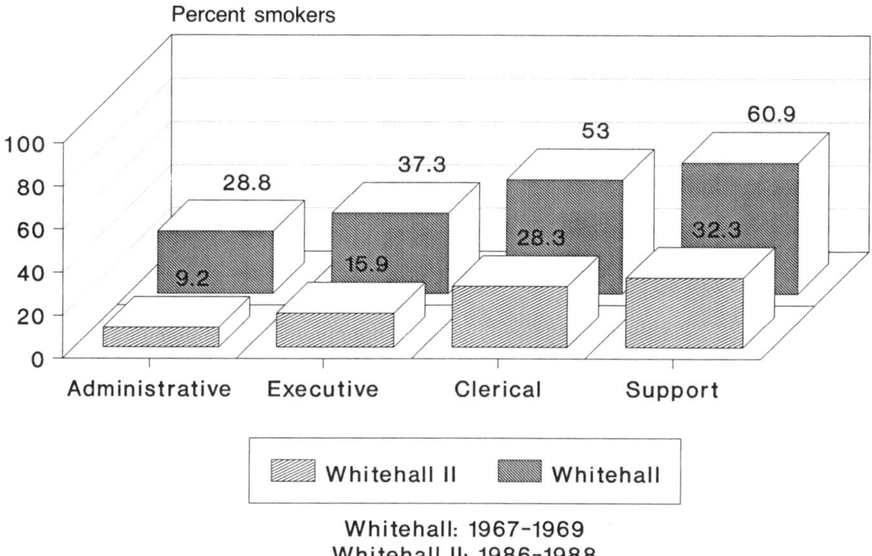

FIGURE 3.12. Prevalence of smokers in men: Whitehall II and Whitehall. *Source:* Marmot et al. (1991).

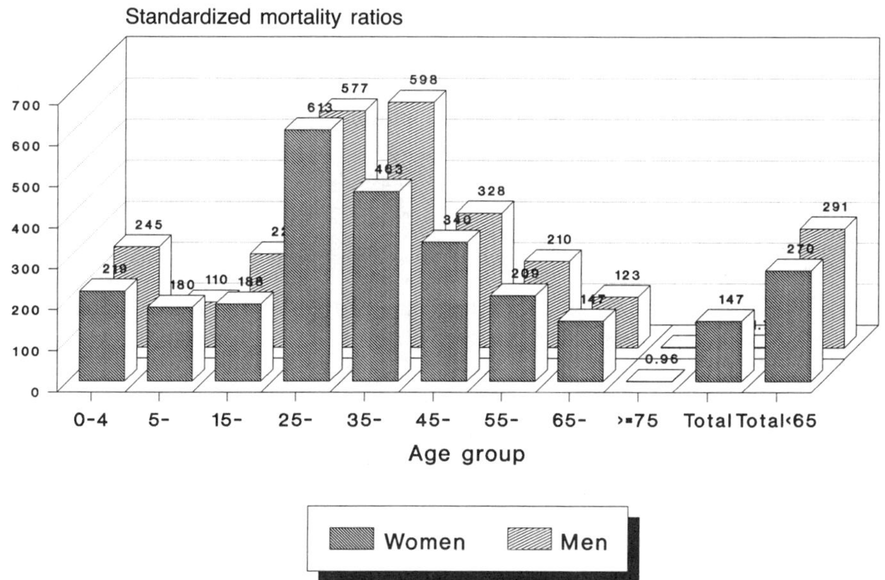

FIGURE 3.13. Standardized mortality ratios for Harlem: U.S. whites = 100 (1979–1981). *Source:* McCord and Freeman (1990).

TABLE 3.16. Standardized mortality ratios and excess mortality in Harlem (US Whites < 65 = 100).

Cause	SMR	Excess (%)
Cardiovascular	223	23.5
Cirrhosis	1049	17.9
Homicide	1424	14.9
Neoplasm	177	12.6
Drug dependency	28310	7.4
Diabetes	543	3.7
Alcohol	1133	3.2

Source: McCord and Freeman (1990).

mortality ratios in Harlem residents are substantially higher than in United States whites: the rate is more than double for most ages, is over six times in those aged 25–34, and is similar to whites only in those aged 65 and above. Deaths in males and females under the age of 65 for drug dependency were over 200 times greater in residents of Harlem compared with the average for United States whites (Table 3.16). Mortality associated with alcohol and violence was raised markedly. Apart from affecting the workload, and therefore, one hopes, the type of clinical education students receive, such figures call out for students to be taught to understand the type of social and economic conditions that give rise to such a health profile.

In the United Kingdom too, health can be shown to relate to ethnicity and race. Recent data on infant and early-life deaths are illustrative; infant mortality in England and Wales was 8.9/1000 in 1988, but for women born in Ireland, Africa (outside of the Commonwealth countries of East Africa), and Pakistan it was 9.6, 15.3, and 14.6, respectively. Substantially higher rates of stillbirths (double in women born in Bangladesh compared with United Kingdom-born women), early and late neonatal deaths, and postneonatal deaths are also apparent for a variety of ethnic groups (Office of Population Censuses and Surveys 1991).

Rates of cardiovascular disease vary in United Kingdom adults by ethnic group. Immigrants from the Indian subcontinent have high rates of coronary heart disease and diabetes (McKeigue et al. 1989). Afro-Caribbeans have high rates of stroke and hypertension, similar to those seen in the United States.

Ethnic differences may have implications for a range of important issues such as uptake of services, perceptions of health, presentation of illness, life-style, cultural practices, differing patterns of disease, and the use of alternative medicine (Donaldson and Odell 1984). Some understanding of these, as well as the way in which many societies marginalize (socially, politically, and economically) ethnic groups will help prospective medical personnel to understand the difficulties and sensitivities necessary to promote health in these sections of our communities.

Geography

Analyses of the geographic distribution of disease are valuable as they raise questions about whether the patterns observed reflect characteristics of ethnic or social groups, variations in the chemical, biological, or physical environment, or differences in the domestic and residential setting (Barker and Rose 1984). In the United States and Australia some of these analyses may be conducted on the basis of state, in Canada on the basis of province, and in the United Kingdom on district or local authority, or where larger areas are required, on region. Reports generated by statutory authorities responsible for the provision of services at these levels of administration are a valuable source of data. In the United Kingdom techniques are being developed for examining areas even smaller than districts and this may prove particularly valuable for medical schools wanting to know about the communities they serve.

Geographic patterns of mortality are well described in the United Kingdom. Standardized mortality ratios, for example, are higher in the north and west, and in Scotland and are lowest in the southeast. The Black Report (Townsend and Davidson 1988) found that geographic differences persist even after controlling for the different social class distribution in these areas. There are notable exceptions that pose questions about etiology. For example, standardized mortality ratios for hypertensive disease are low in the north and northwest, Yorkshire, and Humberside. Reversal of the usual pattern is also evident for malignant melanoma of the skin, cancer of the prostate, breast cancer in women, and leukemia (Britton 1990). Cardiovascular disease mortality has been shown to be higher in areas that formerly had high rates of maternal and neonatal mortality, in which mothers had worse physique and babies were smaller at birth (Barker and Osmond 1986). Geographic variation may shed light on cause and mechanism of disease.

Certain local authority areas have higher than expected standardized mortality ratios for a variety of causes, many of these are inner city areas, areas of high population density and lower socioeconomic status. Health districts with particularly high infant mortality rates have tended to have a high proportion of mothers born in the New Commonwealth countries and Pakistan and above average proportions of fathers in the lower social classes.

There are also significant variations in the provision of care by geographic area and there are good data highlighting the massive variation in medical interventions by area. Park et al. (1989) have shown how physicians respond quite differently to whether a medical procedure is necessary despite having the same information available.

The study of migrants may also be revealing. Migrants from an area leave behind particular environmental circumstances but they still carry their genetic determinants of health and disease. Socially and culturally mediated habits and behaviors will persist to a variable extent and may play some part in future health or disease. The study of new arrivals in a society permits comparison with the current inhabitants in terms of genetic, environmental, and behavioral determinants of health.

Period and Cohort

Analysis of the period or cohort in which deaths take place may be informative. Lung cancer has been the leading cause of cancer death in the United States since the early 1950s; in 1930 it ranked sixth whereas at the turn of the century it was virtually unknown. In 1988 the disease accounted for 35% of all cancer deaths in men; the next closest contenders were colorectal cancer and prostatic cancer—both accounting for only 6% each. In women, lung cancer began to rise dramatically in the early 1950s and is likely soon to overtake breast cancer as the leading cause of cancer death. From the early 1960s to mid-1980s women smokers' lung cancer death rates rose from 23.9/100,000 to 130.4/100,000, while those of nonsmokers remained at 12/100,000 throughout this period (Warner 1989).

Despite rising rates for all-age cancer mortality, declining rates in specific ages are apparent, reflecting declining rates of smoking, particularly in younger men. For example, in those aged 35–44, lung cancer mortality rates declined from about 15 per 100,000 in 1969 to around 10 per 100,000 in 1983 (Davis and Schwartz 1988). Lung cancer rates in those aged 45–54 peaked in 1978–1981 and have since declined rapidly. On the other hand, lung cancer mortality in the older age groups continues to increase. These data are consistent with a cohort effect—different birth cohorts are exposed to a particular set of environmental and behavioral causes of disease (smoking in this case). Successive cohorts may experience a decline in mortality from lung cancer since fewer people took up the habit and more ceased smoking in the past 20–30 years.

International data on cardiovascular disease mortality present a different pattern. Here all-age mortality has declined dramatically in certain countries—the United States, for example, showed marked declines in age-adjusted rates in men aged 35–74 from 1968 when the rate was approximately 800 per 100,000 to around 500 per 100,000 in 1979 (Marmot 1985). The decline is evident for all age groups—suggesting a period effect rather than a cohort effect.

Examination of intranational and international trends may reveal successful health promotion programs as well as raising questions of cause and mechanism of disease. An awareness of the wealth of insights that may be gained from comparative study of health status and interventions should form part of the education of every medical student.

VI. Getting the Balance Right

If a medical school sets as its goal reducing the burden of disease in the population it serves, rather than simply treating cases of disease that came to the hospital doors, its priorities would change. This is illustrated by a set of goals developed by the National Cancer Institute (NCI) in the United States. The NCI set out an agenda for action to prevent cancer and improve survival with the disease. It asserts that cancer mortality can be reduced by 25–50% in the United States by the year 2000 if substantial effort is mobilized to accelerate and consolidate the present favorable trends in prevention and treatment. To achieve this, major changes in diet and a reduction in smoking, as well as improvements in screening and treatment procedures are required (Table 3.17). The NCI estimated that a reduction of 8–15% in cancer deaths could be achieved by lowering rates of smoking and that a further 8% reduction could be achieved by dietary change. Increasing the availability of cervical and breast cancer screening programs would lead to a further reduction of 3% while transferring research results on state-of-the-art treatment would reduce deaths by a further 10–26%.

TABLE 3.17. Cancer control objectives for the year 2000—U.S. National Cancer Institute

Action	Target	Year 2000 objective	Estimated reduction in cancer mortality by year 2000[a]
Prevention	Smoking	Reduce percentage of adults who smoke from 34% (in 1983) to ≤15%	8–15% (depending on when objective is achieved)
	Diet	Reduce average fat consumption from 38% to ≤25% of total energy intake; increase average consumption of fiber from 8–12 to 20–30 g/day	8%
Screening	Breast	Increase percentage of women 50–70 years who have annual physical exam coupled with mammography to 80% from 45% for physical exam alone and 15% for mammography	3%
	Cervix	Increase percentage of women who have a smear every 3 years to 90% from 79% (ages 20–39 years) and to 80% from 57% (ages 40–70 years)	
Treatment	Transfer research results into practice	Increase adoption of state-of-the-art treatment	10–26%

Source: Breslow and Cumberland (1988).
[a]Total mortality reduction equals approximately 25–50%.

The estimate of the potential benefit from improvement in treatment has been criticized as greatly overoptimistic. Even accepting the NCI estimate, however, the potential benefits from change in diet, smoking, and alcohol consumption are at least as great as those from treatment. Bailar (1986) argues that the struggle against cancer is not being won and that more emphasis should be placed on prevention if any progress is to be made.

Another example of integrating different influences on health and health care is provided in the Report of the Ontario Health Review Panel (1987). It provides a service-related agenda for improving health in the future, arguing for a greater emphasis on primary care, improved links between primary and secondary care, developing a community focus for care, encouraging a pluralistic health system, facilitating a health promotion and disease prevention approach, integrating planning, enabling a more efficient mix of professionals to deliver services, and establishing better coordinated services.

We have presented the sort of information necessary to shift priorities in these directions. Medical schools should be playing a part in generating such data, monitoring it, analyzing it, and interpreting it for students and the public. They should be able to access data on a wide range of issues (Fig. 3.1 and Table 3.1) to achieve this.

VII. Using Data to Influence Medical Education

The Ministerial Consultation for Medical Education in Europe (World Health Organization 1989) stressed the importance of complementing the traditional teaching of *disease management* with the acquisition of knowledge, skills, and attitudes related to health promotion, disease prevention, and continuity of care. It was agreed that students should be taught and learn in an environment enabling them to gain practical experience of wider aspects of care than can be provided by the highly specialized services of a university hospital. Health services should be better used as a resource for medical education. The Lisbon Initiative concluded that *"all phases of medical education should take place in appropriate settings which reflect all aspects of health and health services"* (World Health Organization 1989).

There have been a number of attempts to relate medical education more clearly to the needs of the community. Community-oriented medical education recognizes the importance of using teaching resources outside of hospital-based services and of enabling students to identify priority health problems, and through problem-solving exercises, pose solutions. Community-oriented medical schools recognize that leaving the teaching of social and preventive medicine to public health departments without any commitment from clinical departments tends to undermine any move toward population-based medicine. They therefore strive to ensure that preventive, therapeutic, and rehabilitative aspects of both teaching and service are integrated. Finally, they identify some role for the medical school in conducting community-based research, and evaluating the availability, utilization, and access to services in the area.

The World Health Organization has drawn attention to the need for a new form of medical education if programs like *Health For All by the Year 2000* are to achieve any success. Emphasis needs to shift from hospital-based health issues to health promotion and disease prevention, the appropriate use of resources, an appreciation of teamwork, multidisciplinary and multisectoral approaches to health, and the attainment of equity in the distribution of resources and services.

A Network of Community-Oriented Educational Institutions for Health Sciences has been established and has widespread international membership. Recent publications (Richards and Fülöp 1987; Kantrowitz et al. 1987) have described the achievements of its many constituent medical schools, and the difficulties they face in promoting significant change in medical education (Mennin and Kaufman, 1989).

It is certainly useful to collate and present a wide range of data on the health of the community, but how does this influence medical education? It is within the context of the above that population-based data need to be considered. Neufeld (1989) offers a mechanism for its use by referring to the *Priority Health Problems Model* (see Fig. 3.2) developed by a task force of the Network of Community-Oriented Educational Institutions for Health Sciences (1989). The model has four stages:

* Analysis of the health situation;
* Identifying actions for priority problems;
* Designing relevant education programs; and
* Evaluating the outcomes.

The first stage involves assessing the health status and health services of the area concerned. The nature of the data required and their sources have been discussed extensively earlier in this chapter. Establishing a *Uniform Minimum Data Set* would help ensure comparability between different schools. This could be built on existing data sets such as that developed by the United Kingdom Department of Health (Balarajan 1990), but would need to be expanded substantially. Both routine and specifically collected data are required, qualitative and quantitative information should be used, and perceptions of communities and objective evidence of needs should be gathered.

The establishment of a *Health Intelligence and Analysis Unit*, within a school with a clear commitment to influencing the health of the community it serves, would be well placed to collect and monitor such data. How such a unit would function, its relationships within the medical school, sources of funding, mechanism for influencing the curriculum, and other important issues are discussed in Chapter 4 and are therefore not described here.

The second step entails establishing the priority problems. Neufeld has listed a number of guidelines for priority determination. These include assessing the importance of the problem, the factors known to cause it, the presence of "at-risk" groups, the point at which intervention is likely to be most useful, and evidence of the effectiveness and efficiency of the intervention.

The importance of a problem may be reflected by the number of people affected, its costs to the individual and the community, the handicap it places on individuals affected, and its impact on quality of life. As Black and Pole (1975) have commented, even if little service usage is made for conditions like eye and ear disease, these are of undeniable importance. The potential impact of interventions is another major factor determining whether a problem is identified as a priority.

The design of relevant education programs (Step three) follows the assessment of problems and determination of their relative priority. The skills and professional qualities required by future doctors for effective, efficient, humane, and up-to-date professional practice should be clearly stated. Such skills include critical appraisal skills, learning skills, the ability to handle information, health economics, policy analysis, determining health status, "prioritizing" a list of problems, allocating resources and monitoring their impact, and evaluating interventions adopted.

This chapter is not the place to present a medical curriculum that would address such needs. However, it is important to recognize that community-oriented and problem-based learning should be important features. Neufeld (1989) argues that educational planners should carefully select those experiences that provide students with the best opportunity to identify, analyze, and manage problem situations. Teaching throughout medical school should take place at a variety of sites—in people's homes, at district clinics, in primary care settings, in voluntary organizations, in general hospitals, in academic teaching centers, and in laboratories. Different techniques need to be employed including individual and group work, problem-solving exercises, surveys, clinical case conferences, and practical experience. Access to data on the health of the community is required at every level.

Finally, careful evaluation of the interventions, both in educational and health service terms, needs to be instituted.

VIII. Conclusion

This chapter has sought to demonstrate the wide range of population-based data that should be routinely collected, analyzed, interpreted, and published if medical schools are to play a part in monitoring and improving the health of the population. It is argued that this will be beneficial for research, teaching, and the provision of services, and that new opportunities for innovative work in a variety of fields will result from this.

Epidemiological approaches complement and extend the traditional patient-centered approach of medical education (Rose 1986). This is achieved by examining the antecedents and natural history of illness and thereby placing the illness in context and by querying why the illness occurred and how it can be prevented. It enlarges the area of concern from the individual to the community by asking what the health problems, needs, and demands of the population are, and identifying the social, economic, environmental, and life-style determinants of the incidence and prevalence of health and ill-health in the population. Finally, epidemiological insights offer the scientific basis for appropriate interventions and health services planning on the grounds of need and effectiveness (Rose 1986).

A wide range of information is available—its appropriate use is dependent on meaningful questions being asked about causation of disease, determinants of health, and mechanisms of illness. Throughout such endeavors, a focus on inequalities and inequities should underscore our involvement—this sets both a medical and social action agenda. A *Health Intelligence and Analysis Unit* based within the medical school may contribute to the identification of population-health concerns relevant to the school and the community it serves.

Making data on the health of the population more generally available, and ensuring that it is considered when planning research, teaching, and service commitments, will make a potentially significant contribution to shifting the orientation of the medical school toward people as part of a community rather than patients as individuals. It will require, however, to be part of a more general commitment by the medical school to serve its community base, a commitment that needs to be explicitly and publicly stated.

Greater awareness of population health will not, *on its own,* solve health problems, nor will it *alone* produce a better service. It will, however, play a part in ensuring that medical education begins to address the broader range of issues that affect health and illness. Regardless of where they were trained and with which specific population in mind, medical students will have learned population-based skills applicable wherever they choose to practice. Graduates who understand these issues will practice in a different way, with a concern for people and not only patients, health and not only disease, the community and not only hospitals.

References

Adams, P.F., and Hardy, A.M. 1989. *Current estimates from the National Health Interview Survey: United States, 1988.* Washington: National Center for Health Statistics.

Arraiz, G.A., and Wong, T. 1990. Recent incidence and mortality trends of some diseases among females in Canada. *Chronic Dis Can* **11**:22–24.

Bailar, J.C. 1986. Progress against cancer? *N Engl J Med* **314**:1226–1232.

Balarajan, R. 1990. Public health in England: Common data set, 1988. *Health Trends* **22**:47.

Barker, D.J.P., and Osmond, C. 1986. Infant mortality, childhood nutrition, and ischemic heart disease in England and Wales. *Lancet* **i:**1077–1081.

Barker, D.J.P., and Rose, G. 1984. *Epidemiology in Medical Practice*, 3rd ed. Edinburgh: Churchill Livingstone.

Bentsen, B.G. 1986. International Classification of Primary Care. *Scand J Primary Health Care* **4**:43–50.

Black, D.A.K., and Pole, J.D. 1975. Priorities in biomedical research: Indices of burden. *Br J Prev Social Med* **29**:222–227.

Blane, D., Davey Smith, G., and Bartley, M. 1990. Social class differences in potential life lost: Size, trends and principal causes. *Br Med J* **301**:429–432.

Blaxter, M. 1990. *Health and lifestyles*. London: Tavistock Routledge.

Bloomsbury Health Authority. 1989. *Health For All*, Annual report No. 3.

Breslow, L., and Cumberland, W.G., 1988. Progress and objectives in cancer control. *J Am Med Assoc* **259**:1690–1694.

Britton, M. (Ed.) 1990. *Mortality and geography. A review in the mid 1980s. England and Wales. Office of Population Censuses and Surveys*. London: HMSO.

Davey Smith, G., Bartley, M., and Blane, D. 1990. The Black report on socio-economic inequalities in health 10 years on. *Br Med J* **301**:373–377.

Davis, D.L., and Schwartz, J. 1988. Trends in cancer mortality: US white males and females, 1968–83. *Lancet* **i**:633–636.

Dawson, D.A. 1988. Ethnic differences in female overweight: Data from the 1985 National Health Interview Survey. *Am J Pub Health* **78**:1326–1329.

Department of Health. 1989. *Health and Personal Social Services Statistics for England* 1989 Edition. London: HMSO.

Donaldson, L.J., and Odell, A. 1984. Planning and providing services for the Asian population: a survey of district health authorities. *JR Soc Health* **104**:199–202.

Editorial. 1986. The occupational mortality supplement: Why the fuss? *Lancet* **ii**:610–612 quoted by Radical Statistics Health Group, 1987.

Evans, R.G., and Stoddart, G.L. 1990. Producing health, consuming health care. *Soc Sci Med* **31**:1347–1363.

Gillies, P.A., and Elwood, J.M. 1989. Health promotion in the medical curriculum. *Med Education* **23**:440–446.

Goldacre, M.J., and Vessey, M.P. 1987. Health and sickness in the community. In: Weatherall, D.J., Ledingham, J.G.G., and Warrell D.A. (Eds.), *Oxford Textbook of Clinical Medicine*. Oxford: Oxford University Press, pp. 3.10–3.17.

Green, L.A., Wood, M., Becker, L., Farley, E.S., Freeman, W.L., Froom, J., Hames, C., Niebauer, L.J., Rosser, W.W., and Seifert, M. 1984. The Ambulatory Sentinel Practice Network: Purpose, methods and policies. *J Fam Practice* **18**:275–280.

Harlan, L.C., Harlan, W.R. and Parsons, P.E. 1990. The economic impact of injuries: A major source of medical costs. *Am J Pub Health* **80**:453–459.

Harlan, W.R., Parsons, P.E., Thomas, J.W., et al. 1989. *Health care utilization and costs of adult cardiovascular conditions, United States 1980*. National Medical Care Utilization and Expenditure Survey. Washington, D.C.: National Center for Health Statistics.

Jordan-Simpson, D.A., and Dowler, J.M. (1990). Disabled women in Canada. Findings of the Health and Activity Limitation Survey. *Chronic Dis Can* **11**:30–32.

Kantrowitz, M., Kaufman, A., Mennin, S., Fülöp, T., and Guilbert, J.-J. 1987. *Innovative tracks at established institutions for the education of health personnel*. WHO Offset series No. 101. Geneva: World Health Organization.

Knox, E.G. (Ed.). 1979. *Epidemiology in Health Care Planning*. Oxford: Oxford University Press.

Knox, E.G. (Ed.). 1987. *Health care information. Report of a joint working group of the Korner Committee on health services information and the Faculty of Community Medicine*. Nuffield Provincial Hospitals Trust, Occasional Papers 8.

Lamberts, H., and Wood, M. (Eds.). 1987. *International Classification of Primary Care (ICPC)*. Oxford and New York: Oxford University Press.

Last, J.M. (Ed.). 1988. *A Dictionary of Epidemiology* 2nd ed. New York and Oxford: Oxford University Press.

Marmot, M.G. 1985. Interpretation of tends in coronary heart disease mortality *Acta Med Scand* (Suppl.) **701**:58–65.

Marmot, M.G., and McDowall, M.E. 1986. Mortality decline and widening social inequalities. *Lancet* **i**:274–276.

Marmot, M.G., Davey Smith, G., Stansfeld, S., Patel, C., North, F., Head, J., White, I., Brunner, E., Feeney, A. 1991. Health inequalties among British civil servants: the Whitehall II study. *Lancet,* **337**:1387–1393.

Martin, J., Meltzer, H., and Elliot, D. 1988. *The Prevalence of Disability Among Adults*. Office of Population Censuses and Surveys. London: HMSO.

McCarthy, M. 1982. *Epidemiology and Policies for Health Planning*. London: King Edward's Hospital Fund for London.

McCord, C., and Freeman, H.P., 1990. Excess mortality in Harlem. *N Engl J Med* **322**:173–177.

McCormick, A., Rosenbaum, M., and Fleming, D. 1990. Socioeconomic characteristics of people who consult their general practitioners. *Population Trends* Spring:8–10.

McKeigue, P.M., Miller, G.J., and Marmot, M.G. 1989. Coronary heart disease in South Asians overseas: A review. *J Clin Epidemiol* **42**:597–609.

McKeown, T. 1976. *The Role of Medicine*. Rock Carling Series. London: Nuffield Provincial Hospitals Trust.

McPherson, K., Wennberg, J.E., Hovind, O.B., Clifford, P. 1982. Small area variation in the use of common surgical procedures: An international comparison of New England, England, and Norway. *N Engl J Med* **307**:1310–1314.

Mennin, S., and Kaufman, A. 1989. The change process and medical education. *Ann Community-Oriented Education* **2**:101–110.

Miller, W.J., and Wigle, D.T. 1986. Socioeconomic disparities in risk factors for cardiovascular disease. *Can Med Assoc J* **134**:127–132.

National Association of Health Authorities and the Royal Society for the Prevention of Accidents. 1990. *Action on Accidents*. Birmingham: National Association of Health Authorities.

National Center for Health Statistics. 1989. Firearm mortality among children and youth. *Advance Data* No. 178. Hyattsville, MD: National Center for Health Statistics.

National Center for Health Statistics. 1990. *Health United States*. Hyattsville, MD: National Center for Health Statistics.

National Center for Health Statistics. 1987. *Patterns of Ambulatory Care in General and Family Practice: The National Ambulatory Medical Care Survey*, United States, January 1980–December 1981. Hyattsville, MD: National Center for Health Statistics.

Network of Community-Oriented Educational Institutions for Health Sciences. 1989. *Task Force II on Priority Health Problems in Medical Education. Final Summary Report*, September.

Neufeld, V. 1989. Community-based medical education: Some recent initiatives towards making medical education more responsive to national health priorities. *Ann Community-Oriented Med Education* **2**:65–84.

NHS Management Executive. 1990. *Health Services Indicators Package*. Crown Copyright.

Office of Population Censuses and Surveys. 1991. *Mortality Statistics: Perinatal and infants, Social and biological factors, England and Wales 1988*. London: HMSO.

Office of Population Censuses and Surveys. 1990. *The Dietary and Nutritional Survey of British Adults*. London: HMSO.

Office of Population Censuses and Surveys. 1989. *Mortality Statistics: Cause 1987*. London: HMSO.

Office of Population Censuses and Surveys. 1987. *Hospital In-patient Enquiry 1985*. London: HMSO.

Park, R.E., Fink, A., Brook, R.H., Chassin, M.R., Kahn, K.L., Merrick, N.J., Kosecoff, J., Solomon, D.H. 1989. Physician ratings of appropriate indications for three procedures: Theoretical indications vs. indications used in practice. *Am J Public Health* **79**:445–447.

Radical Statistics Health Group. 1987. *Facing the Figures. What Really Is Happening to the National Health Service?* London.

Report of the Ontario Health Review Panel. 1987. *Towards a Shared Direction for Health in Ontario*. Toronto: Ministry of Health.

Richards, R., and Fülöp, T. 1987. *Innovative Skills for Health Personnel*. Report on 10 Schools Belonging to the Network of Community-Oriented Educational Institutions for Health Sciences. WHO Offset Publication No. 102, Geneva: World Health Organization.

Rootman, I., Warren, R., Stephen, T., and Peters, L. 1988. *Canada's Health Promotion Survey*. Ottawa: National Health and Welfare.

Rose, G. 1986. Epidemiology and health care planning: Their place in medical education. *J Royal Soc Med* **79**:631–633.

Royal College of General Practitioners and Office of Population Censuses and Surveys, Department of Health and Social Security. 1986. *Morbidity Statistics from General Practice 1981–2*. Third national study. London: HMSO.

Semenciw, R. 1987. Potential years of life lost by major causes of death in Canada. *Chr Dis in Canada* **8**:7.

Short, P., Monheit, A., and Beuregard, K. 1989. *A Profile of Uninsured Americans*. National Medical Expenditure Survey Research Findings No. 1, National Center for Health Services Research and Health Care Technology Assessment. Rockville, MD: Public Health Service.

Shultz, J.M., Rice, D.P., and Parker D.L. 1990. Alcohol-related mortality and years of potential life lost, United States, 1987. *Morbidity Mortality Weekly Report* **39**:173–177.

Smith, A., and Jacobson, B. 1988. *The Nation's Health. A Strategy for the 1990s*. London: King's Fund.

Townsend, P., and Davidson, N. (Eds.). 1988. *Inequalities in Health: The Black Report (1982)* and Whitehead, M. *The Health Divide (1988)*. Middlesex: Penguin.

University Hospitals Association of England and Wales. 1989. *The early postgraduate years. An enquiry by the University Hospitals Association into the progress and career perceptions of doctors within 6 years of graduation.*

United States Department of Health and Human Services. 1987. *Sixth Special Report to the United States Congress on Alcohol and Health.* Rockville, MD: National Institute on Alcohol Abuse and Alcoholism.

Wadsworth, M.E.J., and Rodgers, B. 1987. Longterm follow-up studies: A critical overview. *Rev Epid Santé Publ* **37**:533–540.

Wadsworth, M.E.J. 1987. Follow-up of the first national birth cohort: Findings from the Medical Research Council Survey of Health and Development. *Paediat Perinatal Epidemiol* **1**:95–117.

Warner, K.E. 1989. Smoking and health: A 25-year perspective. *Am J Pub Health* **79**:141–143.

Wennberg, J.E. 1988. Variations in surgical practice: A proposal for action. In: Finkel M.L. (Ed.), *Surgical Care in the United States: A Policy Perspective.* Baltimore: The Johns Hopkins University Press, Chapter 4.

White, K.L. 1988. *The Task of Medicine.* Menlo Park, CA: Henry J. Kaiser Family Foundation.

Whitehead, M. 1988. *The Health Divide.* Middlesex: Penguin.

World Health Organization, Regional Office for Europe. 1989. *Summary Report: Ministerial Consultation for Medical Education in Europe*, Lisbon, 31 October–3 November 1988. EUR/ICP/HMD 115 (S). Copenhagen: World Health Organization Regional Office for Europe.

Woteki, C.A., Briefel, R.R., and Kuczmarski R. 1988. Contributions of the National Center for Health Statistics. *Am J Clin Nutr* **47**:320–328.

Discussion

Sir Douglas Black

Let me begin in what should perhaps be the accepted fashion, by declaring my own bias, so far as I am aware of it. In essence, I believe that what is needed in medical education is to discover "how the perspective of medicine which takes into account the whole population's health needs and which examines critically the shortfalls in present practice may become part of every doctor's training and practice." The latter passage is from a paper by Donald Acheson (1979), before he became Chief Medical Officer in our Department of Health. I share his concept of a balance between the medicine of individuals and the medicine of populations. And I admit in sorrow that in the traditional medical curriculum the medicine of populations has been relatively—though not absolutely—neglected, to an extent which requires correction after due analysis. My reasons for these views are set out in the concluding chapter of my Rock Carling Lecture (Black 1984).

The Marmot–Zwi chapter is very much in harmony with the objectives of this whole exercise; and one illustration of this is that they go far beyond their brief of "measuring the *burden* of illness" by devoting the greater part of their chapter to the social and environmental *causes* of illness, and how they can be measured—a proper and interesting extension.

I have two marginal criticisms and a personal view on the issues.

- In the section on social class and health, more recognition could have been given to the development over the past decade of better indices of *deprivation* (for which so-called "social class"—really "occupational class"—is a less-than-adequate surrogate); and of *morbidity*, such as the Nottingham Health Profile, which are adding a new (and confirmatory) dimension to the pattern previously established on the basis of the bills of mortality.
- The statement "Teaching and research in a medical school rarely reflect the burden of illness in the general population" remains broadly true but less so than it would have been 20 or 30 years ago. Important factors in causing a change for the better in this respect have been the widespread extension of clinical teaching to "district hospitals," so that no longer is a student's experience confined to institutions of "quaternary referral," the now universal attachment of students to general practitioners for varying periods (though some such periods are still sadly inadequate), and the opportunity given to students by elective periods to witness medical problems and medical care in other societies and settings. Without saying that these changes are adequate to the problem, it should still be recognized that they have taken place.

My personal view is that the undergraduate curriculum should be comprehensive, even at the expense of fine detail, for its essential function is to give the student some comprehension of what is involved in the many modes of medical care, without equipping him for the immediate independent practice of any one of them. It follows that no major theme of health care should be omitted from it, and in particular that a curriculum that leaves the students unaware of the population dimension is a fatally flawed curriculum. But to me the antithesis between the population dimension and the individual dimension is incomplete, and the ideal curriculum should recognize that population problems are aggregations of individual problems. Should the graduate ultimately choose a career in public health or epidemiology, he should still feel confident in facing individual health problems in patients who come his way. If their curriculum has prepared them also for this, they will enjoy a success that (again in the words of Donald Acheson) will depend "on the degree to which their work meets their professional aspirations and is seen to leaven medicine from within rather than to belabor it from without."

References

Acheson, E.D. 1979. Clinical practice and community medicine. *Br Med J* 2:880–881.

Black, D. 1984. *An Anthology of False Antitheses*. (Rock Carling Lecture). London: Nuffield Provincial Hospitals Trust.

Robert A. Spasoff

Marmot and Zwi build a compelling case for medical schools to place greater emphasis on measuring illness in general populations. Their recommended emphasis on the determinants of health will increase the attention paid to health promotion and disease prevention, both of which have been relatively neglected in medical schools.

The neglect of primary care may be less egregious in Canada, where both undergraduate and postgraduate programs are well–developed; the situation is different in the United States, where primary care is defined more broadly (although not necessarily more usefully). One should note some additional useful data sources in Canada, especially the databases generated by the Hospital Medical Records Institute (which offers fairly detailed data on all hospital admissions in several provinces) and several (but unfortunately still not all) of the provincial medical care insurance plans.

More might be made of the economic burden of ill health, since this has fascinating implications. Marmot and Zwi discuss direct costs of health care, but make only the briefest reference to indirect costs, and do not mention lost productivity. Wigle et al. (1990) have estimated that indirect costs roughly equalled direct costs in Canada in 1986 ($50 billion direct and $47 billion indirect), although the ratio of direct to indirect costs ranged from 0.3 to 6.4 among disease categories. Like earlier studies (Fraser et al. 1976), they found major discrepancies between the burden of ill health imposed by various disease categories and the proportion of health research dollars spent on them. Health research expenditures as a percentage of total health care costs for selected categories were as follows:

Infectious and parasitic diseases	3.3%
Nervous system and sense organs	1.3%
Cancer	0.6%
Cardiovascular diseases	0.3%
Injuries and poisonings	0.01%
All categories[1]	0.47%

The relative disregard of injuries and poisonings is particularly striking. Since most research is done in medical schools, this presumably reflects their research activities. And given the organization and priorities of most medical schools, one suspects that the relative emphasis in teaching may not be far different.

---

[1]The percentages for endocrine and metabolic and for blood diseases were larger than any of the above, but were believed to contain large amounts of basic research funding. The total includes $18 billion dollars in direct costs, which could not be assigned to any specific disease category.

One key sentence catches the theme of the chapter: "If a medical school sets as its goal reducing the burden of disease in the population it serves, rather than simply treating cases of disease that came to the hospital doors, its priorities would change." Indeed they would, and in the process the school would have begun to redefine medicine. Medical schools should work collaboratively with local health authorities and planning councils in assembling and interpreting the necessary health data; this should enhance their collaboration in planning educational and service programs, as well as avoiding duplication of effort.

References

Fraser, R.D., Spasoff, R.A., and Prime, M. 1976. *Economic Burden of Illness in Ontario 1971*. Toronto: Ontario Council of Health.

Wigle, D.T., Mao, Y., Wong, T., and Lane, R. 1990. Economic burden of illness in Canada, 1986. *Chronic Diseases Can 1991* **12**:1–37 (suppl).

Thomas S. Inui

The recommendations for a general data set (Table 3.1), inventory of available sources (Table 3.2), and general method whereby such data might be folded into a problem-solving method for an educational/service organization (Fig. 3.2) are all valuable contributions. The general model from which this approach emerges is said to be represented in Figure 3.1, a figure with all the right conceptual boxes but with linkages ultimately inscrutable to me. Like the Sheriff of Nottingham, in the end I was bewildered and defeated by all of the coming and going of arrows.

The contents of the tables and figures that followed were also extremely valuable and presented well. I will refer to this article for data on cross-national comparisons. On the other hand, I admit to some frustration with the section on "Using Data to Influence Medical Education," a section that left me without a clear understanding of how I could convert all this information into new and especially well-considered activities in medical education. Admittedly this was not the authors' primary responsibility.

I am, nevertheless, tempted to suggest that certain approaches to assessing the state of health and health care in populations, had they been adopted by the authors, might have produced data more readily translated into lessons for the medical curriculum. I appreciate their attempts to identify vulnerable or high-prevalence populations for certain disorders, using the traditional approaches of examining and contrasting populations by place, time, race, and socioeconomic status. Where striking differences emerge from such categorical comparisons, would the authors like to recommend further analytic approaches that might help us to understand the basis for these variations? Especially if clinical practice deficiencies account for some of the variations, or if physicians may play a legitimate role in remedying social welfare conditions that account for major variations, this kind of "explanatory epidemiology" seems directly relevant to the medical curriculum.

Would it also be advisable to examine variations in medical practice by professional group and geographic location? These kinds of patterns of practice loom large in the United States, as Wennberg (1987, 1989) and others have observed, suggesting that physicians are affected by substantial "clannishness" when developing their conventions for medical practice. Where these conventions are expensive, useless, or even dangerous, they can and should be revealed by analyses that link medical process with outcomes of care. The professional norms that produce and support such patterns of practice can also be eroded through revelation of the existence of the patterns, directly affecting the educational process for medical students and practitioners.

Next, I wondered whether some concentration on data gathering for what some might describe as "critical process" would be warranted in any such effort. Physicians' activities such as preventive vaccinations, Papanicolaou smears, influenza vaccinations for the elderly, and blood pressure measurement might be viewed as "critical processes," insofar as we have strong evidence linking them to positive health outcomes.

Finally, links to educational activities might be more apparent if a "sentinel event" approach were taken for surveying outcomes. David Rutstein and his colleagues (1976) have advocated this approach. Certain outcomes, they argued, should occur rarely if at all. If these events do occur, there is *prima facie* evidence of "failure" of medical care. Examples of these events might include childhood deafness from otitis media, diabetic ketoacidosis in adulthood, and admission for labor and delivery with no record of prenatal care. Regular monitoring for these events and the development of a complimentary scheme for examining the process of care in the locales, institutions, or particular populations affected in order to determine the locus and nature of the problem would have direct implications for physician education.

We need much tighter linkages between epidemiologic information, medical practice, and medical education. Perhaps more focus on an "explanatory" epidemiology, the epidemiology of medical practice, and on critical process and outcomes would tighten the linkage.

References

Rutstein, D.D., Berenberg, W., Chalmers, T.C., Child, C.G., Fishman, A.P., and Perrin, E.B. 1976. Measuring the quality of medical care. A clinical method. *N Engl J Med* **294:**582–588.

Wennberg, J.E., Freeman, J.L., and Culp, W.J. 1987. Are hospital services rationed in New Haven or over-utilized in Boston? *Lancet* **i:**1185–1189.

Wennberg, J.E., Freeman, J.L., Shelton, R.M., and Bubolz, T.A. 1989. Hospital use and mortality among Medicare beneficiaries in Boston and New Haven. *N Engl J Med* **321:**1168–1173.

General Discussion

Epidemiologic data could and should be more widely used to broaden awareness of the determinants of illness, prevalence, and burden of disease in the community. This information can and should be used to guide changes in the medical school curriculum leading to a more balanced perspective than currently prevails. The broad canvas of determinants of health and disease can with advantage be focused on in each medical school's local environment to identify the burden of unrelieved illness, vulnerable subpopulations, medical management failures (bureaucratic or clinical) measured as "sentinel events," and variable outcomes of different medical interventions, including preventive measures. Prevalence of a condition, however, may not reflect its educational value and should not necessarily dictate the time allotted to its study. The hospital environment, especially the tertiary care hospital, is not representative of the full range of health problems in the population; it is not, however, inappropriate for many aspects of medical education.

Inculcation of an epidemiological attitude in considering the problems of individual patients, and appropriate application of the population perspective, are thought to be more important than assimilation of large amounts of information in all phases of undergraduate, postgraduate, continuing education, and career development. Epidemiology should ideally be seen as a continuing strand within all disciplines rather than solely as a discrete subject. In this sense, epidemiology should *inform* rather than transform the whole medical curriculum from beginning to end, in different ways in different disciplines. Familiarity with the natural history of many diseases is an approach to learning medicine that still has much to offer by conveying a wide perspective, including the epidemiological and social dimensions.

No one questioned the need for all graduates to have the basic skills of statistical competency and to be computer literate for keeping abreast of the medical literature, managing their practice, and doing research.

We require more thought about the vital problems addressed and further exploration of the ideas being advanced with respect to

- Determining the most effective ways to harness epidemiological concepts, skills, and information to improve medical education;
- Adopting an epidemiological approach to the systematic study of many more conditions, especially common conditions, than are presently investigated;
- Developing the most effective ways to integrate the epidemiological resources of universities with those of other bodies (i.e., Health Departments and Authorities) in order to foster the university's responses to the needs of the community, and benefit teaching and research;
- Monitoring the extent to which epidemiology is currently informing the curriculums of medical schools; and
- Understanding what students want and what excites their interest in population-based medicine.

4
The Potential and Organization of Health Intelligence Units

VICTOR R. NEUFELD and ROBERT A. SPASOFF

I. Introduction

Is the role of the university in society simply to generate, interpret, and transmit new knowledge? Or will universities come out of the "ivory tower" and join in meaningful partnerships with community leaders and governments, to resolve society's present and future problems? Medical schools are part of the university, so these questions apply. As they are also linked with the health care system in carrying out education and research, questions about the mission of the medical schools, the health of the people, and the allocation of resources to deal with the determinants of health are interrelated. Medical schools require a capacity for the analysis and interpretation of health information in order to deal adequately with these issues.

In this chapter we

- Provide the rationale for the creation of a *Health Intelligence Unit* (HIU) within each medical school;
- Define the roles and functions of such a unit;
- Briefly describe two emerging institutional HIU examples, along with a recent province-wide medical education project which has as a starting point the analysis of societal health needs and expectations;
- Discuss our experience to date, commenting on the potential for the generalizability of the HIU concept to other institutions and for other purposes; and
- Propose some future directions and recommendations.

II. Rationale

Why should a medical school have a health analysis and interpretation capability? We believe that the need is evident. Academic planners may lack awareness, interest, and competence in data-based academic planning and in community health status assessment. Academic planning (concerning education and research programs) then occurs in a "vacuum," without reference to the needs of the population, as indicated by health data and health trends, or to a systematic analysis of resources, both fiscal and human. Attempts to use available health data for educational planning and research are likely to be frustrated by the lack of systematically collected data that have been evaluated for quality and applicability, and then synthesized and displayed in an understandable fashion. Too often there is no systematic planning at all!

In a 1982 address to Canadian academic and health systems leaders, Kerr White (1983) said:

Is it too much to suggest that every vice-principal or vice-president presiding over a health sciences center should have attached to his or her office a dynamic and creative intelligence service? This service should keep him or her abreast of the health status of the surrounding community, of changes in status, in comparison to other geopolitical jurisdictions. It should inform him or her of new ideas that bear on health matters beyond those likely to be encountered by the contemporary faculty of his or her university, and it should strive to assess new scientific and technological innovations as they reach the points of advocacy, diffusion, or potential application. The intelligence service would not undertake all these tasks, but it might stimulate interest in pursuing them and it might act as a catalyst and even a coordinator and synthesizer of available, credible, and useful health information.

There are two basic assumptions as the above challenge is addressed in this chapter. The first is that "supply-side" thinking has been too dominant a paradigm within the medical school, and that more "demand-side" thinking is needed, to create an appropriate balance. In this metaphor supply-side thinking is primarily concerned with the creation, assimilation, and application of new knowledge and technology. Its manifestations are the increased quantity of knowledge, increased specialization, and fragmentation, and the increased availability of a wide array of investigative, diagnostic, and therapeutic technologies—in effect, the current health care system. This has resulted in education and research largely dominated by "experts," in crowded curriculums, in mounting pressure for access to the curriculum from specialized groups, and in lectures by a "parade of stars." "Demand-side" thinking begins with an analysis of expectations, needs, and trends based on data regarding determinants of health status. These include such factors as heredity, the physical and social environments, and life-style (Lalonde 1974). A fourth determinant, the health care system itself, is a supply-side factor. The manifestations of demand-side thinking are the documents prepared by governments, groups, and agencies that advocate directions and policies, and statistical reports about the health and disease of populations. The potential impact of demand-side thinking on medical education will be seen in increased attention to "important" health problems, to the cost-effectiveness of interventions, and to the definition of a broader range of physician roles and competencies.

The second assumption in this chapter is that the impact of the HIUs to be described will be dependent on the goals and objectives of the groups and institutions involved. Clear statements concerning the mission and objectives of medical schools will provide the basis for clear thinking about the role of health information in influencing the activities of the partner institutions—medical schools, communities, and governments.

III. Definition

A *Health Intelligence Unit* (HIU) is a unit (group, department, institute, center, program) within an academic health institution designed to

* Monitor community health status; and
* Assess, in light of the available information, the need for specific educational programs;

and undertake such *functions* as:

* Collecting and evaluating available data, and summarizing them into a "prioritized" and understandable form;
* Evaluating available evidence on the trends, causes, and treatments of important ("priority") health problems, and the resources available and required to deal with them;
* Preparing summary statements for academic (and possibly health systems) planners; and
* Disseminating analyzed and summarized health information.

Some special contributions of the university (medical school) component of this university-community partnership might include

* Methods development in data analysis;
* Translation of the analysis into educational programming and presentation; and
* The conduct of "spin off" research using the assembled data, e.g., ecological research on the causes of health problems.

We refer to unprocessed facts as "health data," which may be analyzed to yield "health information," which may in turn be interpreted to yield "health intelligence." Since only the last category is likely to lead to rational decision-making, we shall refer primarily to health intelligence and to *Health Intelligence Units* (HIUs).

The "community" in "community health status" refers to the population for which the medical school and its institutions accept responsibility. This may be fairly obvious in the case of political jurisdictions with but a single medical school, but much less so in cases where there are several medical schools in a single city. Even in the former case, the relatively free mobility of physicians means that a high proportion of any medical school's graduates will not serve that school's target population. Nevertheless, each medical school should identify a target population and design its programs to meet the needs of that *entire population*, not just those who find their way to its teaching hospitals. This ensures that graduates of the school will develop a population perspective and that research activities and health services provided will similarly address the needs of an entire general population. Furthermore, the needs of communities in developed countries are usually not very different, so physicians prepared to meet the needs of one such whole community should also be able to meet the needs of others.

IV. Three Initiatives

We present three examples of the HIU concept at work; two of these are institution-based—McMaster University and the University of Ottawa, while the third is an Ontario-wide collaborative medical education project.

Health Priorities Analysis Unit (HPAU) at McMaster University

In 1987, McMaster University was selected to become Ontario's Educational Centre for Aging and Health, a province-wide resource established to increase the number and proportion of skilled health professionals who are committed to providing exemplary care for aging individuals, and to developing collaborative educational approaches to understanding the processes of aging and improving the health of the elderly, including methods of program evaluation. A health intelligence unit, called the *Health Priorities Analysis Unit* (HPAU), was designed as an integral part of this initiative. Its initial task was to assist with the classification, validation, and analysis of data sets related to the health of the older population, for use in planning education and service programs. As the HPAU has evolved, it has assumed a somewhat broader role within the faculty of Health Sciences and has strengthened its links with the community by locating its offices adjacent to those of the Hamilton–Wentworth Department of Health Services, a Teaching Health Unit of McMaster University. The current objectives of the HPAU are to

- Monitor health in a regional municipality (Hamilton–Wentworth, population 500,000);
- Ensure a population or community health focus in health science education programs; and
- Develop community health indicators that have relevance in education, research, and service.

Several activities illustrate how the HPAU is attempting to fulfil its objectives.

- *Fact Book on the Health Status of the Residents of Hamilton-Wentworth.* This 100-page document was developed to provide educators, health planners, and service providers with easy access to community health information that is routinely collected by service providers and others for the Hamilton–Wentworth Region and for the province. This should facilitate the communication of health reports and study results in the Region, and provide an overview of some of the available community health information, while enabling the reader to locate the original source before drawing conclusions. Five hundred and seventy copies of the Fact Book have been distributed to the District Health Council, health education planners, and health and social service managers and providers. A flyer describing its availability was distributed to 3200 individuals, including all the Health Sciences faculty and medical and nursing students.
- *An Education Resource on the Use of Alcohol.* This package included a collection and analysis of available data related to the use and abuse of alcohol in the Hamilton–Wentworth region, with some comparisons to the rest of Ontario. The report features a description of the "burden of illness" using selected indicators, a critical review of the role of physicians in reducing the alcohol-related burden of illness, and a listing of specific suggestions to education planners. The package also included a selected bibliography and relevant data displays. It is now used in the undergraduate medical education curriculum, and has been made available for postgraduate education as well.
- *HPAU Infowatch Newsletter.* Three issues of a newsletter, *Infowatch*, have been published and distributed to Health Sciences Faculty, students, and selected individuals and groups in the community. The most recent issue reported on a survey of the health of senior citizens in the North Hamilton district. The survey was done to assist an academic family medicine unit locating in North Hamilton to plan its education, research, and service activities.
- *Community Health Forum.* The HPAU was responsible, as a collaborative effort between the university, regional government, and various community groups, for organizing a day-long forum entitled "Developing and Sustaining a Healthy Community in Hamilton–Wentworth." This was probably the first of a series of similar events.

Community Health Research Unit (CHRU) at the University of Ottawa

In 1986, a Teaching Health Unit was developed, linking the Ottawa–Carleton Department of Public Health and the University. In 1989, this led to the development of a Community Health Research Unit (CHRU), jointly sponsored by the university's Department of Epidemiology and Community Medicine and by the Health Department, with a mandate to carry out applied community health research. One of the research themes of the CHRU is Community Health Information. The CHRU is developing a computerized community health database for the Regional Municipality of Ottawa–Carleton (population 650,000), to serve as the basis for planning and priority setting for the Region. It will describe and evaluate the occurrence of health and health problems, as well as assessing the impact of various risk factors in the population. This very new project has the potential to serve as the basis for future curriculum planning, though the mechanisms are still being developed. The prospects are improved by the fact that the codirectors of the CHRU are also centrally involved in "Curriculum 2000," a major curriculum revision at the medical school.

Educating Future Physicians for Ontario: The EFPO Project

In the past 3 years, the province of Ontario has focused attention on the health care it provides to its 9.7 million citizens. Three major reports are being used in a major rethinking of the health care system (Ontario Health Review Panel 1987; Panel on Health Goals for Ontario 1987; Minister's Advisory Group on Health Promotion 1987). The most notable result of this work has been the formation 2 years ago of the Premier's Council on Health Strategy. Chaired by the Premier, and based on the realization that the health of the people is a product of many different determinants (of which the health care system is only one), the Council is forging a strategic plan for the improved health and quality of life for Ontario residents (Premier's Council on Health Strategy 1989).

This is the context in which a major collaborative effort in medical education was launched in July 1989. Initiated by a philanthropic foundation, Associated Medical Services, and recognizing that medical education must be more responsive to the needs of Ontario society, the province's five medical schools have embarked on a project entitled *Educating Future Physicians for Ontario* (EFPO). The initial funding agency was joined in supporting the project by the five universities involved, and recently by the provincial Ministry of Health. The overall goal of the project is to modify the character of medical education in Ontario so that it is more responsive to the evolving needs of Ontario society. The objectives are to

- Define the health requirements of Ontario society as they relate to the training of physicians;
- Foster faculty development to meet the expanded needs of medical education, including curriculum change, problem solving, clinical epidemiology, and continuing medical education;
- Develop a mechanism for the evaluation of medical students that will assess both knowledge and competence;

- Support the development of education programs for medical students in Ontario that are based on meeting defined societal needs; and
- Generate a mechanism and process for the development of leadership in medical education that will sustain the changes initiated by the project.

A major component of the project is clarification of roles for future physicians. This component can be characterized as a "health intelligence" component, charged directly to translate the analysis of health needs and expectations of Ontario society into a statement of roles and competencies of future physicians. Several working groups have been launched to examine health needs in detail, to assess the public's and health professionals' expectations of future physicians in responding to those needs, and to identify appropriate educational strategies. The findings of this component will contribute directly to the other components of the project, which focus on faculty development, assessment of competence, and leadership development. It is noteworthy that the leaders of the two HIUs described above are also leaders of this component of the EFPO project.

A community advisory committee brings perspectives from a wide variety of societal health interests and areas to the project. All five Ontario medical schools are represented in the overall project steering committee, the component executive committees, school-specific liaison committees, and a variety of related activities. The work will be carried out collaboratively by participants from all five medical schools. The project has the full support of the five deans; in fact, the Council of Ontario Faculties of Medicine has assumed direct responsibility for the project, with the EFPO Steering Committee as its operational arm. This Committee and the various working groups interact closely and regularly with the five leaders of undergraduate medical education and their committees. Four of the five medical schools were in the process of initiating substantial changes and innovations in their curriculums at about the time the EFPO project began, and the latter is being designed to support and expand these changes.

V. Experiences to Date

The *Health Intelligence Units* described above are very early in their development; there has not been time for significant successes or failures to occur. Questions about the generalizability of their experiences cannot be answered at this time. Nevertheless, it may be useful to define some of the key questions being asked, and describe the early experiences of the two units and the EFPO project in response to them.

- *What is the impact of the HIUs on their institutions: the institutional mission, policies, and programs?* It is probable that the HIUs are largely the products of their institutional environments. That is, both were already committed to the importance of population-based education and research, and it is this commitment that, in part, led to the formation of the HIUs. Both schools developed mission statements in 1990, that emphasize the institution's obligation to respond to their community's health needs.

The McMaster statement reads in part, "the faculty of Health Sciences has committed itself to contribute to the quality of life of the communities it serves by fostering excellence in health education, research, and service . . . We shall pursue: the development and critical evaluation of new knowledge about the biological, behavioral, social, and environmental bases of health and disease, and about the usefulness of preventive, therapeutic, and rehabilitative maneuvers; . . . development and critical evaluation of new knowledge relevant to the continued evolution of an optimal health care delivery system; . . . application of knowledge . . . to support leadership in the implementation of the services and systems for the benefit of the local, national, and international communities that we serve."

While the *Health Priorities Analysis Unit* and its associated faculty members participated vigorously in the strategic planning process, it cannot be said that the HPAU directly influenced the new mission statement. Similarly, the Ottawa statement reads in part: "Physician graduates of the faculty will be well prepared to address the present and future health needs of the Canadian population . . . The faculty will provide exemplary, scientifically-based health services to the population of Ottawa and its catchment area." The development of the mission statement predates the actual establishment of the Community Health Research Unit, but the two planning processes were interrelated.

- *Has the systematic and clearly presented analysis of health information influenced institutional priorities and policies?* Again, the units are a product of their environments. There has been a strong emphasis in both institutions on communitylinked academic programs. It is significant that these were the two academic health sciences centers chosen about 1985 by the Ontario Ministry of Health to initiate and demonstrate the *Teaching Health Unit* concept. This involved a formal affiliation agreement between the University and the Regional Public Health Department, somewhat on the teaching hospital model, to facilitate population-based research and educational activities, and to strengthen public health services. The *Health Intelligence Units* described above have not yet directly influenced new institutional priorities and policies. They are, however, now supporting the general institutional direction toward population-based academic activities.

- *Have the units directly influenced the institution's educational programs?* At McMaster University, a "priority health problems" model was developed starting about 1986 (MacDonald et al. 1989). In fact, the word "priority" in the name *Health Priority Analysis Unit*, was derived from this experience. The model involves an analytic approach to the assembling of health information from several relevant sources, the analysis of this information, and the assignment of "prioritization" criteria. The resulting list of priority health problems is then used as a guide in the design of the undergraduate medical curriculum based on the case-study method. The list is also used in the assignment of patients to students in various clerkship rotations. Some of these strategies are now being tested in postgraduate residency education programs. Formation of the HPAU followed much of this work; it now supports the education programs through the preparation and dissemination of focused educational packages (such as the package on alcohol use and abuse, described earlier).

In Ottawa, the chairman of the medical education Curriculum Committee and the Assistant Dean for Undergraduate Education led a move in the early 1980s to develop new educational objectives for the school—objectives that would be based on the health status and needs of the population (Rosser and Beaulieu 1984; White 1984). They assembled data on the reasons for which people visit family doctors, and used these to develop a list of "common conditions." This was supplemented by a list of conditions considered "important" because they illustrate significant medical concepts or are life-threatening and susceptible to medical intervention. The undergraduate educational objectives ultimately adopted were based on these "Common and Important Conditions." Although the lists themselves were somewhat controversial, the principle of basing curriculum on health needs was established. The "Curriculum 2000" project now underway in the medical school continues this approach and has a strong community thrust.

In summary, the HIUs are beginning to have an impact on the educational and research programs of these two medical schools—especially at McMaster. The output of the Units can guide the development of the curriculum, regardless of the method of instruction. Potentially, it can guide the choice of lecture topics, of case studies or problems, and of community visits—in each case demonstrating the relevance of the educational program to the needs of the community. Presentation of "the facts" regarding the community's health needs should do much to counteract uninformed turf protection and expansionary drives based on the special interests of disciplines and departments.

- *Who specifies the questions, and the work agenda for these Units?* The HIU should be closely linked to the Dean's Office and to any office of institutional planning that may exist, and more specifically to curriculum planners. It should take much of its direction from them. But the units should have several masters. Although this chapter is concerned with the contribution of HIUs to the medical school's planning, it makes little sense for them to be sponsored solely by the medical school. Other organizations like District Health Councils, Public Health Units, Social Planning Councils, and perhaps the Planning Departments of local or regional governments have similar information needs. It seems reasonable, therefore, for the Units to be sponsored by a coalition of such organizations which would share the costs and jointly set the work agenda. In addition to improving efficiency, such coalitions would strengthen the medical school's linkages to the larger community and thereby improve its community orientation. Of course, these arrangements also contain the seeds of conflict, since the various sponsors will have somewhat different priorities.

In Hamilton, the unit is a component of the university's faculty of Health Sciences. However, it has always had a community Board, and there is strong representation from the community in the development of the unit's priorities and plans. In addition, the unit is increasingly linked to the various regional health agencies and projects, such as the Department of Public Health, the Social Planning and Research Council, and the District Health Council. The newer Ottawa unit is the product of both the medical school and the Public Health Unit, although university "ownership" so far extends to only one department. The questions to be pursued and the work agenda are influenced by both sponsors, as well as by an Advisory Committee drawn from other community agencies, but the linkages to the curriculum planning process are not yet well developed.

Recently, the provincial Ministry of Health has issued a set of *Mandatory Health Programs and Services Guidelines* to be implemented by the province's 42 *Public Health Units* (Ontario Ministry of Health 1989). Included are general standards on *Community Health Status Information*, with the objective of "ensuring that the Board of Health addresses the health needs of the residents of its health Unit." For example, there is a requirement to produce, at least once every 5 years, a community health status report to include such areas as reproductive outcomes and risk factor prevalence. A similar report on local environmental risk areas is also to be produced every 5 years, with annual updates that include data on landfill sites, contaminated sites, and so on. In Ontario, therefore, there is now a statutory basis for tackling important problems and a work agenda for all Public Health Units. And since both HIUs are closely linked to their local Departments of Health Services, they will undoubtedly be involved with the carrying out of this provincial health agenda.

• *Will the units be involved in monitoring socioeconomic trends?* This is already happening on a selective basis. For example, in Hamilton, the *Fact Book on the Health Status of Hamilton–Wentworth Residents* includes socioeconomic data. As new local community health and relevant socioeconomic information becomes available it will be addressed both through *Infowatch* newsletters and incorporation into the next edition of the "*Fact Book.*" This publication is evaluated through a survey of a stratified random sample of "*Fact Book*" recipients; the findings result in content and format modifications of the subsequent editions.

In Ottawa, the assembly and analysis of community health information is a central goal of the *Community Health Research Unit*. A major component of this effort deals with social and economic variables drawn from the Census—data needed for planning, priority-setting, and research.

- *To what extent can the role of the local Health Intelligence Unit be complemented by provincial or national groups to address issues relevant at these levels?* The local Unit should draw on relevant data from provincial, national, and even international sources for analysis, interpretation, and use as they apply to the local health circumstances. This requires the development of communication channels to assure awareness of and access to appropriate data. Where there are several medical schools in a province or state, their HIUs should not work in isolation, but should form a network for purposes of data acquisition, methods development, and comparability of results, as well as for intellectual stimulation. Other models, such as the Canadian Task Force on the Periodic Health Examination (Morgan 1979), might function as HIU "equivalents" to make general recommendations or interpretations, but assessment of the "fit" of these recommendations to local health issues must be done locally. The concept of continuity in the flow of such information among analysis Units at national, regional, and local levels might be worth developing further. The Directors for both the HIUs described here are members of the Advisory Committee to the Ontario Health Survey.

- *How can we assure "demand" for the contributions of Health Intelligence Units by institutional leaders (education program chairs, Deans, and health planners)?* Every effort should be made to develop the Units as working partners with community, education, and research programs and with health services planners. Clearly stated objectives by each partner will help to guide the activities of the Units, increasing the likelihood that their products will be useful to their medical schools and other health care institutions.

- *How can the formation of such Units be promoted in medical schools where the environment may be less supportive of this orientation?* Reports of the successful functioning of existing embryonic Units should help, as should peer pressure from education and professional leaders become convinced that medical schools should develop programs that address directly the community's health needs. Help with funding the Units should be forthcoming from governments and from collaborating agencies should reduce financial impediments to their creation.

- *What resources are required for operating such a unit?* The units described in this chapter are in early stages of development and functioning, with very limited faculty and support personnel—on the order of 4–6 staff each. Except for the core faculty members, all costs are currently drawn from research funds from outside the University—obviously not a stable source of support in the long run. Medical schools should contribute to the support of such units, both through assignment of faculty members to them part-time and through some contribution of staff and computer support.

White (1989) estimated the annual cost of operating a Health Care Analysis and Intelligence Center at around US $600,000; this is for a core staff consisting initially of two clinical epidemiologists, one health economist, one health statistician, and one medical sociologist, plus 10 support staff. Few schools will be able to bear the total costs of supporting a Unit, so external sources must be found. Since the benefits of the Units accrue to a variety of community (and possibly provincial) agencies, all members of the local coalitions should contribute support. The benefits of a properly functioning network of HIUs to educational, research, and service planning would seem to be so great that governments should consider providing financial support. White (1989) suggested (in the context of a province with only one medical school) that it would be appropriate for the provincial health insurance plan to allocate 0.1% of its annual expenditures for this purpose, analogous to the Research and Development allocations of industry.

VI. Future Directions and Recommendations

The experience in the early days of these projects is exciting and promising, although it is yet very limited. Their potential lies in three general directions:

- Where universities, and medical schools in particular, have a stated mission of contributing to the improved health status of a specified community or a defined population, a Unit devoted to the analysis and interpretation of health trends and information can become a key activity within these institutions. Much remains to be learned about the structures and strategies required to ensure maximum impact of these Units on the values, policies, and programs of the institutions. This area is in itself a useful focus for "operations research."
- Several Units located in institutions in the same geopolitical jurisdiction represent a potential "research network." Collectively they could influence academic programs in the several institutions they represent. To some extent, the EFPO project may become an example of this.
- Most important, these Units have the potential to be the bridge in evolving partnerships between the University, the communities served, and the health care systems. The partnerships share the common goal of improving the health of the people. The University has a distinctive contribution to make in the achievement of this goal, through its educational mandate and its research capability. A *Health Intelligence Unit* can be a key link in this collaborative effort.

Two specific recommendations are offered:

- A major incentive fund should be established to encourage medical schools to establish and test various models for *Health Intelligence Units*, to foster collaboration among the institutions involved, and to disseminate the results of their collective experiences.

• The establishment of a well-functioning HIU should be included in the accreditation criteria for undergraduate and postgraduate medical education.

Acknowledgments. The authors gratefully acknowledge the substantial contributions of Larry W. Chambers and Richard J. Pickering.

References

Lalonde, M. 1974. *A New Perspective on the Health of Canadians.* Government of Canada.

MacDonald, P.J., Chong, J.P., Chongtrakul, P., and Neufeld, V.R., Tugwell, P., Chambers, L.W., Pickering, R.J., and Oates, M.J. 1989. Setting educational priorities for learning the concepts of population health. *Med Education* **23**:429–439.

Minister's Advisory Group on Health Promotion (S. Podborski, Chairman), 1987. *Health Promotion Matters in Ontario.* Toronto: Ministry of Health.

Morgan, P.P., 1979. The periodic health examination. *Can Med Assoc J* **121**:1–2.

Ontario Health Review Panel (J. Evans, Chairman), 1987. *Toward a Shared Direction for Health in Ontario.* Toronto: Ministry of Health.

Ontario Ministry of Health, 1989. *Mandatory Health Programs and Services Guidelines.* Toronto: Ministry of Health.

Panel on Health Goals for Ontario (R. Spasoff, Chairman), 1987. *Health for All Ontario.* Toronto: Ministry of Health.

Premier's Council on Health Strategy, 1989. *A Vision of Health*: Health Goals for Ontario. Toronto: Premier's Council.

Rosser, W.W., and Beaulieu, M. 1984. Institutional objectives for medical education that relates to the community. *Can Med Assoc J* **130**:683–689.

White, K.L. 1983. Health care: Limits and opportunities for health science centers. In: Squires, B. (Ed.), *Proceedings of the Conference on Health in the 80's and 90's and its Impact on Health Sciences Education* (Montebello, Quebec, 1982), Toronto: Council of Ontario Universities.

White, K.L. 1984. The mission of medicine. *Can Med Assoc J* **130**:680–681.

White, K.L. 1989. *Towards a New Beginning*: Review of the College of Medicine. Saskatoon: University of Saskatchewan.

Discussion

Lord Butterfield

A wholly acceptable case has been made out by Neufeld and Spasoff. Over the last 40 years medical schools in the United Kingdom have had to accommodate their educational curricula and developments to the National Health Service (NHS) developing all around them and controlling the nation's hospital building programs, the development of regional specialties and therefore of specialist posts, the distribution of community-based family practitioners, and the remuneration of doctors and other health professions. Those concerned with the training of students have tried to ensure they are exposed to the nation's health statistics as the basis for recognizing important social problems.

This part of the curriculum has been met by university departments concerned specifically with community medicine that have blocks of teaching time in the final years of the medical courses. Certain schools have set up and run associated general practices. Community medicine, occupational medicine, and public health measures have therefore all retained students' attention both in the teaching program and through examination questions in the final qualifying medical examination. The success of these programs has varied from school to school and it is hoped that a recent survey of medical schools may throw some light on the reascns for differences. Postgraduate opportunities in all these fields of activity in the community are associated with training programs and specialist diploma examinations. There has also been the establishment of a variety of specialist institutions and colleges.

Liaison arrangements very similar to those put forward by Neufeld and Spasoff have also been operating in medical schools in the United Kingdom. University staff often sit on national, regional, and district NHS Authorities and NHS administrators and doctors have frequently worked in and with departments of community medicine. Members of such departments have been appointed individually or have been seconded as administrators in the NHS at regional and district levels. Indeed in the 1980s, consideration was given at the new medical school at Cambridge to the possibility of establishing an alternative curriculum for training doctors to encourage them to see themselves as having direct responsibilities to the community at large rather than being introduced initially to the excitement of caring for individual patients. There can be no doubt that most medical students leaving their pre-clinical laboratories yearn to start grappling with the personal difficulties, the diagnostic problems, and the sorts of treatment available for the individual patient, in preference to studying cold health statistics. Aware of the potential threat to time in the curriculum, clinicians have not been slow to point out that patients must not be treated as statistics but as individuals!

It will be important to consider all the impedances likely to arise to schemes as logically and socially desirable as those set out by Neufeld and Spasoff. In this connection experiences in the United Kingdom may again be useful. For example, support for the alternative curriculum at Cambridge was blocked in large part by financial constraints on the appointment of the staff needed to carry it out. Another impedance was the fact that it seemed inescapable, if a social contract-oriented curriculum were to have any chance of success, that the students be exposed to it first before becoming engrossed in the excitement surrounding the care of individuals so brilliantly displayed by the teaching clinicians!

The establishment of the *Health Intelligence Units* suggested must not only have an impact on the Deans and leaders of the medical schools but must have the ability to attract students to their activities including the ablest of students. Ways and means of achieving this will have to be thought through. At Nottingham University's Medical School one way was to involve the students in the social aspects of care of patients from the very first week of their medical training, but there are, of course, other means of achieving the same ends.

It will also be important that detailed consideration and thought be given to ways and means of getting governmental licensing authorities to open the way for schools to set up the proposed educational programs and encourage a new attitude of social responsibility for health care. It may well be that proposals about the accrediting and licensing of schools to train a nation's doctors should depend on the presence in the schools of liaison committees and *Health Analysis and Intelligence Units* as is proposed. But there will be inevitable resistance and it is my view that time could be usefully spent discussing strategies to achieve the stated objectives described in this chapter. Recent reorganization of the National Health Service makes it a responsibility of the newly formed Regional and District Health Authorities to discover the health needs of their relevant population and then finding ways and means to meet them. In this way training programs for postgraduates in the United Kingdom and other countries should be made much more relevant to their population's needs.

The United States Department of Health and Human Services has launched a "Healthy People 2000" project. This national endeavor aims to encourage the establishment of a network of persons interested in fostering better health for all citizens by any means available, including the political will in cities, towns, districts, and neighborhoods. An important aspect of the development has been the formation of working links between the Department of Health and bodies such as the National Civic League. Similar "Healthy People 2000" projects are being developed elsewhere in the world, particularly in Canada and some cities in the United Kingdom and elsewhere. This global movement, fostered by the World Health Organization, offers unique opportunities to strengthen proposals in medical schools such as those suggested by Neufeld and Spasoff. Integration between medical schools' efforts and those going on in the public arena could provide ready-made support for the educational programs now adumbrated. Such developments chimes strongly with the phrases in specific recommendations designed to reassure the public that medical schools are indeed responding to their health problems. I believe the ideas advanced by Neufeld and Spasoff provide a unique opportunity to encourage giant strides forward in many countries.

Harry S. Jonas

The present Liaison Committee on Medical Education (LCME) standards for accreditation of medical education programs leading to the M.D. degree in the United States and Canada call for a curriculum that enhances student concerns about the effects of social and cultural circumstances on the health of their patients. It is clear that many medical schools, particularly in the United States, have not substantially emphasized this important area.

This chapter presents a concept that is both logical and sensible. The question immediately raised by the authors is why medical schools have not utilized information relevant to the health problems of the community in developing their educational programs? One reason is that most United States programs have difficulty in defining the community for which the medical school accepts responsibility. Is it the region immediately surrounding the medical school, the area within a given radius, or the entire state? Academic medical centers often accept referrals from widely diverse geographic areas.

Medical centers in the United States also serve different population groups within the same community boundaries. For example, a single institution may provide a substantial amount of health care to both an affluent suburban population as well as to financially disadvantaged inner city residents with vastly different life-styles, health care needs, and demands. If a school's curriculum and entire educational experiences are based primarily on the assessed needs of the surrounding community, there is a risk that such an education might not provide students a firm foundation in all the broader aspects of medical care. I would agree with the authors that a high proportion of any medical school's graduates may not serve that school's target population. Data from the 1990 LCME Annual Medical School Questionnaire show that an average of only 45% of United States medical school graduates enter residency programs in the same state as their medical school.

These explanations, however, should not prevent medical schools in the United States from implementing a concept similar to that which the authors propose. In the past few years in the United States there has been a new emphasis on educational outcome, bringing into sharper focus both the institutional as well as the individual physician's responsibilities to the community. There is wide diversity among the United States' medical schools; some are public, some private, some in highly urbanized areas, others not. They differ greatly in availability of resources, financial and otherwise. These diverse schools in the past have had difficulty in articulating their respective objectives and in relating those objectives to the community.

Historically in the United States, the gathering of data about the health status of various population groups has been vested primarily in the hands of local, state, and Federal health officials, all with substantial budgets and personnel resources. A more logical approach would be to more fully integrate the efforts of this existing network of city, county, and state health departments and those of our Federal government with the capacities of academic medical centers. This would eliminate unnecessary and costly duplication. In this era of sharply limited medical school budgets, I am concerned that a school's resources could be significantly diluted to establish an effective *Health Intelligence Unit*, unless other sources of support can be obtained from government agencies and schools of public health that already are engaged in such activities. The important issue here is not so much who is responsible for gathering data on community health status, but whether or not and how those data are to be incorporated into the curriculum.

A real tragedy for the United States system of medical education in recent decades has been the separation and isolation of schools of medicine and schools of public health—within the same university. One strong recommendation I would offer is that schools of medicine and schools of public health cooperate fully to address the health needs of the community.

The authors state that the health services system is dominated by "supply-side" thinking independent of societal expectations, needs, and trends. Change might be more likely if the health care system could be subjected to "demand-side" manipulation.

Finally, if the LCME were to make the presence of an *Health Intelligence Unit* a requirement for accreditation, the mere presence of such a Unit is not sufficient without also requiring that the impact of the Unit on programs leading to the M.D. degree be documented.

Much earlier in this century Sir Eric Ashby observed that "[t]he great American contribution to higher education has been to dismantle the walls around the campus—one of the rare inventions in the evolution of universities. It is one which has already been vindicated by history. Other nations are beginning to copy the American example."

Somehow we have modified that American educational concept by building giant academic medical centers and put up mini-Berlin walls around our medical schoolhouses. Perhaps the time has come for the academic walls around medical schools in the United States (and in other countries) to come down also. This chapter has described a concept that may help move us in that direction.

Lionel E. McLeod

The authors address a problem important to all health professional faculties—the relevance of their programs to the communities served. In medical schools, the potential and promise, the kudos, and the sheer elegance of basic biomedical research have diverted attention away from the importance of the health status of the community. Rebalancing and resetting educational priorities are urgently required if community and political support is to be strengthened.

Neufeld and Spasoff present a model by which this rebalancing might be achieved. Their model requires the cooperation and collaboration of senior echelons of university administration and appropriate governmental agencies. Unfortunately, not all universities, or in Canada, provincial governmental agencies, recognize or have the will to bring about change. Working with those that are receptive could begin a national network, perhaps patterned on the model used by the *Canadian Institute of Advanced Research*

(Toronto), especially its *Population Health Program*. For success, at least three or four provinces must become involved. The Federal government should be petitioned to facilitate the process, set overall objectives and standards, and ensure the cooperation of Statistics Canada—the nation's statistical agency. Uninterrupted support of at least 7 to 10 years would be essential and should be followed by a critical review of accomplishment measured by identifiable modification in curricula and student experience.

The author's brief reference to resource allocation provokes a further consideration, one with significant overlap in expertise requirements, the need for governmental cooperation, and expected outcomes. The medical schools, educating tomorrow's physicians, must grapple with the impact of cost containment and maintenance of high quality contemporary health care. The teaching clinician, to be a forceful role model, must acquire new expertise and skills in evaluating the outcomes of care and the appropriate place of new technology.

For an effective response to both the need for evaluating technology effectively and bringing evaluation expertise to the teaching wards, outpatient clinics, and offices, another kind of *Health Intelligence Unit* would be extremely helpful. Ability to establish protocols and collect and analyze information will be critical to success. New communication skills and strategies to bring about change will also be required. This second kind of unit must be positioned differently. To be effective, it must be positioned in close relation in the center of the patient care enterprise. Staffed by experts in experimental design, clinical epidemiology, and biostatistics, it must attract the "scholarly" teaching clinician and students. Everyday discussion of clinical decisions and their information requirements must include pertinent information generated by such Units.

The expertise required for both kinds of Units is in very short supply in Canada. A national inventory should be completed and followed by a plan for the rapid implementation of training programs. While the very best young people should be the population target for training, consideration should be given to able clinician scientists ripe for a career change. Only those who have retained or can quickly refresh their clinical skills should be encouraged to take training.

New funding will not be found easily despite the fact that an overall program would represent a minuscule fraction of today's health care costs. The savings generated by success would quickly repay the investment in startup and operating costs. Because it is essential that faculties of medicine ascribe wholeheartedly to the changes these Units would signal, a program of incentives and matching funds might represent a useful starting point.

General Discussion

Although participants saw great merit in the concept of the Units described in this chapter, some questioned the use of the term "intelligence." This was countered by pointing out that just as there was a need to transform raw *data* into useful *information* through thoughtful aggregation and analysis, so there was a need to interpret the latter as *intelligence* in the context of political, social, economic, and health-related contexts for practical use by those in a position to do so. It was in this sense that the term *intelligence* is used, not in the contemporary association of that term with military and some civilian applications.

The advantages of diversity were stressed; perhaps all medical schools do not need such a Unit when the health information required is readily available from other sources such as tumor registries and Health Maintenance Organizations. However, few of these bodies can produce data from general populations, in contrast to special subpopulations or groups of patients. Some thought that the Units might best be based in the community rather than in the academic health sciences center.

The range of functions of the *Health Intelligence Unit* was debated; some favored a relatively narrow educational and research orientation. In this mode the Unit could act as a "sensor" for limited sets of problems, undertaking specific time-limited surveys. Others argued for a broader mission with potential for impacting clinical services, as well as education and research, by monitoring common, as well as more serious, problems.

Perhaps the most important issue discussed was the need to clarify the links between health data, curriculum changes, and implementation of the school's goals and objectives. How is the loop to be closed between data collection, analysis, interpretation, and changes in the content, context, and format of medical education? And how is the impact of these changes on the health status of the population to be evaluated? Continual iteration of these loops over years and decades would be required. There is much to be said for starting modestly with feasible and achievable projects so that the dangers of overwhelming faculty and students can be avoided and both concepts and methods internalized gradually. Among those who might be most influenced by the products of a *Health Intelligence Unit* are the Deans, especially as the information affects faculty recruitment and student admission policies.

The *Health Intelligence Unit* concept, as well as many other ideas discussed, was seen as especially important in Canada where it was observed that "unless the medical schools start planning for the future and become advocates for change, the government(s) will be happy to rewrite their social contracts. Moreover the drive to regionalize health care planning in Canada requires the availability of good data on health status and its determinants."

5
Population-Based Medicine: A Case Study from a Traditional School

Mutya San Agustin

I. Introduction

In the United States, physician education developed within and was formed by two institutions: the medical school and the teaching hospital, the first emphasizing basic science and second emphasizing, supervised clinical experience (Swanson 1984; Ebert 1985; Dasco 1989). Within those settings excellent institutional competencies were developed: undergraduate and postgraduate teaching by full-time faculty and attending physicians with faculty appointments employed a full range of teaching techniques, student participation in laboratory and clinical research, a variety of teaching modalities (lectures, seminars, grand rounds, and bedside teaching), and close supervision built into the learning process (Abbott 1989). The medical schools and teaching hospitals were constructed to accommodate the needs of students with libraries, classrooms, ongoing medical records, laboratories, and ever increasing technology. As part of the process patients were expected to submit themselves to the needs of education, persuaded through economic necessity, or by the belief that the best patient care was provided in teaching hospitals (Schroeder et al. 1989). These patients were regarded as "teaching material." The poorest allowed their bodies to be used for the educational process in return for free care. In addition, expectations of patients were in large part dependent on what services were made available. In practice, the three institutional aims of patient care, education, and research were often impossible to identify separately.

This whole elaborate structure was based almost exclusively on the inpatient service. "Throughout the 20th century medical students have learned about the natural history and physiologic manifestations of disease, diagnostic, and therapeutic rationales, and the nuances of physicianhood through interactions with patients in hospital wards" (Wooliscroft and Schwenk 1989). The outpatient service was viewed as an appendage, a sop to charitable impulse, as a service to the poor, and a source of "interesting" patients, not as an essential site for medical education (Roemer 1981). The community around the hospital was more or less ignored except as changes in the population brought new diseases into the hospital.

A powerful establishment with a strong interest in its own preservation developed around this inpatient-based system of physician education (Ginzberg 1985). Funding and regulatory agencies, often as the result of effective lobbying by those who wished to preserve and strengthen the status quo, favored inpatient care so that although many critics have argued for more training in primary care, and for more extensive and appropriate ambulatory care clerkships, few well-organized sites existed for either activity (Alpert and Charney 1973; Seidel 1975; Petersdorf 1975; Perkoff 1986). To develop different institutional competencies on any large scale required profound changes in medical schools, teaching hospitals, financial agencies, and those government departments concerned with health care policy (Smith 1985). Those concerned with national or regional health care policy were among the first to recognize the need for more effective training related to the health status of particular communities, large or small.

In the United States, the rapidly growing supply of physicians will produce a doubling in their ratio from 140 physicians per 100,000 population in 1965 to 280 per 100,000 population by the year 2010 (Singer 1989; Tarlov 1983, 1988). In addition, since reimbursement systems reward subspecialization, further maldistribution across the specialties has resulted in a preponderance of subspecialists. Nearly half of the nation's physicians were in a primary care specialty in 1963; by 1986 only 34% were in a primary care specialty (Barnett and Midtling 1989).

The United States is frequently described as the only developed country, apart from South Africa, that has neither national health insurance nor a national health service (Navarro 1989); 37 million of its people are thought to lack access to medical care (Dickman and Milligan 1987). This is not true, however, of New York City, which has long accepted responsibility for providing medical care to all who live within its borders, or enter its borders in search of care. For many years the City offered free medical care to the poor through a network of hospitals, nursing homes, and clinics as well as through subsidies to private charitable institutions. In recent years the City has used whatever state or Federal monies were available to help pay for these services but it has always been prepared to use local tax money (Ginzberg 1986).

The City's first priority was to provide both inpatient and outpatient care to those who could not afford to purchase it from other sources either from their own funds or from insurance. For more than two centuries, the City has operated hospitals in one form or another. The present bureaucratic structure had its origins with the New York State legislature's 1970 decision to create the New York City Health and Hospitals Corporation (HHC). This was to become a $2.4 billion public benefit corporation to meet the medical and health care needs of New Yorkers; it is a semiautonomous arm of the City of New York. As such it is vulnerable to all the vagaries of city politics and fiscal crises. The HHC now operates 11 municipal hospitals, including North Central Bronx Hospital (NCBH), four long-term care facilities, the City's Emergency Medical Care Services, four free-standing clinics in housing projects in low-income neighborhoods, and 31 satellite clinics. Ties to the city government are defined by law and are maintained by agreements between the City and HHC (New York City HHC 1984). Municipal hospitals have long been part of the physician education system in New York City; they provide large numbers of internships and residencies as well as indigent patients—the "teaching material."

During the late 1950s, the municipal hospitals were in crisis; their buildings and equipment were outdated, dilapidated, and shabby. They were unable to provide adequate professional supervision or to attract the most qualified residents. To solve this problem a contract system was created by which private, nonprofit teaching hospitals and medical schools would provide the medical staffs for the municipal hospitals, including residents and their supervisors (Ginzberg 1986).

The North Central Bronx Hospital (NCBH) is a modern 420 bed municipal hospital located adjacent to the Montefiore Medical Center (MMC), in the Northwest corner of the Bronx. MMC under a contract with the HHC is responsible for all professional services at NCBH, including qualified attending staff and support services related to direct patient care activities. Residents contract with HHC for their training and rotate through NCBH for varying lengths of time depending on clinical service requirements. As part of this affiliation contract with the City, MMC provides NCBH with an on-site administrative staff and full-time directors of its clinical services. NCBH also has a separate administrative staff that is approved by and responsible to the HHC.

MMC is a not-for-profit hospital founded in 1884 with a long history of social commitment and of caring for the poor. The medical center is operated by a self-perpetuating board, composed largely of descendants from the nineteenth-century philanthropists who established a charity hospital for chronically ill indigent immigrants. Today most of MMC's patients pay their bills through some form of health insurance. For many years it had an activist director who gave strong support for the creation and development of the NCBH's Department of Ambulatory Medicine (Levenson 1984). Over the years, by way of contrast, the departments of pediatrics and of internal medicine have offered either support or opposition according to the priorities of their changing chairmen.

MMC is affiliated with the Albert Einstein College of Medicine (AECOM), a part of Yeshiva University, and is affected by the policies and financial status of that entity. The medical school was founded in the 1950s. Some of its departments were strongly influenced by the social activism of the 1960s and that decade's concern for improving the community's health but the school also has a strong tradition of commitment to the basic sciences and biomedical research. During the 1970s the relationship between MMC an.. the AECOM grew closer and most of the clinical departments were unified. As a result, the chairmen of these very large unified departments supervised empires that sprawled across a medical school, four hospitals, and related programs in other hospitals, nursing homes, and community-based clinics, etc. Together they serve a population of well over a million.

NCBH's catchment area includes communities suffering from the plight of the urban poor, and neighborhoods slowly deteriorating as services and businesses move to wealthier areas. It serves an ethnically heterogeneous population considered representative of many other large urban settings in the United States. Although most patients live in the local community, the Department of Ambulatory Medicine attracts a significant number of individuals and families residing beyond its service area. These patients come from other areas where health manpower is traditionally short and where they might, in better circumstances, be expected to utilize local institutions for their health care needs. The majority of the patients are the medically indigent; they are ineligible for either of the two U.S. government medical insurance programs (Medicare for the elderly and Medicaid for the poor) and do not have third party insurance coverage (United Hospital Fund 1988). In recent years, crime, drug abuse, and homelessness have adversely affected the health of the population. Mental health problems, child abuse and neglect, sexually transmitted diseases (STDs), and AIDS seem inextricably linked in a community where they are imposed on an already debilitated population with inadequate resources to meet essential needs. Added to these problems is a high rate of teenage pregnancy. Certain other conditions also are predominant in the population; these include asthma, lead poisoning, and tuberculosis (NYC Department of Health 1987). Compounding these problems has been lack of access to medical care and advice, as well as lack of knowledge about health care, parenting, family planning, and medical resources. NCBH serves an economically deprived population of about 300,000; 50% are Black, 45% Hispanic, and 5% White (United Hospital Fund 1988). Soon after its opening, the hospital had the highest inpatient occupancy rate of any New York municipal hospital and 190,000 outpatient visits a year: 48,527 were for adult primary care, 37,397 for pediatric primary care, 40,111 for obstetric–gynecological care, 11,314 for medical subspecialty consultations, and 62,520 for surgical subspecialty consultations. In a recent year, 55,109 adults and 28,007 children came to the Emergency Room (North Central Bronx Hospital 1989).

The Department of Ambulatory Medicine at NCBH was established as an outcome of the reorganization of the ambulatory care clinics at Morrisania City Hospital also in the Bronx, and another of the HHC's municipal hospitals. The outpatient department of Morrisania City Hospital exemplified many of the difficulties encountered in trying to provide exemplary patient care and teaching in a traditional setting. Patient care was fragmented, episodic, and disease-oriented, and follow-up was inadequate. The clinic's facilities, staff, and programs were unable to cope with the volume of service demanded and unprepared to provide first-rate care and resident education. Supervision of residents in the clinics was inadequate. Graduating physicians were oriented primarily toward inpatient services and unfamiliar with the needs of the outpatient population (San Agustin et al. 1976).

With the closing of Morrisania City Hospital in 1976, NCBH opened. The structure of the ambulatory care services at NCBH emphasized a comprehensive primary care program. A separate Department of Ambulatory Medicine was established with a full-time director responsible for program planning, implementation, and coordination of all the hospital's ambulatory care components (Appendix 1). We chose to operate the Department of Ambulatory Medicine at NCBH not as a self-contained autonomous program but as an integral part of these other components of MMC and AECOM. Interacting with them at many levels, our Department aimed at influencing their programs of patient care and physician education. While developing this functionally independent department, the Director of the Department of Ambulatory Medicine developed on-going interactions with the chairmen of the clinical departments (medicine, pediatrics, surgery, obstetrics–gynecology, and psychiatry) concerning program-planning and staffing of specialized clinical services. This functional independence facilitated the establishment of priorities for the different ambulatory care components while minimizing the conflicts of interest (San Agustin 1978).

At NCBH the Department of Ambulatory Medicine gradually has developed patient care, educational, and research programs that are population-based and related directly to the needs of the community served by the hospital. This was not an easy task. The Department of Ambulatory Medicine is but one department in a huge hospital. The latter, in turn, is not a free-standing autonomous body but part of a complex network of public and private not-for-profit institutions. Each has its own agenda, set of priorities, and sources of funding. Under these circumstances the development of competencies that foster population-based approaches becomes essential not only at NCBH but at all the diverse partners in the enterprise. The Department of Ambulatory Medicine at NCBH has been the catalyst for many changes within this complex. These changes have made it possible to develop the essential institutional competencies required to serve a neighborhood of poor people dependent for both inpatient and outpatient care on services provided by a hospital owned and operated by a municipal government. While the focus of this Department is on ambulatory care, it has fostered the integration of the inpatient and outpatient services, and directed both toward meeting immediate and long-term community needs. This patient care program has, in turn, provided the basis for the establishment of a program for undergraduate and postgraduate education that trains physicians to provide inpatient and outpatient primary care firmly grounded in a knowledge of the community. These physicians are also trained to work productively with the specialists and subspecialists in the Department of Ambulatory Medicine. All are trained to meet the same standards of responsibility and responsiveness to the community (San Agustin 1978). Additional controls and incentives are provided by the New York State Department of Health, which actively regulates and funds much of health care within the State. In addition the Department encourages certain forms of physician education through funding mechanisms for residencies. The Federal government also played a major role in funding and regulating both patient care and physicians' education.

The New York City Department of Health monitors the provision of certain health services within the City including some at NCBH. We were not fortunate enough to have the ongoing cooperation of a school of public health but much of the assistance that we might have sought from such an institution was provided by the Department of Epidemiology and Social Medicine, one of the unified departments of MMC and the AECOM. This department supplied much helpful epidemiological information and community-based statistics on, for example, substance abuse and the prevalence of HIV infection in women and children in the Bronx. It also operated several programs serving drug abusers so that it was able to provide first-hand knowledge of drug use within the community as well as counseling and consultation services for NCBH patients.

II. Institutional Competencies for Population-Based Education in the Department of Ambulatory Medicine

In the United States, particularly in New York City, significant changes in the last three decades conspired to bring into prominence its hospital-based ambulatory health care arrangements: there was increased access to care for the elderly and poor brought about by the introduction of Medicare and Medicaid and a subsequent burgeoning of health care expenditures; there were decreases in the length of hospital stay as a result of the introduction of payment based on Diagnosis Related Groups (DRGs); there was an increase in the services offered in the outpatient clinics; greatly increased specialization was coupled with geographic maldistribution of physicians; primary care practitioners were in short supply everywhere but especially in depressed neighborhoods; and expansion of health insurance brought expansion of new modes of practice, i.e., Health Maintenance Organization's (Ginzberg 1986).

These tumultuous changes highlighted the role of the Department of Ambulatory Medicine as gatekeeper to the health services system and as a barometer of the needs of the population served (Reagan 1987). The Department's reorganization of services became the model and focal point for institutional change. Just as there was a shift of patients from the inpatient to the outpatient services, so there needed to be fundamental changes in medical education (Rogers and Gastel 1988; Feltovich et al. 1989; Rosenblatt 1988). The latter is inextricably intertwined with the way in which medical services and practices are organized and as such provide the environment in which education occurs. Law students do not learn in the courtroom and engineers do not have classes on construction sites, but medical students receive the great bulk of their clinical education in the largest and technologically most advanced hospitals in the nation (Ebert 1985). In the United States, primary care is performed by graduates of departments of family medicine, by general internists, by ambulatory pediatricians, or, by some reckonings, obstetrician–gynecologists (Starfield 1986; Schroeder 1984).

At NCBH the same physician who cares for the patient in the outpatient setting follows the patient into the hospital if he or she is admitted. Since about 80% of the inpatients at NCBH are admitted from the Department of Ambulatory Medicine (the remaining are transfers from other hospitals or satellite clinics), this system involves the essential principles of integration of the inpatient and outpatient services, and of continuing and comprehensive care for each patient. The program at NCBH also is predicated on the principle that the standard of ambulatory service is equal to that on the inpatient service. Experiences in a variety of settings have shaped the program. These included a community-based health clinic, a shabby out-of-date and overcrowded outpatient department in an old, neglected public hospital, and a new city hospital with outpatient areas built to program specifications. Whatever the clinical setting, certain institutional essential competencies were planned for NCBH.

The first was institutional autonomy; the Ambulatory Department has a Director with power, rank, and salary equal to other clinical directors in the hospital; it has a separate budget with full fiscal authority, as well as the power to hire and fire attending medical staff, and to assign medical students and residents for training in primary care. The Director is directly responsible for the planning, organization, direction, and control of patient care, and for the development and execution of all educational programs on the service. This dual responsibility for patient care and education institutionalizes authority for prompt responses to perceived needs and changes in a world of constrained resources, and assures balance and equity.

Second, it is believed that superior or even adequate ambulatory care can exist only where teaching and supervision are integral parts of the service (Taylor et al. 1984). Teaching in the outpatient service has its unique problems, foremost of which are time limitations and the need to respect patient autonomy (Girard et al. 1984; Kroenke 1986). Whether ambulatory care is based in a hospital or in a community facility, it needs to be an essential part of both the medical school's and the teaching hospital's structures, held to the same standards, and taught by similarly qualified faculty. The latter are required to meet the standards set by the different clinical departments and the medical school; they have the same opportunities for promotion as other faculty so that they are seen by the residents as the peers of other teachers (Greer 1990; Skeff 1988).

The third essential institutional competency is the provision of a physical site and support services adequate for both good patient care and for teaching. The physical site may be regarded as a resource, not a competency. But, given the inadequacies of most hospital-based sites for the provision of comprehensive ambulatory care of high quality, the provision of adequate facilities for teaching exemplary ambulatory care must be regarded as a rare institutional "competency." To support first-rate teaching, an ambulatory facility has certain basic requirements: a floor plan that promotes efficiency while adapting to the needs of patients, students, and their teachers, adequately-sized waiting rooms that convey warmth and friendliness, private examining rooms for all those providing care, and a separate conference room for teaching medical students and residents (Nardone and Webb 1989; Arneill and Nuelsen 1978). Other necessities include adequate support services, an efficient medical records system, on-site laboratory space for performing selected procedures, i.e., gram stains, properly maintained equipment used routinely, i.e., ophthalmoscope, otoscope, and blood-pressure apparatus, examining tables appropriate for gynecologic examinations in each examining room, and provisions made for keeping track of patients' compliance and appointment keeping.

The fourth institutional competency is the capacity to define the population served and to specify its major health problems. These measures are essential for modifying services to appropriately respond to the population's perceived needs. This competency is not the sole responsibility of the Department of Ambulatory Medicine or even of the teaching hospital alone. It involves a much larger group that includes the medical school, the Department of Health, as well as local, regional, and national governments (Rogers 1982; Nutting 1986). The Department of Epidemiology and Social Medicine provides the Department of Ambulatory Medicine with important information about the health status of a community with high rates of homicide, substance abuse, lead poisoning, child abuse, and low birthweight infants. The most immediate, relevant, and reliable information for managing our resources and responsibilities, however, is gathered by the Department of Ambulatory Medicine itself. Since NCBH provides most of the primary and emergency care for the surrounding population it encounters virtually all their health problems. Most hospital inpatient services necessarily are restricted in the kinds of patients admitted, but the ambulatory services accumulate examples of a much wider range of health problems. For example, detailed collection and analyses of data on patients with asthma, sickle cell disease, and lead poisoning, etc. have provided a sound basis for planning the care of these patients, and for training physicians in their appropriate management.

The fifth institutional competency is capacity to assure that its services are of high quality. Standards as rigorous as those in the inpatient setting had to be established for ambulatory care and guidelines had to be set for accreditation of the ambulatory site for patient care and teaching (Daley et al. 1988). Government regulations and those of the Joint Commission for Accreditation of Hospitals provide detailed rules for the operation of inpatient services. Much less detail exists for outpatient services. Therefore, the Department of Ambulatory Medicine devotes considerable effort to the design and testing of protocols and procedures to maintain standards and assess quality.

The sixth institutional competency is the capacity and the ability to undertake research in the ambulatory setting. Such research, in the past, has had a low priority. As patients have become more enlightened and third party payers more involved in the care provided in offices and clinics, and as more questions are raised about their organization and effectiveness, research in ambulatory care has come into its own (Starfield and Pless 1973). The Department of Ambulatory Medicine conducts research, alone and in cooperation with other departments on issues related to the management of specific diseases, the effectiveness and efficiency of health services, the cost-effectiveness of interventions, and the adequacy of responses to community health problems. All six of these competencies are integral parts of the Department of Ambulatory Medicine's program; several others require the support from the medical school.

III. The Health Care System of the Department of Ambulatory Medicine

Primary Care Model

At present the Department of Ambulatory Medicine comprises five functional areas: four primary care teams (PCTs); medical and pediatric subspecialty consultative services within the PCTs; specialty clinics in surgery, ophthalmology, otolaryngology, dentistry, psychiatry, dermatology, and allergy; emergency medical services with medical, pediatric, surgical, and psychiatric components; and employee health services.

The Department is located on the first four floors of NCBH and occupies 57,500 square feet of floor space. The emergency medical service is housed on the first floor, and occupies 13,234 square feet of floor space. A total of 44,136 square feet is allocated to the PCT and specialty clinics, located on the second, third, and fourth floors.

Primary Care Teams

The four PCTs replaced the traditional general medical/pediatric clinics and screening/walk-in clinics. Each PCT consists of an adult and pediatric component that provides family-oriented medical care. The adult or pediatric component is composed of three to four full-time attending physicians, two full-time nurse practitioners, residents, and medical students from the AECOM and support personnel, including registered nurses, nurses aides, clerks and, social workers. Each PCT is an independent unit with the adult and pediatric components located physically adjacent to each other, to facilitate the provision of total health care and coordination of services to all members of a family.

The primary care physicians are full-time attendings in the Department of Medicine or Pediatrics at MMC, some with additional training in a subspecialty such as gastroenterology, cardiology, endocrinology, pulmonary, hematology, or infectious diseases. They are jointly recruited, interviewed, and appointed by the director of the Department of Ambulatory Medicine and the chairman of the relevant clinical department (medicine, pediatrics, surgery, obstetrics–gynecology, and psychiatry). For their daily work, the physicians are directly responsible to the Director of the Department of Ambulatory Medicine. They provide an equivalent of 3 days per week for direct patient care and 1 day for research and/or subspecialty consultative services for the PCT. In addition each team attending physician spends 1 day a week as a preceptor to the medical students, residents, and nurse practitioners. During these supervisory sessions the attending has no direct patient care responsibilities.

The team attendings provide continuous medical care for both acute episodic and long-term illnesses in a manner not unlike that of a private physician. When a PCT's patient requires hospitalization, the primary care physician follows the patient into the hospital wards to assure continuity of care. This integration of inpatient and outpatient care is facilitated by a single medical record for each patient that combines all outpatient, emergency visits, and previous hospitalizations. Each team physician has a 2-month rotation as an inpatient ward attending physician to enhance continuity of medical care and education.

Patient Flow

Patients are registered in a PCT as referred from the emergency medical services, surgical clinics, and inpatient wards, and from self-referrals (Appendix 2). New patients coming to the hospital are seen by a triage nurse outside the Emergency Room (ER) area. Triage is defined as a brief assessment of patients to determine the type and severity of the medical complaint. This triage system, staffed by trained nurses, operates on weekdays, from 8 AM to 3:30 PM. During this time only patients presenting with true emergencies and those patients considered inappropriate for enrollment in a PCT are treated in the ER. Therefore, the ER is better able to take care of patients whose problems constitute significant emergencies. Patients are triaged directly to a specialty clinic only when specifically referred by a physician outside the institution or if the chief complaint obviously requires a specialist (i.e., surgeon, dentist, or obstetrician–gynecologist). Patients without a regular source of care, with nonurgent medical complaints are triaged directly to a PCT. New patients referred to a PCT on their first visit are seen by one of the team providers who then assumes continuing care for the patient in all subsequent visits. Patients registered in a PCT usually are seen in follow-up visits at scheduled appointments. When patients present themselves to their team without an appointment to see the same provider, they are seen by another member of the team. For those patients who miss appointments, team members call the patients or in some situations send a postcard asking them to reschedule the appointment.

The PCT's operate on weekdays from 8:30 AM to 5 PM. After 5 PM weekdays and on weekends, PCT patients are seen in the ER and referred for follow-up care to the original team provider. For PCT pediatric patients, a telephone consultative service is available for their parents or guardians to minimize unnecessary visits to the ER after clinic hours.

Medical Subspecialties

The system of medical subspecialty consultations within the PCTs was designed to ensure continuous and comprehensive patient care by the team provider. Under this system, all patients requiring consultations are seen by the respective subspecialist in the team's area and not in separate subspecialty clinics. All consultations require a complete medical work-up prior to referral. Often the primary care attendings and residents are present to personally present the case to the subspecialist. In this manner, the consultant is able to communicate findings and recommendations directly to the referring resident, attending, or preceptor through discussion, followed by a note in the medical record. Patients requiring more specialized diagnostic services are referred to the MMC subspecialty clinics. All referred patients are given return appointments to the teams at NCBH to ensure follow-up by the team providers.

In summary, this referral system enhances continuity of care and provides essential experience in the management of subspecialty problems and the use of appropriate consultative services.

Special Programs

Special programs are developed by the Department of Ambulatory Medicine to respond to the needs of the community. These needs are identified through several processes: information supplied by the Department of Epidemiology and Social Medicine, observations of outpatients and inpatients, requests from community agencies, and requests from primary care physicians who identify problems in the community. Several illustrations follow.

- A severe epidemic of cocaine addiction occurred in the surrounding population; large numbers of women of childbearing age were using the drug, and many pregnancies were being exposed to cocaine, with potential harm to the mother, fetus, and newborn infant. In 1989, over 400 of the 3600 babies delivered at NCBH were known to have been exposed to cocaine, and possibly at high risk for developmental/behavioral problems, congenital infections such as syphilis and AIDS, and child abuse and neglect. Until a special program started, the vast majority of babies exposed to cocaine born at the hospital did not return there for pediatric care, and were unlikely to be receiving adequate follow-up by providers elsewhere. In addition, these families had other medical and social needs that required attention.

  In May 1989, a group of concerned PCT pediatric attending physicians in the Department of Ambulatory Medicine initiated the Early Family Outreach Program (EFOP). It was designed to direct specific services to families affected by cocaine addiction. The primary focus was to identify cocaine-exposed pregnancies at birth (or in the prenatal period, if possible) and to offer early assessment and follow-up of cocaine using mothers and their children.
- The Adolescent Pregnancy and Teen Mothers program provides prenatal care to adolescents up to 17 years of age and follow-up of adolescent mothers and babies for 2 years after delivery. The number of pregnant adolescent girls who came to the hospital prompted development of a special program for them. In

the course of ten years the program has served 1625 young girls. Over this period there has been a gradual lowering of the average age of the patients from 16 to 14 years. The program provides follow-up care to both adolescent mother and baby after birth, assuring continuity of care to these teen mothers and their babies, as well as helping them to cope with their new responsibilities.

- Other special programs include the Child Protective Services that addresses problems of child abuse and neglect and the telephone consultative service for pediatric patients that reinforces continuity of care, especially after office hours and during weekends for pediatric patients. In addition, certain diseases have occurred with enough frequency to merit routine screening in the PCTs. These include lead poisoning, tuberculosis, and STD. Another program involved setting-up special treatment rooms for asthma management by the PCTs and in the ER.

- The potential benefits of health education, especially in health promotion and disease prevention, prompted establishment of other programs with specific objectives: the Breast-Feeding Advocacy Program addressed the problem of infant nutrition; the HIV counseling program is provided for the growing AIDS-stricken population—mainly IV drug users and their sexual partners, many of whom were women and their offspring; and a Health Education Program for parents and their children under pediatric care in the PCTs required the hiring of a Health Educator. The latter helped to identify high priority health education issues and introduced specific interventions, i.e., accident prevention, promotion of parenting skills, and school outreach activities to provide information for junior and senior high school students in the Bronx on pregnancy, STD, AIDS, etc.

    All of these programs are funded by Federal government, New York State Department of Health, or HHC grants. They were established to provide consultative services to the PCTs as well as to provide comprehensive and continuous care to those patients who need them.

Quality Assurance

Evaluation has long been built into inpatient care through in-hospital committees, accreditation agencies and local, regional, and national governmental supervision. At NCBH it has been built into ambulatory care.

Because so many decisions must be made quickly, Emergency Room medicine is particularly liable to error. The charts and the laboratory data are reviewed daily so that mistakes in patient management can be identified quickly. ER attending physicians from medicine, surgery, and pediatrics, and physician's assistants assigned to the ER review the charts each day, looking for individual and generic errors. Patients are recalled if necessary and the person who has given the inappropriate care counseled by the attending physician doing the audit. This is an excellent teaching and learning experience. All the laboratory data generated each day are reviewed by the physician's assistants. Abnormal results are noted, the charts pulled, and the patients called if necessary, either to the ER or a clinic. The charts of all patients who die within 48 hours of admission to the hospital from the ER are audited each month.

A pediatric protocol project was established in 1984 at NCBH to monitor the quality of care delivered in the pediatric ambulatory component. It is a computer-assisted quality assurance system that uses protocol guidelines and data from structured patient charts to produce regular reports that expand the pediatricians' ability to monitor care. The protocol guidelines describe standard management for common acute-care problems of children seen in the Emergency Room and related clinics (Brezenoff and Farrell 1984).

Research

To determine the impact of the reorganization of the ambulatory care services numerous studies have been undertaken. One project analyzed the results of the reorganization of ambulatory services in terms of reductions in the admission rates for selected diseases in the 18-month period before and after the reorganization (San Agustin et al. 1976). Another study reported on the impact of the triage system on the utilization of the ER by new patients and registrants with nonurgent medical complaints and without known regular sources of care (San Agustin et al. 1984). A third investigation examined the effect of the Pediatric Protocol System as a quality assurance instrument focusing on the short- and long-term health outcomes of asthma (Fund for the City of New York 1990).

These studies document the favorable impact of the new health care arrangements in the Department of Ambulatory Medicine. There was a statistically significant decrease in admission rates for the selected diseases studied i.e., diabetic coma-acidosis, severe hypertension, congestive heart failure, cerebrovascular accidents, and severe asthma. The triage study demonstrated that patients with no regular source of care who arrived with nonurgent medical problems, especially in the pediatric group, could be referred directly to a PCT at their initial visit rather than having to be seen in the ER. It also showed that the earlier a patient was assigned to a specific primary care provider, the better the compliance in keeping follow-up appointments. Thus, the triage system made it possible for patients with no regular source of care to be registered at their first encounter and assigned to a single identifiable practitioner within a PCT at NCBH. In addition, it was observed that during triage hours more pediatric patients had their first encounters in a PCT whereas for adult patients the ER was more often the site of first encounter. This finding reinforced the move for extending PCT services into the evening hours and weekends.

Specific programs also looked into the characteristics of their defined populations to find solutions for recurring problems. It is important in programs dealing with adolescent pregnancy to identify the risk factors leading to unplanned pregnancies. A pilot study conducted by the Adolescent Pregnancy Program at NCBH explored various aspects of the life experiences of an adolescent that could be contributing factors to an unwanted pregnancy (Quijano et al. 1985). Data included biopsychosocial and educational aspects. The findings of the pilot study pointed to scholastic difficulties and academic failures as a significant risk factor. Results of this study led to a second investigation that reexamined the role of the family. Specifically, it focused on the teenager's perceptions on parental bonding, and whether a particular pattern might impair their psychological and social development, thereby placing them at risk for later psychosocial problems including precocious pregnancy (Cobliner et al. 1989). The results showed that a particular pattern of parental bonding or style, where there is care but inadequate protection, might place the teen at risk. As the Adolescent Pregnancy Program expanded, it included health services for nonpregnant sexually active teenagers. Linkages also were established with various educational, vocational, and employment agencies in the community. A "Peer Outreach Program" was instituted to provide ongoing medical evaluation in a school and to attempt to overcome some of the barriers to obtaining health care by using peer involvement and influence (Demeny et al. 1985).

IV. Medical Education

Postgraduate Medical Education

In the United States, government and private foundations have financed the establishment of primary care residency programs through medical schools and teaching hospitals. In 1979, funding was approved by the United States Department of Health and Human Services for the Primary Care Residencies in General Internal Medicine and in General Pediatrics at MMC-NCBH. These training programs are administered by the Department of Ambulatory Medicine in collaboration with the Departments of Medicine and Pediatrics. The PCT model in the Department of Ambulatory Medicine serves as the major ambulatory training site for the residents. First-year residents are assigned to a specific PCT where they remain as integral members during their 3 years of training.

The residents are able to provide continuing longitudinal care for a large group of patients. They provide preventive care as well as care for patients with a variety of chronic illnesses and for those with emotional, behavioral, and developmental problems. Each resident acquires a panel of patients for continuing follow-up care by drawing on the inpatient, nursery, or emergency medical services. During their ambulatory care rotation the residents spend 50 to 60% of their time with a PCT. In addition, they devote one 4-hour session a week to their PCT during the rest of the year while assigned to the inpatient rotation, the nursery, and specialty electives. Many procedures have been established to ensure continuity of patient care during the 3 years of their training. Schedules at all sites are produced 3 months in advance. Each session has an assigned preceptor to maintain continuity in teaching. The continuity clinics and appointment system are so organized that the resident can take appointments from ward discharges and Emergency Room patients. In addition, residents on cross-site rotations are able to continue to see ward or Emergency Room patients at their continuity clinics. Residents are assigned families, as well as individual patients.

The educational goals of the ambulatory medicine training are achieved through continuity experience in medicine, a carefully defined subspecialty curriculum, innovations in ambulatory rounds (Paccione et al. 1989), and the creation of a series of interactive seminars emphasizing contributions from the residents and integration of epidemiologic principles with clinical medicine.

Curricular Goals

The curriculum for the primary care residency program includes the following goals:

- Clinical: To provide clinical training in ambulatory medicine and pediatrics with the same rigor and vitality experienced in the inpatient setting, to focus this training on practical patient care issues, not restricted by didactic lecturing, to involve the resident as much as possible in the educational process, to broaden residency training beyond general pediatrics and general internal medicine in preparation for possible careers in other areas such as gynecology, ENT, ophthalmology, etc.
- Psychosocial: To produce physicians who are knowledgeable, motivated, and skillful in the recognition and management of the psychosocial dimensions of pediatrics and internal medicine, and skilled in medical interviewing, and in the major diagnostic and therapeutic interventions of office-based practice.
- Clinical Epidemiology: To enable the physician to develop special expertise in the principles of clinical epidemiology, decision-analysis, and biostatistics in order to assess the medical literature intelligently and apply findings to patient care, ask challenging clinical questions and design feasible research protocols to answer them, and use decision-making principles in clinical practice.
- Community: To enable the physician to integrate the principles of community-oriented care with clinical practice, work comfortably with community and home health care resources, become familiar with different systems of health care, and be aware of the major issues in health policy affecting our society and our profession.
- Law and Ethics: To enable the physician to acquire a foundation in health law and work through and develop an awareness of the ethical issues in modern medicine. The primary focus of the program is an examination of both the law as it relates to the provision of health care and the moral and ethical concerns that transcend discussion of case law and regulatory stat-

utes. The overall objectives of this program are to sensitize residents to a range of troubling issues and provide them with the background and critical analytic skills necessary to resolve such issues.

- Quality Assessment and Cost Containment: To provide training and experience in quality assessment and promote cost-consciousness and the critical use of diagnostic tests as a major theme in appropriate ambulatory practice.

Curricular Activities and Evaluation

Activities for the acquisition of population-based skills are integrated into the total ambulatory care rotation of the residents. These include didactic seminars, community site visits, home visits, and involvement in a research project.

The didactic seminars are conducted at different points during the 3 years of training. Topics deal with communication and interviewing skills, clinical epidemiology, and community-oriented primary care. Particular attention is given to the Bronx community and its resources. Part of the curriculum involves visits to various health care facilities in the Bronx, such as alcohol treatment programs, methadone maintenance programs, home health agencies and visiting nurse services, the Ritter–Scheuer Hospice, homeless shelters, community health centers, and a nursing home (Home for the Aged). The purpose of these visits is to provide residents with "first hand" experiences of the resources in the community from which their patients come. The program is also designed to demonstrate the practical importance of employing a comprehensive approach to the medical, psychological, and socioeconomic factors in their patients' illnesses and the benefits of coordinating a multidisciplinary teams in the provision of health care in the community. Each visit is preceded by required readings and discussion of didactic material covering the medical problems and treatment settings to be encountered. It is then followed by a discussion of the primary care residents' own patients and possible approaches to more effective utilization of community resources in their management.

This experience is further broadened by the Home Visit Program for second year residents. The latter perform home visits at least once a month with their own patients for whom they consider such a home visit would be clinically useful. Among the reasons are treatment compliance and the existence of psychosocial problems requiring closer assessment etc. Evaluation of residents includes videotaping and direct observance of patient interviews, as well as review of clinical encounter forms. The latter strategy is used to determine whether the residents successfully delegate assessment and patient management plans that include such critical aspects of the population's living environment as housing, employment, economic status, community structure, social support arrangements, as well as formal and informal community resources.

The principles of clinical epidemiology and decision-analysis permeate the entire curriculum. They are introduced in a structured series of seminars during "protected" elective time at the end of the residents' first year, at the beginning of the second year, and integrated with the residents' clinical experience throughout their ambulatory care rotation. Aside from lectures, other activities include journal clubs, diagnostic test rounds, resident-conducted seminars, and research.

Residents are encouraged to pursue a research project during their training. In this they are guided by a PCT preceptor and allotted "project time" during their ambulatory care rotation months. Projects undertaken by the residents reflect issues they frequently encounter during training. Examples include precipitants of asthmatic attacks, patient follow-up intervals, HIV counseling practices, and "Do Not Resuscitate" issues. These research projects are supported in part through the primary care residency grant.

Undergraduate Education

Medical students from AECOM are assigned to its various clinical departments, other than the Department of Ambulatory Medicine, in the school's affiliated teaching hospitals for their clinical rotations, most of which have a traditional inpatient orientation. The exception is a required 2-month clerkship in Ambulatory Medicine in the fourth year of medical school introduced at AECOM in the 1970s. Some of the third-year clerkships such as pediatrics and obstetrics–gynecology also include a small percentage of outpatient time. The internal medicine clerkship for third-year AECOM students, until recently, had been exclusively inpatient-based. Some Department of Ambulatory Medicine faculty with long-standing involvement in the Department of Medicine's inpatient and outpatient teaching activities worked closely with the Associate Deans for Educational Affairs and for Student and Graduate Medical Education to develop and evaluate a well-structured, supervised ambulatory care component for the third-year internal medicine clerkship. As a result, the outpatient components of the third-year medicine clerkship at all AECOM teaching hospitals now consists of a half-day every other week for each student. A faculty position is supported by AECOM to provide for observation of students' history-taking and physical examination skills in caring for ambulatory patients, to supply feedback to students while working with them on mastering diagnostic and clinical management skills in the PCTs.

The 2-month ambulatory care block in the fourth year exposes students to office-based primary care practice in a variety of AECOM affiliated sites including the PCTs at NCBH. Also included are rotations in several ambulatory subspecialty clinics and a didactic core curriculum in ambulatory medicine. At NCBH fourth-year students spend the 2-month rotation in a PCT, 4 or 5 half-day sessions each week, working in the role of junior physicians with close faculty supervision. The students acquire patients from clinic "walk-ins" or referrals from sites that do not have primary care services. A triage nurse first screens these patients to determine whether they are suitable for evaluation by a student. The students then assume the role of primary care physician, elicit a history, do a physical examination, and present the patient to the supervising attending physician. A joint "bedside" consultation follows, and finally a discussion in which problems, diagnoses, and management plans are clarified. Whenever follow-up is indicated, the patient becomes part of the student's "panel" of patients, and is normally presented to the same faculty supervisor on each return visit. At the end of the rotation such patients are cared for by the attending physician who has supervised their care to that point. The students are thus given experience in

- Evaluation and management of common problems in a primary care setting;
- The importance of continuous care;
- The principles of health maintenance; and
- Approaches to team management.

Most students respond positively, with frequent comments reflecting their appreciation of the combination of clinical responsibility and close supervision they are given. Many students indicate that this is their only medical school experience of such positive, close interactions with clinical faculty. Although this intensive 2-month block in the fourth year offers some opportunity to experience continuity of care first-hand, it occurs too late in the medical school curriculum to affect most students' career choices. The PCT staff of the Department of Ambulatory Medicine is working to develop a longitudinal ambulatory care experience from the first year onward for all AECOM medical students.

V. Financing

Prior to the reorganization of the outpatient clinics at Morrisania City Hospital, each clinical department (internal medicine, pediatrics, psychiatry, surgery, and obstetrics–gynecology) was responsible for both inpatient and outpatient services. The budget for each clinical department reflected both components. When the separate Department of Ambulatory Medicine was established the affiliation administration of NCBH, supported by the President of MMC, segregated the outpatient component of each clinical department's total budget to make up the Department of Ambulatory Medicine's budget. However, additional money was required to develop the Department's new primary health care system and the HHC as well as MMC committed the necessary funds. The Department of Ambulatory Medicine's budget supported several residency positions in the Emergency Medical Services and the PCTs. In addition, Federally funded Primary Care Residency Training grants provided other residents' salaries as well as several faculty positions and other educational costs.

In its 16 years existence, the Department has been able to elicit additional support for its clinical care, teaching, and research activities through government and foundation grants. This has made possible the continuing expansion of its programs.

VI. The Role of the Medical School

Over the years the Department of Ambulatory Medicine's struggles at North Central Bronx Hospital in the light of its philosophy and goals has had successes and failures. Many of the latter resulted from the absence of substantial commitment or interest on the part of the medical school and its collective faculty. On the other hand, the Albert Einstein College of Medicine was a relatively new school, struggling for peer recognition and financial viability. It was forced to make difficult choices in determining priorities and programs. The faculty elected to emphasize the basic sciences and biomedical research and to use traditional tertiary care hospital settings for teaching. A medical school whose fundamental philosophy was grounded in community and population-based medicine would have offered a much more supportive educational environment. When the Department of Ambulatory Medicine was established the medical school provided no tangible support. On the other hand, it did not place obstacles in the path of the Department's creation or growth. As long as the chairmen of the clinical departments agreed, the medical school continued to accept its existence as an integral part of the departments of internal medicine, pediatrics, surgery, psychiatry, and obstetrics–gynecology. Later, the medical school established programs that incorporated rotations for third- and fourth-year students in the Department of Ambulatory Medicine, modified the standard curriculum to include an introductory course on Community Medicine, and supported the faculty position for a part-time primary care internist in the Department of Ambulatory Medicine to teach ambulatory medicine. Such actions were helpful but many of the educational weaknesses in the Department of Ambulatory Medicine result from the absence of much stronger support from the medical school:

- The Department of Ambulatory Medicine is an integral part of the structure of NCBH incorporated in the constitution and by-laws of the Medical Board of the hospital as a separately established clinical department.

  The Department of Ambulatory Medicine, however, is *not* part of the formal structure of the AECOM.
- The Department of Ambulatory Medicine has a separate budget and a full-time Director with equal power, rank, and salary with other directors of the clinical departments at NCBH.

  The Director of the Department of Ambulatory Medicine, however, does not have equality of power, rank, and salary where those are dependent on recognition by the medical school.

- The faculty members of the Department of Ambulatory Medicine undertake inpatient teaching rounds at North Central Bronx and Montefiore Hospitals.

  The attending primary care physicians have not, however, received promotions in the medical school commensurate with their experiences and achievements. A further indicator of the medical school's priorities is the overt discrimination experienced by the Department of Family Medicine at Montefiore Medical Center. Not one of its attending physicians has been given a faculty appointment.

- The Department of Ambulatory Medicine has been the site for active, long-term residency training programs approved and funded by the U.S. Federal government.

  The medical school, however, has not directly recognized the Department of Ambulatory Medicine as a site for teaching undergraduates primary care medicine. A well-organized primary care practice site in a hospital-based Ambulatory Care Department, not unlike an inpatient setting, is an ideal site for teaching medical students and residents.

  If community-based settings such as private practices and/or community-based health centers and other clinics are available, both medical students and residents can be placed in such facilities. However, appropriate linkages still need to be established between these entities and the Department of Ambulatory Medicine with its base in a teaching institution providing secondary and tertiary services. In addition, faculty appointments should be provided for physicians teaching in these ambulatory settings.

- The population to be served by the Department of Ambulatory Medicine, in effect, was "defined" by the Health and Hospitals Corporation when it decided where to build NCBH. MMC played an active role in this decision by donating the land on which the hospital was built. Some community groups opposed the site. The medical school was uninvolved.

  For many years, the medical school's Department of Epidemiology and Social Medicine has studied the community and pinpointed a wide variety of problems. On the other hand, the medical school's faculty has *not* accepted any collective responsibility for them.

- From its inception, a strong factor in the Department's success and reputation has been its clinical leadership.

  In general, however, most departments of ambulatory care are treated as purely administrative entities, directed by administrators without clinical credentials, and judged for accreditation purely on administrative efficiency. As a consequence they lack academic status and respect.

- Increasing superspecialization in medicine, abolition, in the United States, of the general internship, and early specialized residency training immediately after graduation from medical school, make the Department of Ambulatory Medicine an essential site for training in general internal medicine and general pediatrics where young physicians encounter a case-mix of unselected patients with general medical and related problems.

VII. Conclusion

The Department of Ambulatory Medicine at North Central Bronx Hospital has never been a free-standing, self-sustaining entity. In the complex world of modern medical care, probably no enterprise of any size or significance can or should aspire to complete autonomy. From its inception, the Department has depended for its existence, survival, and progress on the support of the City, State, and Federal governments and of the Montefiore Medical Center and the Albert Einstein College of Medicine. The weakest link has always been the medical school. This was probably inevitable, not because of the special characteristics of a particular medical school but because of the generic nature of American medical schools as they have developed in the twentieth century. Whether privately or publicly sponsored, whether funded by taxes or philanthropy, medical schools emphasize the basic sciences and biomedical research in curriculum development and related endeavors. They emphasize the training of research scientists, clinical specialists, and subspecialists. They respond to the imperatives of the scientific research community, not to the problems that afflict the people who live in the communities where the schools are physically located.

Medical schools have become increasingly dependent on governmental funding, whether from research and training grants or payments for patient care, at the same time governments have allowed the medical schools to set their own agendas. Many legislators are aware of the need to shift priorities, including the role to be played by population-based education and research, but until governments are prepared to use their financial power to require medical schools to place much greater emphasis on the population's perceived health care needs, little is likely to change.

From its inception the Department of Ambulatory Medicine has been supported by the New York City government to provide more primary care for the City's poor, by the U.S. Federal government to train more primary care physicians, and by the New York State government to change the priorities and content of physicians' training within that State (Appendix 3).

In large United States' cities, for complex historical reasons, hospitals provide most of the ambulatory care received by the poor whether they have Medicaid or do not have health insurance. Where community-based clinics exists, they function most effectively when linked to a teaching hospital. At the same time, the training received by most physicians provides little in the way of population-based perspective or skills. The reorganization or creation of Departments of Ambulatory Medicine along the lines of that established at the North Central Bronx Hospital could provide suitable sites for teaching population-based medicine. Active and positive commitment by medical school faculties is essential for such training programs to achieve their full potential.

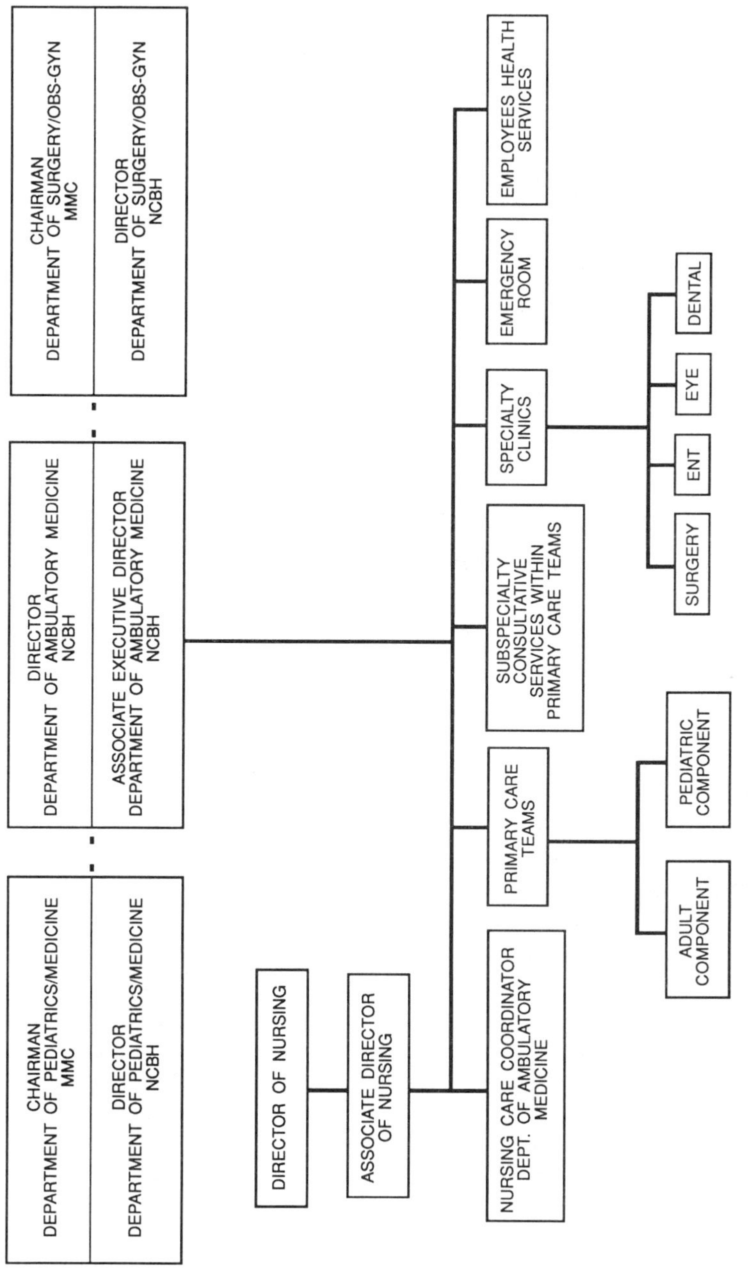

FIGURE 5.1. Table of organization: Department of Ambulatory Medicine North Central Bronx Hospital.

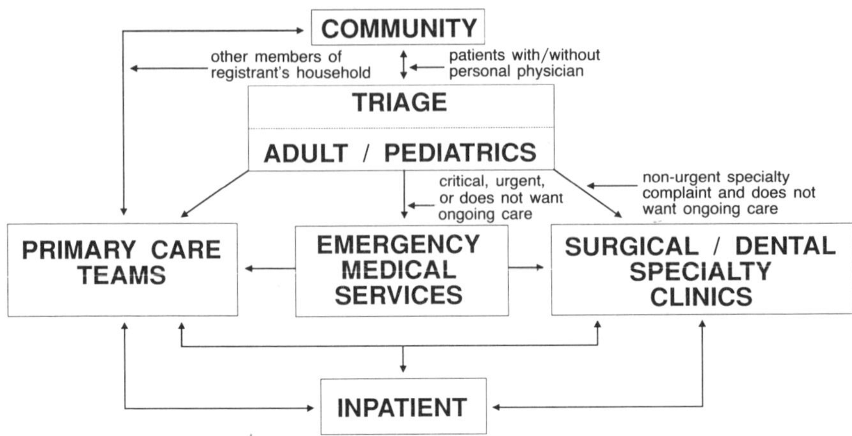

FIGURE 5.2. Patient flow chart—Department of Ambulatory Medicine North Central Bronx Hospital.

Appendix 3: New York State Department of Health Initiative for Graduate Medical Education

New York State established a Commission of Graduate Medical Education that, in early 1986, promulgated strong recommendations bearing on the future training of physicians in that State. It pointed out that New York State, with 7.8% of the population of the United States and 11.2% of the medical school graduates, housed 14.7% of the residency programs in the country. These figures indicated that the State was training almost twice as many physicians as were needed to serve the people of the State, a significant expenditure of expensive resources. When these residency programs were looked at in terms of specialties and subspecialties the figures were even more startling. While New York State produced only 5.4% of the physicians trained in family medicine, it produced 26% of the experts in nuclear medicine, 17.2% of all the surgeons, 17% of the neurologists, and so on through a long list of specialties that constituted a majority of the residency programs concentrated in New York City. The Commission made several recommendations, the most controversial being those which advocated an overall gradual cut of 30% in the number of residency programs in the State and the direction of a majority of the approved programs toward primary care training.

The New York State Council on Graduate Medical Education subsequently concluded that effective administration of graduate medical education required collaborative relationships among a medical school, its affiliated hospitals, and other teaching sites. The Council set forth a list of criteria that such a "consortium" should meet to fulfill the basic goal of increased primary care training and service. To facilitate the formation of graduate medical education consortia, the Council recommended that demonstration projects be developed to test their feasibility and to explore alternative financing mechanisms in collaboration with the New York State Department of Health (New York State Council on Graduate Medical Education 1988).

Acknowledgments. In the development of this chapter, the author gratefully acknowledges the assistance of Dorothy Levenson and Bernadette Madrid, and the staff of the Department of Ambulatory Medicine at NCBH.

References

Abbott, L. 1989. Medical student education in ambulatory care. *Acad Med* **64**:S9–S15.

Alpert, J.J., and Charney, E. 1973. *The Education of Physicians for Primary Care.* U.S. Dept. of Health, Education and Welfare. DHEW Pub. No. (HRA) 74–3113.

Arneill, B.P., and Nuelsen, P.H. 1978. Functional components of the ambulatory care facility. *J Ambul Care Manage* **1**:23–40.

Barnett, P.G., and Midtling, J.E. 1989. Public policy and the supply of primary care physicians. *J Am Med Assoc* **262**:2864–2868.

Brezenoff, S., and Farrell, G. 1984. The Pediatric Protocol System: Improving the quality of outpatient health care. *Public Papers of the Fund for the City of New York* **3**:1–8.

Cobliner, W.G., Quijano, E., and San Agustin, M. 1989. Family dynamics: An important risk factor in teenage pregnancies. Paper presented at the 19th International Congress of Pediatrics, July 28, Paris.

Daley, J., Gertman, P.M., and Delbanco, T.L. 1988. Looking for quality in primary care physicians. *Health Affairs* **7**:107–113.

Dasco, C.C. 1989. Factors influencing ambulatory care education in the U.S. Department of Veterans Affairs. *Acad Med* **64**:S4–S8.

Demeny, D., San Agustin, M., Quijano, E., Davis, A., and Maclin, G. 1985. *J Adolescent Health Care* **6**:206–210.

Dickman, R.L., and Milligan, S. 1987. An end to patchwork reform of health care. *N Engl J Med* **317**:1086–1088.

Ebert, R.H. 1985. The medical school revisited. *Health Affairs* **4**:47–59.

Feltovich, J., Terrill, A.M., and Soler, N.G. 1989. Teaching medical students in ambulatory settings in Departments of Internal Medicine. *Acad Med* **64**:36–41.

Ginzberg, E. 1985. Academic health centers: A troubled future. *Health Affairs* **4**:5–21.

Ginzberg, E. 1986. *From Health Dollars to Health Services.* New Jersey: Rowman & Allanheld.

Girard, D.E., Elliot, D.L., Linz, D.H., and Cooney, T.G. 1984. The general medicine clinic: Making the ugly duckling fly. *Arch Intern Med* **144**:2217–2219.

Greer, D.S. 1990. Faculty rewards for the generalist clinician teacher. *J Gen Int Med* **5**:S53–S58.

Kroenke, K. 1986. Ambulatory care: Practice imperfect. *Am J Med* **80**:339–342.

Levenson, D. 1984. *Montefiore: The Hospital as Social Instrument*. New York: Farrar, Strauss & Giroux.

Nardone, D.A., and Webb, D.W. 1989. Administration in ambulatory care. *Acad Med* **64**:S28–S34.

Navarro, V. 1989. Why some countries have national health insurance, others have national services, and the United States has neither. *Int J Health Serv* **19**:383–404.

New York City Department of Health. 1987. *Vital Statistics by Health Areas and Health Center Districts*. Bureau of Health Statistics and Analysis. New York.

New York City Health & Hospitals Corporation. 1984. *Annual Report*. New York.

New York State Commission on Graduate Medical Education. 1986. *Report of the New York State Commission on Graduate Medical Education*. New York.

New York State Council on Graduate Medical Education. 1988. *First Annual Report*. New York.

North Central Bronx Hospital. 1989. *Annual Report of the Department of Ambulatory Medicine*. New York.

Nutting, P.A. 1986. Community-oriented primary care: An integrated model for practice, research and education. *Am J Prevent Med* **2**:140–147.

Paccione, G.A., Cohen, E., and Schwartz, C.E. 1989. From forms to focus: A new teaching model in Ambulatory Medicine. *Arch Intern Med* **149**:2407–2411.

Perkoff, G.T. 1986. Teaching clinical medicine in the ambulatory setting: An idea whose time may have finally come. *N Engl J Med* **314**:27–31.

Petersdorf, R.G. 1975. Issues in primary care: The academic perspective. *J Med Educ* **50** (Part 2):5–13.

Quijano, E.C., Cobliner, W.G., San Agustin, M., and Joseph, M. 1985. Life experience of the teenager and its role in unwanted pregnancy. Paper presented at the American Public Health Association Annual Meeting, November 17–21, Washington, D.C.

Reagan, M.D. 1987. Physicians as gatekeepers: A complex challenge. *N Engl J Med* **317**:1731–1734.

Roemer, M.I. 1981. *Ambulatory services in America: Past, Present and Future*. Rockville, Maryland: Aspen Systems Corporation.

Rogers, D.E. 1982. Community-oriented primary care. *J Am Med Assoc* **248**:1622–1625.

Rogers, D.E., and Gastel, N. (Eds.). 1988. *Clinical Education and the Doctor of Tomorrow*. New York: The New York Academy of Medicine.

Rosenblatt, R.A. 1988. Current successes in medical education beyond the bedside. *J Gen Intern Med* **3**:S44–S61.

San Agustin, M., Goldfrank, L., Matz, R., Suberman, C., Hamerman, D., Bloom, R., and Pitter, D. 1976. Reorganization of ambulatory health care in an urban municipal hospital. *Arch Intern Med* **136**:1262–1266.

San Agustin, M. 1978. Primary care in a tertiary care center. *Ann NY Acad Sci* **310**:121-128.

San Agustin, M., Madhaven, S., and Fassig, J. 1984. *The Role of Triage in Emergency Room and Primary Care Practice within a Hospital Based Ambulatory Care Setting*. North Central Bronx Hospital, Department of Ambulatory Medicine.

Schroeder, S.A. 1984. Western European responses to physician oversupply: Lessons for the United States. *J Am Med Assoc* **252**:373–384.

Schroeder, S.A., Zones, J.S., and Showstack, J.A. 1989. Academic medicine as a public trust. *J Am Med Assoc* **262:**803–812.

Seidel, H.M. 1975. Organization of model systems for primary care practice and education: Problems and issues. *J Med Educ* **50:**23–28.

Singer, A.M. 1989. Projections of physician supply and demand: A summary of HRSA and AMA studies. *Acad Med* **64:**235–239.

Skeff, K.M. 1988. Enhancing teaching effectiveness and vitality in the ambulatory setting. *J Gen Intern Med* **3:**S26–S33.

Smith, C.T. 1985. Health care delivery system changes: A special challenge for teaching hospitals. *J Med Educ* **60:**1–8.

Starfield, B., and Pless, B. 1973. Research in ambulatory pediatrics. In: *Advances in Pediatrics*, Schulman, I. (Ed.), Vol. 20, Chicago: Yearbook Medical Publishers.

Starfield, B. 1986. Primary care in the United States. *Intern J Health Serv* **16:**179–198.

Swanson, A.G. 1984. Medical education in the United States and Canada. *J Med Educ* **59:**35–56.

Tarlov, A.R. 1983. The increasing supply of physicians, the changing structure of the health services system, and the future practice of medicine. *N Engl J Med* **308:**1235–1244.

Tarlov, A.R. 1988. The rising supply of physicians and the pursuit of better health. *J Med Educ* **63:**94–107.

Taylor, C.M., Kornblatt, J.E., and Kindig, D.A. 1984. Lessons learned from the urban health network program. *J Ambul Care Manage* **7:**12–24.

United Hospital Fund of New York. 1988. *New York City Community Health Atlas.* New York.

Wooliscroft, J.O., and Schwenk, T.L. 1989. Teaching and learning in the ambulatory setting. *Acad Med* **64:**644–648.

Discussion

Sir David Innes Williams

The author reports the establishment within a district general hospital of a Department of Ambulatory Medicine that provides primary care for an indigent, ethnically mixed population where there is a high incidence of drug abuse, homelessness, teenage pregnancy, and sexually transmitted disease. Given its particular remit it has evidently been a successful development and has provided the basis for a popular residency program, but the author believes that it has been undervalued by the Medical School, with inadequate exposure of undergraduates to its service and little influence by its staff on educational policy; the result, the author believes, of an orientation of the Albert Einstein College of Medicine towards basic science and specialization at the expense of commitment to the local community.

The author poses the following questions for discussion:

- Is a hospital-based Department of Ambulatory Medicine the best model for primary health care of an indigent population and therefore a proper vehicle by which the Medical School can demonstrate its concern for the community?

Such a system is at variance with mainstream thinking in Britain, where within the National Health Service primary care is the business of independent general practitioners working from their own premises and undertaking home visiting as *required*. There is no doubt, however, that the British system has not been entirely successful in the inner city context where there is a smaller proportion of settled families and more homeless immigrant and transient inhabitants. Recruitment of dedicated general practitioners in these areas has been difficult and their premises are often deplorable and heavy use is made of the local casualty department (Emergency Room). In these circumstances a centrally located whole-time salaried General Practitioner service has been suggested as a possibility, so far rejected, but if the Bronx system is demonstrably effective it might be considered further.

- Is a Department of Ambulatory Medicine the best place for education in primary care?

  The concentration of services in good and spacious accommodation immediately adjacent to the Medical School campus, allowing ready collaboration with specialist clinical units and such academic departments as epidemiology, has enormous advantages for teaching which cannot be matched by the dispersed and often unsatisfactory premises of independent family practitioners. It has further advantages for the students over Emergency Room experience since it can provide continuity of care in both acute and chronic illness. However, although its contribution is valuable, it can scarcely be sufficient: primary care (general practice or family medicine) requires a greater involvement in home and family circumstances than is possible from the ambulatory medicine department and an almost exclusive concern with the indigent cannot prepare the student for practice in less deprived, more "normal" communities. This raises a general point about the Medical School's commitment to the local community: it must not become exclusive of wider horizons. Education in scientific medicine should produce doctors who can adapt to a range of practice circumstances and therefore promote free interchange between different countries. Too great a concern with the local community only could, in developing countries, turn out doctors unable to take up posts in the more advanced health care systems. It will be necessary to strike a balance between local concern and broader education.

- Given the need in the United States for a greater proportion of primary care physicians, should undergraduate experience of this discipline be given earlier and more prolonged curriculum time?

  Sufficient exposure to enable the student to make an informed career choice is obviously essential, but the objective of producing at graduation the "undifferentiated physician" is an ideal that should not be abandoned. On this basis specialist training can be built and for this purpose primary care medicine is as much a specialty as hospital-based disciplines.

- Given the importance in primary care of teamwork involving nonmedical staff, should a part of the undergraduate course be undertaken concurrently with the education of nurses, midwives, psychologists, pharmacists, and the like?

    That suggestion is usually made by those who would downgrade the status of the physician and should not be taken up by medical schools. Very few teams work without a captain, and the doctor's training should equip him to understand the role of the other professions and to adopt a leadership position.

- How should the teachers of primary care, whose role in medical education is undisputed, attain the power and status now attached to staff in basic science and hospital specialist disciplines?

    The obvious answer is by research output, and in the field of primary care research it may best be combined with some other discipline such as epidemiology. In default of research excellence, we must descend from matters of principle to the level of guile and expediency. The existing hierarchy will not be easily shifted, but experience has shown in hospitals and colleges that less prestigious subjects can raise their status by the initiatives of individual leaders who may be assiduous committee men and women prepared to take on management chores that may be despised by the high flyers but ultimately lead to power and influence, who may be charismatic teachers who gain such respect from students that they cannot ultimately be ignored by the establishment or who act as guide and counselor to staff and student alike, thereby gaining knowledge that can, even without breach of confidence, be put to good effect.

Arthur Kaufman

The author presents a comprehensive review of how a public, community hospital in the Bronx established an integrated, community-oriented health service that has become an important training model for primary care residents and senior medical students. There are many appealing features in the North Central Bronx Hospital (NCBH) program. It offers a training center model that lends itself to a population-oriented approach due to both its location within and its mandate to serve a defined geographic population. This approach is difficult to emulate in a university teaching hospital, with its large and, at times, ill-defined catchment area. There, learners are drawn more readily to the complexity of the inpatient's illness, reinforced by the high technology and subspecialist role models, than to the equally complex sources of illness in the surrounding communities. Thus the NCBH can more easily provide its learners with community and population-oriented role modeling precisely because it is removed from its research-oriented, mother institution.

It is also important that NCBH's innovations in medical education are intimately linked to innovations in the provision of health services. This coupling exposes learners to a viable model for future community-oriented practice. Such a model is lacking at most innovative, community-oriented, medical schools around the world. There, faculty energy has focused inwardly on that which it can more easily control—its own curriculum. Unfortunately, graduates of these institutions find a practice environment that is inhospitable to the unique skills and orientation gained in their training programs.

There are some areas of the NCBH program that should be strengthened to more effectively address population health. For example, high quality ambulatory care offered within the medical center, so thoroughly detailed by the author, is unlikely, by itself, to have a major impact on the community's health. That health status is more reflective of the population's economic and social circumstances, its habits and life-styles. Thus, outreach programs into the community, such as that cited for teen pregnancy reduction, come closer to having a wider health impact. Such community-based activities occur but appear not to dominate the learning experience of the residents or the students affiliated with NCBH. Nor are skills needed for working effectively with the community to improve its own health likely to be learned within the medical center, even one as progressive as NCBH.

There is an emotional undertone running throughout which I found moving. It is a mixture of pride and resentment. On the one hand, there is pride in having forged such a comprehensive, integrated model of community-oriented care, under considerable financial and bureaucratic constraints. On the other hand, there is resentment in being somewhat marginalized within the power structure of the Medical School. This is a familiar struggle for all of us pushing for greater public accountability by our biomedical, research-oriented institutions. We lament that the health of the surrounding communities that "feed" the medical school's training programs seems such an afterthought in institutional planning. Far more should be made of this issue. The most creative, population-oriented program models are occurring outside their institutions, in the community. They are developing precisely because they are in the community and at the fringe of their established, conservative, academic centers. Thus, a more difficult struggle must now occur to foster comparable, population-oriented change within the traditional academic center itself. The guerilla movement in the mountains must descend and confront the conventional army in the city if the revolution is to be won. While the role of the medical school occupies relatively little room in this account, I think it is the most important question medical schools must now address. The struggle for a primary focus on population health within our traditional medical schools will require, I believe, two strategies hinted at by the author.

Institutional change in the short run is most likely to be driven by either lust or fear—a "lust" for alternative revenues or a "fear" of losing accreditation should a population orientation not be a centerpiece of academic educational and service efforts. The overpowering influence of current government support for biomedical research and of conservative medical school and residency accreditation policies can only be counteracted by alternative governmental funding priorities and by enlightened accreditation policies. Population-oriented interest groups must therefore educate and collaborate with community forces, local, state, and national legislators, and with medical school and residency accrediting bodies to create a favorable climate for change.

Progressive academic forces must also couple their short-term strategies with the more durable, long-term reward of graduating students and residents who are change agents for a population orientation in their academic centers and in their future practice communities. To do so, graduates must be equipped with appropriate experiences and political skills in their training programs. Students and residents must, therefore, be encouraged to become partners in the reformation of their medical schools and teaching hospitals, helping shift their learning venues from the classroom and hospital into the community where the population lives.

Mamoru Watanabe

The author describes what appears to be a very well-conceived, desirable, and successfully integrated program for the training of primary care physicians, and a system for providing primary care, responsive to the health care needs of that community and population, to the poor people of New York (Bronx). The major conclusion appears to be that the medical school (Albert Einstein College of Medicine) has provided the weakest link and this reflects the generic problem of Western medical schools that traditionally have emphasized basic science and biomedical research accomplishments. While there may be some validity to this observation, it would be useful to have a response from the medical school (AECOM) to know what the constraints are that prevent or preclude greater support for not only this Department of Ambulatory Medicine, but for the concept of medical education in the ambulatory setting, or for a population-based, socially responsive educational curriculum. This response might allow us to find some common grounds for dialogue and offer solutions that would lead to a greater participation of medical schools in these ventures.

As the Dean of a Canadian medical school in Calgary, where the health care system is different, and where the community we serve and its health care needs and issues are not totally analogous, at least in magnitude, it would be foolhardy for me to offer a defense on behalf of medical schools in the United States, but some of the questions that come to mind are the stated mission and philosophy of the medical school and its University, its history and evolution, its role and success in shaping health care policies, affiliation with other institutions or programs, such as the Department of Family Medicine, the administrative structure, and the constraints of the funding system. If medical schools in the past have been, in fact, unresponsive to community needs, is there an evolving climate and a mood that favors change?

The NCBH program has now been in place for 16 years and, while there are useful evaluations of the program itself, it would be helpful to know what graduates of this program are doing and where they are located. Do they remain in the Bronx, go to equivalent large urban centers with similar health care issues, remain in primary care, or enter career streams that require different educational experiences? Does exposure to this program alter the behavior of these physicians and has their competence been evaluated over a longitudinal period?

Prior to the creation of the Department of Ambulatory Medicine, the individual Departments were responsible for both inpatient and outpatient services. Have the problems of that administrative structure, which presumably necessitated the change, disappeared? Would a return to the previous administrative structure lead to greater support from the medical school? What is the relationship, if any, between the Departments of Ambulatory Medicine and Family Medicine?

In Alberta and Canada, physicians are almost equally distributed between family or general practitioners and specialists, so there is no shortage of primary care physicians. With the introduction of a universal medicare system, clinics catering to the indigent population have either never existed or have essentially disappeared from teaching hospitals. The bulk of primary care is, therefore, delivered by family physicians in private office settings. On the other hand, teaching hospitals, constrained by budgets and pressures to be more cost-effective, have closed beds and moved programs, where possible, into ambulatory settings. These tend to be specialized tertiary programs requiring sophisticated technology and personnel. The University of Calgary has always supported ambulatory experiences for both medical students and residents, whether in a private office setting or in hospital clinics, and the medical school supports both a Department of Family Medicine and an Ambulatory Care Center. Our community responsibility deals more with providing our graduates with the necessary skills, knowledge, and competencies required for rural practice. Clerkship experience in family medicine is mandatory for our final year students and both medical students and family practice residents are encouraged to obtain training and experience in a rural setting. Although our programs may differ, we would do well to adopt the curricular goals of the primary care residency program described by the author.

General Discussion

It was recognized that the value system of most contemporary medical schools may "deform" not only the educational and research agendas but also the concept of "quality." The latter has both an individual and a population dimension. If the venue for assessment of "quality" is restricted to tertiary care hospitals, the much larger concern for the "quality" of the health status of those without care or for those cared for by generalists in the community remains unassessed. There are those concerned that the medical school may have less power to control the curriculum and less influence on the students experiences when they are assigned to ambulatory clinics, group practices, health centers, and other community-based health facilities. However, strategies for evaluation of both teaching and patient care can be implemented. The impact of a community-based experience on the students should make the medical school's risks supportable. Perhaps one measure of success of the program will be found in the graduates' ultimate commitment, in residency and practice, to primary care and a population perspective.

Clinical research should be encouraged in these community-based ambulatory health care facilities. It is one means of enhancing understanding and improving the management of important primary care problems and should enable the faculty to respond more effectively to the health and health care needs of the entire population.

Some counseled against going to extremes and "deforming" medical education in another direction by overemphasizing community-based medical education so that other equally important aspects were neglected. Balance was needed, above all.

6
A Community and Population-Oriented Medical School: Newcastle, Australia

JOHN D. HAMILTON

I. Introduction

Newcastle is the commercial and industrial center of the Hunter Valley, which was first explored by Europeans almost 200 years ago. The city started as a convict station established to mine large coal deposits in the lower valley. Coal mining is still a major industry together with steel making, aluminum smelting, and primary chemical manufacture, farming, and fishing. Bushwalking, vineyards, and beaches are the basis of a growing tourism and leisure industry.

The population, mostly of Anglo-Saxon origin, is relatively stable with low levels of migration into the region. Current demographic, social, and health profiles for the Hunter Valley Health Area are provided in Appendix 1. Although there has been a recovery in the steel industry in recent years, unemployment is still higher than in other areas of New South Wales. Major industrial decisions are made in Sydney and Melbourne, not in Newcastle.

The health services of the Hunter Valley have always had strong associations with the community. In the early years, Miners Unions and other community groups provided financial support and volunteers to hospitals. Local health insurance schemes were established; individuals were protected for a subscription—"a penny a month"—when the Royal Newcastle Hospital first opened. Hospitals were staffed mainly by honorary consultants.

During the 1950s, its Medical Superintendent began to restructure the Royal Newcastle Hospital. He introduced full time staff specialists, outpatient clinics, and strong postgraduate training programs for the specialty colleges. His intention was to persuade the government to establish a full medical school in Newcastle.

By 1958, the clinical facilities at the medical school at the University of Sydney were overburdened and there was vigorous pressure to establish a second medical school in New South Wales. Despite strong representations from Newcastle, the decision was made in favor of Sydney, and the new school was established at the second university in Sydney, the University of New South Wales.

The University of Newcastle started as a college of the University of New South Wales in 1952. It became an independent university in 1964. Although the hospital and community generally still pushed for a medical school, the new University opposed this development as too expensive; its main priorities were to establish engineering and science faculties as more appropriate to an industrial region. However, the University's opposition disappeared once these faculties were operating, fortunately in time to make submissions to the Karmel Committee, which was set up by the Government in 1972.

This Committee, headed by Professor Peter Karmel, was mandated "to enquire into and make recommendations to the Australian Universities Commission on the need for new or expanded Medical Schools in the light of likely trends in the delivery of health care in Australia over the next 20 years." Because of their earlier unsuccessful bid, various groups in the Newcastle community had already spent a great deal of time thinking and consulting about these matters. This spadework enabled them to prepare substantial submissions, each reflecting a broad community commitment and a well-informed understanding of the needs of medical education.

The Newcastle Chamber of Commerce, speaking for the community at large, referred to the general community awareness of the need for a medical school and the benefits that would accrue to the community from such a school. It highlighted the strength and breadth within the community structure on which a school could be built. The University of Newcastle expressed its preference for an emphasis on general practice and on community medicine that would "allow Newcastle to make a significant contribution to national as well as regional needs. . . . Students would be exposed to the experience of working amongst a wide community spectrum, a microcosm of the Nation."

The Royal Newcastle Hospital welcomed the opportunity for innovation, and for students to have a wide exposure to general practice. The relation between the hospital and the community created "the opportunity to engage in a course concentrating on social medicine and later family practice. . . . The medical profession is sufficiently progressive to consider changes in the curriculum and in teaching methods." This submission highlighted the community-based teaching facilities already available in the region, i.e., the general practice network, community and child health clinics, industrial medicine dispensaries, psychiatric services, and a domiciliary geriatric care service that was itself a pioneering model of worldwide repute.

The Central Northern Medical Association, representing the profession, proposed innovations in the curriculum derived in part from regular consultations with the Royal Australian College of General Practitioners. These included early clinical contact, integration between clinical and basic sciences, group learning, communication skills, and problem-solving skills.

"The best doctor possible must be community-oriented . . . with responsibility in preventive medicine . . . and [able to] take time and effort to understand mankind" (Submissions to the Karmel Commission 1972). The Association pointed to a number of initiatives in population health already existing in the area. These included the Perinatal and Obstetric Death Survey, set up by the Newcastle Obstetrical and Gynecological Society, which has resulted in a system of perinatal monitoring and quality assurance for obstetric care. All these submissions presented a strong case for the establishment of a medical school in Newcastle.

In its 1973 report, the Karmel Committee recommended two new schools, the first at Newcastle and a second in due course at James Cook University, Townsville. This latter has not materialized. Among the reasons for advising a new school was the opportunity for innovation that it perceived was difficult in the conservative, established schools. Their Report dealt at length with the matter of community medicine, Community Medicine departments, and General Practice. It accepted that there was a need to encourage doctors to enter general practice and to prepare them for it. However, it felt that there should be more to community medicine than this.

It is necessary to evolve a new philosophy in respect to general practice in the medical curriculum. Training in general practice as such is vocational and is best carried out after graduation. . . . Exposure to the problems of human beings in the community is part of the orientation of the student in his scientific training and his future life's work. . . . Teaching of medical problems in the community setting therefore begins in the earliest years of the course so that the student may relate his scientific learning to the problems of living and being ill in the community itself.

University Departments based on the philosophy of human health and disease in the community itself will have greater impact on the student than those based narrowly on the object of training doctors to become general practitioners. The student who is community–minded and interested in people and their problems should thus become more stimulated to practice medicine in a community setting as a general practitioner than he would if towards the end of his course he was merely instructed in some of the practical aspects of general practice.

The time now appears right for a significant development of Departments of Community Medicine which will demonstrate the problems of community health care in practice. In addition to helping to stimulate interest in general practice, such a philosophy of training will also assist those students destined to become specialists or medical scientists, giving them a greater appreciation of community problems and needs so that they will practice their own vocation with greater understanding. . . . If . . . departments of Community Medicine embrace multiple responsibilities: General Practice, Epidemiology, Preventive and Occupational Medicine, a comprehensive intellectual discipline can be established. (Karmel 1973)

It was clear that Karmel intended initiatives in Community Medicine to be more than training for general practice. Many people to this day still have difficulty grasping the broader scope of our curriculum despite clear public statements such as this in 1977 from the *Newcastle Morning Herald*:

Wl.en Newcastle was chosen for the site of the third medical school . . . most people thought Community Medicine was basically the training for general practice . . . but . . . Community Medicine, by definition, is concerned with the study of health and sickness of populations. It uses the tools of epidemiology, demography, sociology, statistics, and other sophisticated methods to throw up a profile of a region's health and its problems and even lifestyles.

The Karmel Committee Report observed "[Community Medicine] is often almost unrepresented in any way in existing departments and its teaching requires facilities and an organization outside the medical school and hospitals" (Karmel 1973). Issues of community health were rarely incorporated into the mainstream of curriculum. Government did take the point and provided funds to set up a Chair of Community Medicine in each Medical School.

In 1973, at the time the Newcastle school was recommended by Karmel, traditional medical education was based on separate preclinical and clinical courses. There were some experiments in integration, but in Sydney there was major resistance to innovation: "Criticism of moves towards educational reform were freely voiced and even modest educational progressions were likely to be labelled as eccentric" (Maddison 1977).

II. Early Days of the Faculty

The first step in the establishment of the new medical school was the appointment of key individuals. The Vice-Chancellor of the University of Newcastle was to retire at the end of 1974. Consequently, a new Vice-Chancellor and a new Dean of Medicine would launch the medical school at Newcastle together.

The Dean

The University established a Search Committee for the foundation Dean. Its external advisor was David Maddison who was then Professor of Psychiatry and Dean of the University of Sydney Medical School. He had already become frustrated by the resistance of that traditionally structured school to change and had written extensively about the problems and limitations of the existing pattern of medical education (Maddison 1977, 1978). From his experience in psychiatry, he recognized the need for a perception of the social origins of health and illness, the importance of communication, and the need for the curriculum to generate a more appropriate style of learning.

The new medical school at Newcastle would present a unique opportunity to implement new ideas from its inception. Maddison was disappointed that early candidates failed to recognize that opportunity. The Search Committee seized the initiative and invited him to offer himself as Dean. Before making that offer he needed to know who was to be the new Vice Chancellor and whether he would support him.

The Vice-Chancellor

In 1972 Don George, while Professor of Electrical Engineering at Sydney, was commissioned by the Federation of Australian University Staff Associations to report on academic staff structures and University governance in Australian universities. He documented the problems caused by the rigid structure of academic departments and highlighted the need for checks and balances in the interplay between academic authority and academic freedom. He was ready to try a new approach to university administration.

Don George and David Maddison had been colleagues at Sydney University, and each recognized the contribution the other could make to change in an academic institution. It was therefore fortunate that, as David Maddison was thinking of becoming Dean, Don George was being invited to become Vice-Chancellor. Apparently, they assured each other of a commitment to innovation in curriculum and university administration. That commitment was essential to allow the medical school to adopt a radically new approach.

After his appointment as Dean, David Maddison undertook a 2-month study tour of overseas medical schools that were attempting new approaches to medical education. These included the schools at Beersheva in Israel, Southampton in the United Kingdom, Maastricht in the Netherlands, and McMaster in Canada.[1]

His private notes (Maddison 1975) indicate that he was seeking the answers to many questions:

- How can a community assist in student selection?
- How can we choose students with appropriate backgrounds and attitudes?
- Should a faculty be involved in the administration of health services?
- How can we encourage the development of Community Medicine?

David Maddison chose to establish a Department of Community Medicine, which would nurture general practice although some advised against a separate department for Community Medicine feeling that other departments would avoid their community responsibilities.

- How can we avoid independent power bases in basic sciences?
- What about behavioral sciences?

"Behavioral sciences," he wrote, "are completely fundamental for the whole of medical practice and therefore should establish their own independent existence in the Medical School."

Maddison examined problem-based learning in Nottingham and observed it in action at McMaster. He was reassured by the students' ability to func-

---

[1] These schools, together with Newcastle and others in developing countries, subsequently formed the global Network of Community-Oriented Educational Institutions for Health Sciences, an organization committed to innovation and a community orientation in health education.

tion in this new way, the sophistication of their learning, and their grasp of basic science. As far as research was concerned he planned "multidisciplinary research with perhaps some applied components eventually being translatable to improve the health of its regional community." He noted the importance for students of critical reasoning and the necessity for them to consider ethical issues. This study tour focused Maddison's thinking, and many of the ideas gained during the tour were developed in the new curriculum at Newcastle. It also established contacts and resulted in recruitment of some of the key foundation staff.

Foundation Faculty

The University as a whole welcomed the faculty of medicine and, indeed, hailed it as a mark of its own maturity. However, some sectors objected strongly when the faculty assumed responsibility for its entire curriculum rather than drawing on the courses provided by other faculties. The advertisement for the first three Chairs, those in Medical Education, Behavioral Sciences in Relation to Medicine, and Medical Biochemistry, drew an immediate protest from some sections of the University. The Professors of Education, Psychology, and Biological Sciences were at the Vice-Chancellor's door to protest that these were their areas of responsibility. Maddison, however, was adamant that if the Medical School was tethered to the priorities of other faculties it would not be able to undertake the innovations required to implement the Karmel recommendations. The faculty of mathematics took a positive view and its support was key to strong collaboration in Biostatistics.

It is worth reflecting on the background of some of the first appointees to the medical faculty, for although David Maddison provided strong leadership and acted as a mentor, individual appointees played a crucial role in the orientation of the faculty and its curriculum. Prior to their arrival, Maddison had set up a Consultation Committee of local practitioners who had already laid the groundwork on which this school would develop and the new appointees joined that Committee. There is a hazard in picking out for special mention any of the early staff even just to illustrate a point; for every one of them made a contribution and that will be illustrated later.

- Charles Engel (Medical Education) came to Newcastle after extensive educational experience in WHO and the British Life Assurance Trust. His main contribution to the initial workings of the faculty was the proper ordering of its educational thinking. He acted as a stimulus to the documentation and evaluation of the curriculum.
- Tony Vinson (Behavioral Science in Relation to Medicine) worked in Newcastle to develop social indicators while he was on the staff at Macquarie University. This study provided some of the background data for the Group Medicine strand of the curriculum (later Population Medicine).

He had a strong commitment to social change and fulfilled Maddison's expectation of "skills, knowledge and influence which would clearly be required if any practical sense was to be made out of the commitment to be of use to a graduate with a sophisticated understanding of social and community process and who would also display a high level of sensitivity and skill in all matters pertaining to the doctor/patient relationship" (Maddison 1985).

- Stephen Leeder (Community Medicine) had a background in clinical medicine at Sydney and in epidemiology at McMaster University and St Thomas's Hospital. He matched Maddison's requirement: "Community Medicine would need for this position to be concerned with the identification and resolution of the total health needs of a defined population . . . with the factors affecting the prevalence, mode of presentation and response to treatment of all episodes of illness within a defined population. . . . It is essential the Professor possess a high level of credibility in epidemiology, demography, and statistics and be prepared to commit a substantial proportion of his discipline's resources to active involvement in prevention at the individual level and in relation to social and community issues" (Clarke et al. 1981).

- Rufus Clarke (Anatomy) had a strong commitment to innovation in medical education. This was tempered by his experience of a new curriculum in England that failed to achieve its potential through lack of clear educational principles. He became the first Chairman of the Undergraduate Education Committee at Newcastle and played a crucial role in the development of a curriculum that drew on contemporary thinking in medical education and focused on the learning process.

Troubled Times

Maddison provided personal leadership to the faculty and introduced many to the concepts of group tutorials, problem-based learning, and interactional skills. To support integration in the curriculum he proposed an administrative matrix based on function with no formal departmental structure.

Being given a mandate to construct an innovative program does not assure absolute freedom to carry it out. David Maddison wrote that the most "important constraints [were] the characteristics, attitudes, and expectations of the parent university . . . ,—the attitudes and expectations of the local medical profession . . . , the level of funding provided, [and] the characteristics and qualities of the existing health services" (Maddison 1977).

The first years were troubled. The political climate at the national and state level had changed since the Karmel Report. A new conservative government was not committed to the community health developments and the community clinics proposed by its predecessor. The recommendations of the Karmel Committee and the orientation of the new medical school were seen by some politicians as left-wing and also as hostile to private medicine.

Some Newcastle clinicians found that the startling innovations in this new school were not quite what they had anticipated, and there was some resentment when the first Professors were appointed from outside Newcastle. Foundation staff recall an atmosphere of substantial hostility, and practitioners in the City complained that the faculty, which started with open consultation, soon retreated into its castle. The state government failed to provide the health service with extra funds to support the hospitals in their involvement with the school and for the first 5 years there was a strong concern that the medical school would be closed or converted to a clinical school for another University.

David Maddison died suddenly in 1981. Geoffrey Kellerman, Professor of Medical Biochemistry, led the faculty for 2 years and the faculty stayed true to its principles. He also established much trust in the political field by his personal diplomacy. A solid foundation of educational principle, experience, and creative leadership was essential to weather these storms.

III. A Community-Oriented Curriculum

This section will describe the early steps, particularly as it relates to a community and population perspective and finally the curriculum as it has evolved in 1990.

Working Papers

The Consultation Committee and foundation staff wrote 15 Working Papers to lay down fundamental principles of curriculum, faculty governance, student selection, and so on. A review of this shows how good they were as a foundation, both as documents and as vehicles for consultation within and without the faculty. They have held true to the needs of medical education and in the main the faculty has held true to them.

Student Selection

Maddison felt strongly that decisions concerning student entry into the medical course should be influenced by the community. The Admissions Committee included six community representatives (the Lord Mayor, a senior trade unionist, a business executive, a social worker, and two medical practitioners), three of whom were women. It was decided that multiple entry criteria were preferable to the single criterion of academic achievement. This would select a wider diversity of students to the benefit of them all: "Heterogeneity should enhance the learning process and, in the long run, the benefits to the community" (Working papers 1972–1977).

This desire for "heterogeneity" was also an attempt to find, over time, the qualities necessary to make a "good doctor" and it was felt that a broad base of students was more likely to lead to the producing of "good doctors." Applicants all have to have a good academic standing, and then take several tests that assess motivation, empathy, and problem-solving abilities. Those ranked best take part in a structured interview, assessing similar qualities. The interviewers are a pair—one from the faculty and one from the community. Subsequent analysis shows the interview predicts success in the course; the single most important criterion is motivation (Powis et al. 1988).

Over the years the process has been refined but not altered radically. There is no barrier to those without experience in science and we admit mature-aged candidates. Aboriginal students are admitted through a special program. This not only responds to the severe problems of poor health in aboriginal communities but also enriches the experience of the whole class. Sixty-eight students enter each year.

Educational Objectives

Maddison knew how important it was to have educational goals, in order to avoid regression towards the mean:

One outstanding lesson which I derived from my Sydney experience was the absolute necessity to spell out, in reasonable detail, the objectives towards the achievement of which the educational program would be directed, and to ensure that these objectives received a substantial measure of agreement from the foundation staff. (Maddison 1977)

A major priority for the foundation staff was the development of the education program. Forty-five objectives for the program were constructed. In these the concern with social, community, and preventive issues was made explicit, by stating, for example, that the graduate will

- Demonstrate positive, consistent and informed attitudes towards the prevention of illness and the maintenance of health . . . . ;
- Demonstrate awareness that major changes in individual and community health are likely to depend as much or more on change in the behavior of people as on the manipulation of the physical environment;
- Manifest a positive attitude toward the concept of the physician as an educator, for example of patients with regard to their illness, of the public in matters of health . . . and will show an appropriate level of ability and confidence in this role (Clarke et al. 1981).

Studies of a Community

Although the curriculum outlines and the Undergraduate Program Objectives were written in 1976, it was not until the end of 1977, a few months before the first students were to arrive, that there was a concrete plan for how students should get to grips with community medicine. In retrospect, having students study the community from within seems a simple and obvious solution but, in 1977, it seemed a new and startling approach. Stephen Leeder wrote that the curriculum should

provide the students with an opportunity, in their groups of eight, to move out into the community, each student group having its own predetermined community locality in which students can work. The intention...would be to enable students to begin to develop skills in approaching the community, talking to people within it, assembling information with respect to its structure, understanding something of the community, and generally developing insights which are fundamental to a sociological and epidemiological understanding of the way in which the community functions. (Working Papers 1975–1977)

With this foundation, students were expected to discover for themselves the basic health needs of their chosen community and the features that might have a bearing on these health needs. They were to suggest preventive strategies and ways in which the community could deal with its needs. The written reports of the groups were assessed.

The greatest problem with this early project was the fact that, although there were precedents in developing countries, it was totally new to Australian medical education. Knowledge about the nature of the community programs in Newcastle was limited and it was difficult to find tutors or role models. Hence, in the early days the students complained vociferously about the lack of guidance from tutors, and sometimes, even about a tutor's lack of understanding about what was to be achieved by the students. Some students could not see the relevance of the community-based project to the learning of medicine. Social scientists were frustrated that tutors had no framework of reference for sociological terminology and concepts to assist the students. In retrospect they suggest that it would have been best to emphasize social action rather than social theory. In truth there was social action, for students were obliged to set up a program responding to a need in this community; safe play areas and help for single mothers are examples.

Despite the problems, it was felt that the community perspective gained was invaluable to students.

It is our belief that only a continuing, practical exposure to the realities of community organization, needs, and health care provision can achieve our long term objectives. We do not consider it likely that [students] will understand the dynamics of various groups within the community (including those in the community who provide health care and those who administer health care organizations) unless [they] have repeated opportunities for task-oriented contact with such groups. (Working Papers 1975–1977)

But student agitation was strong and in later years the community project was replaced with a smaller community-oriented but disease-based research project. A number of students reflecting with hindsight on the experience now recognize it was more valuable than they had thought at the time. The best experience was, naturally, in the more disadvantaged communities, where problems were stark and the plight of some families shocked them and challenged them. A good and informed tutor was a great support. A tutor unskilled, insecure, or dismissive of this experience could ruin it. It may well be that it was the staff rather than the students or the experience itself that failed—no surprise to innovators in education.

Review and Revision

Commencing in 1982 the curriculum was reviewed, using a Delphi survey and wide discussion. This section will describe those outcomes of the review that relate to population health as a preparation for describing the curriculum as it is now, in 1990.

Domains of Learning

Originally the curriculum had been largely organized by both content and types of learning. It was now considered that it could be better organized according primarily to distinct domains of learning. Five were defined and the educational objectives were rearranged (but not substantially changed) to match them (Appendix 2). The curriculum of each Domain will be described later:

Domain 1: Professional Skills
Domain 2: Critical Reasoning
Domain 3: Identification, Prevention, and Management of Illness
Domain 4: Population Medicine
Domain 5: Self-Directed Learning

The Nature of Community Medicine

Community Medicine in this faculty had three major but interdependent themes.

- Population Medicine: The population-based aspect of Community Medicine that deal with the health of large communities.
- The Medical Care of Individuals in the Community: This occurs through general practice, other community services, and occupational medicine.
- Clinical Epidemiology: The application in clinical settings of the methods and perspectives of classical epidemiology. It deals with the evaluation of effectiveness of interventions, assessment of prognosis, the interpretation of clinical and laboratory tests, and the investigation of aetiology (Dickinson et al. 1985).

These themes are woven into much of the curriculum, especially in Population Medicine, Critical Reasoning, and General Practice.

The need for a population framework to individual care
In all settings, and not just in the community, the care of individual patients must be informed by information about epidemiology, risk factors, prognosis, benefits, risks, and costs of prevention and intervention. This has not been a familiar approach

for many specialist clinicians and despite a high profile of epidemiology at grand rounds and other educational events it is still difficult for clinical teachers in the wards to keep these aspects of care prominent in the student experience.

The need to attend to the personal needs of patients
Criticisms of doctors have been voiced in Australia as elsewhere, with familiar themes: that they do not understand the needs of individuals or communities, and the importance of family, culture, and occupation; they do not inform them or involve them adequately in decisions; they ignore preventive health needs and the role of nonmedical community resources in health care.

The need to base health care on the ethical values of the community
The faculty had always recognized that while the ethical basis of medical care must be informed by the quantitative and qualitative study of health and disease, it is a superordinate frame of reference whose definition must include a full contribution from the community itself. Advancing technology, competitive claims on resources, and changing social values required us to come to grips with these issues.

The benefit of the faculty's experience and research in the community
The aspects of population health described above could have been derived from largely theoretical discussion. What was especially important at Newcastle was that over the years we had established our own data base and insight on which developments in curriculum, research, and clinical service could be built. Many examples will be described later. Prominent were the population-based epidemiological studies of illness and risk factors in the WHO MONICA study, the studies in general practice of substantial deficits in preventive care and attention to psychosocial factors, the development of hospital bioethics committees, and the exploration of issues of health and illness in employment.

The Curriculum in 1990

The five Domains of Learning run in parallel through each year. In describing these Domains the population perspective will be emphasized. It is convenient to start with Domain III for this provides the main organizing structure for the content of this curriculum.

Domain III: Identification, Prevention, and Management of Disease

This Domain uses problem-based learning from clinical problems. In the first 2 years this is done in regular tutorials, with problems provided on paper, but illustrated, to allow students time to develop their strategies for learning and to explore the basic sciences in particular. They follow a sequence organized by body systems. In their third year the experience shifts to clinical postings in the minor specialties and a term in a country hospital. The fourth and fifth year consist mostly of clinical clerkships in the major specialties, reinforced by a continuing program in applied basic sciences. The problem-solving method of the tutorials are now applied to the management of real patients.

A Population Dimension in Domain III

Many of the original clinical conditions for Domain III were chosen because they were common, dangerous, or preventable. However, since they are presented as individual cases, it is important to see how a population perspective is established. This is best done by describing one of the original problems that is still in use.

A Problem of Impaired Development: This problem is based on a child with phenylketonuria whose screening test was lost. The family now faces the problem of delayed intellectual development and the difficulty of feeding a complicated diet to a child with disturbed behavior—a medical and social catastrophe. The problem is introduced by a video recording of a painful discussion among the parents, the pediatrician, and nurse that demonstrates resentment, blame, and family conflict over responsibility. The students discuss the video and identify a set of hypotheses about what has happened (for the diagnosis is not spelled out) and from this define their own learning goals. Only then is further information about the child made available to help refine their hypotheses and clarify their learning goals. This is the process of problem-based learning, deliberately following the hypothetico-deductive sequence of a clinical encounter or a scientific investigation. The issues that emerge for study include, of course, a wide range of issues of population health will be identified for study now and for reinforcement in more detail later in the course. These include issues of parental coping and family breakdown, social policy or the provision of community facilities for long-term care, the economics of care versus prevention, the role of screening tests and public and individual responsibility for them, interprofessional cooperation ethics, and genetic counseling. In the early years of the course these issues were spelled out ahead of time as learning goals backed by reading material. This preempted the students' own opportunity to identify the issues for themselves, so they are now given only to the tutor as a guide and are shared only later with the students so they can check that they have explored the main issues. Talks geared to the issues of the problem studied, selected recordings and videos, and above all the library, are the main resources for learning—and also, of course, from other students through joint study and discussion and from the diversity of their own experience. The tutor facilitates but does not dominate discussion and must avoid preempting discussions by giving the answer!

Domain I: Professional Skills

Students who are studying clinical problems in a tutorial must see real patients and learn appropriate clinical skills. This intensive program starts in the first months. It is geared it its content to Domain III. It includes communication skills, counselling and preventive care techniques and continuing contact with families experiencing illness, disability, and pregnancy. Some of the experiences are in long-term attachments in general practice, which provides its own perspective on health care of patients with early and defined problems. Alongside the problem described above, the students will learn how to assess psychomotor development and to recognize its normal range and will discuss family issues with parents of children at a special education center.

Domain IV: Population Medicine

Students are led through a series of concepts as they undertake their own research studies, either from the literature or within the community. They work in tutorial groups with tutors generally experienced in community matters, and often from other health professions. The Domain relies heavily on the concepts of statistics, epidemiology, the social sciences, and the methodology of population-based research. "Population" may refer to a geographic community or a group with common problems, needs, or risks.

In brief the concepts year by year are:

Year 1: Studies of the burden of illness on individuals, families, and communities. Each group studies a different problem (e.g. abortion, smoking, cerebral palsy). Seminars by alternative health practitioners, increasingly popular to the community, have recently been arranged at student request.

Year 2: A study of a single topic of major public health importance (e.g. AIDS and mental health). Each group studies a distinct aspect (epidemiology, public perception, impact of health education, costs of options for care), prepares a research protocol, and completes a pilot study. Each group presents results of the study and the background literature review to the whole class, usually with great style; all groups have to learn from the others, to build a comprehensive picture of the topic.

Year 3: A study of largely preventable diseases from a population perspective (e.g., glaucoma, melanoma, and gonorrhoea) chosen to capitalize on the clinical experiences and specialty postings of Domain III.

Year 4: The evaluation of health care programs, including screening, secondary prevention, programs for disadvantaged groups, and domiciliary care. These add a community and population perspective to the largely hospital-based experience of Domain III and the health counselling skills of Domain I.

Year 5: The study of the population perspectives of 10 major diseases (e.g. cancer of the breast, asthma, diabetes, etc.) linking clinical epidemiology, clinical medicine, and public health to establish the population framework for the care of individual patients.

Domain II: Critical Reasoning

This Domain provides the intellectual capacity to interpret and assess the application of the scientific method to medicine and biomedical research. It enables students to make rational decisions and decide between conflicting evidence. Since much of that evidence is in published papers, these are the main subjects of study and students are assessed on their ability to critique papers and to apply their conclusions to the rest of their work.

The Domain builds an understanding of a sequence of concepts, drawing heavily on biostatistics. The concepts are studied generally through exercises to analyze papers that may relate to any of the other Domains. But there is a particular affinity with Population Medicine and the two Domains have become closely coordinated in recent years.

The skills of this Domain are of importance to many aspects of learning and form one of the most important foundations for continuing learning.

Domain V: Self-Directed Learning

This Domain develops the skills of independent learning, essential not only for success in the curriculum, but also for subsequent continuing education. Students learn by study tasks with open access to the library and staff. Emphasis is on marshalling and appraisal of evidence, and clearly makes use of skills in Critical Reasoning.

An elective program is administered through this Domain. In the final 2 months of Year 3 and Year 5 students arrange their own elective, its objectives and supervision. Many choose to work in developing countries so adding a global perspective to their view of medicine.

What Happens After Graduation?

Our own studies of interns from all schools in New South Wales have demonstrated a falling away of preventive and psychosocial skills during the intern year. Interns are, in large hospitals, coping with acute medical crises and tend to be socialized to the style of medicine practiced by the traditionally trained doctors with whom they are working. A major challenge for Newcastle is to ensure that the community-based knowledge, skills, and attitudes, acquired in the undergraduate program, persist through the intern years and into practice. A new program for interns and junior medical officers, described below, is designed to do just that. We need to develop clinicians as role models, both as individual clinicians and in population health. We need to train our clinical staff to present population aspects as an integral part of clinical medicine.

Finally, and most importantly, we need more information about whether the program works. Only two studies to date have attempted to explore whether graduates from Newcastle are different from those from other medical schools in Australia. Both studies looked at interns. The first used videotapes of interns' consultations with both real and simulated patients in a hospital setting (Gordon et al. 1989). The second uses ratings from supervising clinicians (Saunders et al. 1982). Neither study found marked differences between graduates from different medical schools on questions of clinical competence and knowledge. However, the supervising clinicians in the second study found that Newcastle graduates were better at talking to patients and their families, and at analyzing and solving their problems.

Continued empirical evaluation of the program is one of our most important challenges, if we are to improve our existing program and encourage other schools within Australia to adopt this approach.

IV. Academic Disciplines

A full range of Disciplines has been established at Newcastle, each committed to an integrated curriculum under the governance of the Undergraduate Education Committee, and to developing a community orientation to its research. Our total academic staff is only 48, with some 16 additional faculty on external funds. The Disciplines are therefore small. Pediatrics and Reproductive Medicine, for instance, have each managed with a Professor, Senior Lecturer, and Professional Officer. The largest group is Medicine with six academic staff. The clinical Disciplines are strongly supported by staff specialists who contribute to teaching and, in some cases, research.

Disciplines of this size could not function effectively as isolated departments. It is a strength of the faculty that members from different Disciplines have formed research clusters and so build up a critical mass. These include the Neurosciences Group, the Clinical Immunology Group, the Reproductive Endocrinology Group, the Musculoskeletal Group, and the Primary Health Care Group. The close working relationships built in shaping an integrated curriculum have been transferred most effectively into the research arena. Younger staff take substantial leadership roles in both curriculum and research and it is important to emphasize that their commitment has been crucial to our achievements.

The following brief review of the Disciplines will emphasize those aspects of their work that relate to a community perspective.

Community Medicine

This Discipline now contains the following components:

Clinical Epidemiology: This has become a particular strength in Newcastle, formalized through the creation of the Centre for Clinical Epidemiology and Biostatistics, directed by Professor Richard F. Heller, Professor of Community Medicine. Salary and other support are provided by the Rockefeller Foundation, through the International Clinical Epidemiology Network (INCLEN), and by the Australian Government through the Public Health Grant recommended by the Kerr White Report (White 1986). The main aims of the Centre are research and the training of graduates in epidemiological research. Local specialist clinicians are now enrolling and this will enhance their teaching capacity.

Biostatistics: Biostatistics is a necessary supporting Discipline for clinical epidemiology. A Chair of Medical Biostatistics was established in the faculty of mathematics, following close research collaboration with Medicine. Additional staff are appointed to the medical faculty through the Public Health Grant.

The combined research capacities in Clinical Epidemiology and Biostatistics have provided for substantial epidemiological studies of health risk factors for cardiovascular disease and, in conjunction with other Disciplines, studies of the epidemiology of asthma and chest disease in adults and children as they relate to environmental exposure and industrial pollution. This central core of skills has strengthened the epidemiological capacity of all the Disciplines and has brought to the hospital-based clinical services an epidemiological approach to education and clinical Grand Rounds. The international connection through INCLEN and other associations has broadened our research contacts.

General Practice: This has been nurtured within the Discipline of Community Medicine and is now ready for independence. At the start there were two part-time Fellows, drawn from local general practice. Their first priority was to ensure that working problems represented real-life presentations in a community context. There are now two full-time General Practice staff members. Both play comprehensive educational roles in the faculty. Sandy Reid, originally in practice, was a member of the original Consultative Committee in 1975 and is now Associate Professor of General Practice and also currently Chairman of the Undergraduate Education Committee. In addition, 200 general practitioners in the Hunter Valley allow students into their offices and cooperate in research studies of patterns and quality of care by the Primary Health Care Research Group staff from General Practice and Behavioral Science. Practitioners have allowed video cameras to record their daily practice routine, a mark of the trust that has been built up, largely as a result of conscientious communication and of working with the faculty in undergraduate education. A new development is the Department of Primary Care at the new John Hunter Hospital (see below), designed to establish effective continuity of care between hospitals and General Oractice—of special importance as hospital stays shorten.

Health Economics: The Rockefeller Grant supports a health economist who facilitates a systematic approach to health economics for undergraduates as well as postgraduates. Health services in Australia are provided by both public and private sectors and the country faces financial limits to its capacity to provide the expensive and expanding medical technology now available. The need for balanced investment in curative and preventive care requires undergraduates to develop insights into health economics.

Health Social Sciences: One academic position is supported by the Rockefeller Foundation. Responsibilities include interacting with clinicians and links also are being forged with other social scientists working on health issues in Australia.

Environmental and Occupational Health

Starting with a single position in Community Medicine this Discipline is now set up on its own, with support by the Australian Public Health Grant. Major research initiatives have been built in cooperation with Unions and Management. The Hunter Occupational Health Service backed by an industrial hygiene laboratory provides a consultancy service on clinical and environmental problems in industry. This Discipline has now taken over the training of all Occupational Health and Safety Officers and this will establish contacts throughout the industries of the Hunter Valley.

Behavioral Science in Relation to Medicine

This Discipline has concentrated on population-based studies of health-related behavior in the community as a whole, and the quality of preventive health care in general practice. With members in General Practice it has set up the Primary Care Research Group that has now a good record of research into the efficacy of intervention in preventive care and health promotion in relation to smoking, cancer prevention, drugs and alcohol, women's health, and AIDS. The Area Health Service has now capitalized on this by appointing the Head of the Discipline, Professor Rob Sanson-Fisher, as Area Director of Health Promotion, together with Drug and Alcohol and Women's Health Services. This now brings a rigorous academic capacity to the evaluation of health promotion to better shape policy and practice and to improve training and career development through a Diploma and Masters Degree in Health Promotion based on the core program in Epidemiology—the first such in Australia.

Clinical Pharmacology

This Discipline has been strong in both its clinical and basic sciences staff. Professor Tony Smith is an experienced clinician who has set up a 24-hour Drug Advisory Service to provide consultation to practitioners and pharmacists on the side effects and interactions of drugs. The Discipline operates a clinical toxicology service and manages all patients who have attempted suicide through drug overdose. It provides leadership in the pharmacy and therapeutic committees in the teaching hospitals.

Studies in the use and side effects of pharmaceutical drugs in the community and the educational and research links with the Centre for Clinical Epidemiology and Biostatistics provided impetus for the recent development of Pharmacoepidemiology, which studies the patterns of use, efficacy, and side effects of over-the-counter and prescribed medications. It is one of the themes of the INCLEN program and has been identified by the Australian Government as a major tool in its search for a rational approach to therapeutic drug regulation. A Masters Degree program in Pharmacoepidemiology has been set up based on the core program in Clinical Epidemiology. The Discipline also has strong consulting relations with the Commonwealth Government, which is considering setting up in Newcastle a Drug Evaluation Unit as its technical arm.

Pediatrics

This Discipline has played a major role in expanding health services not only in the hospitals but also in the community and has facilitated the appointment of an academic Chair, the Area Director of Community Child and Family Health. This is intended to take our academic access well into the Community health service. Population-based research studies are in training on genetic aspects of lipid metabolism, the epidemiology of childhood asthma and environmental risk factors, and aspects of social deprivation resulting in failure to thrive. It has stimulated our own thinking on curriculum developments on nutrition and we now have the most comprehensive and integrated curriculum on nutrition in Australia.

Reproductive Medicine

This Discipline has played a major role in the care of high-risk pregnancy, prenatal diagnostic services, and, with pediatrics, in perinatology. It has highlighted the ethical issues in reproductive technology. Research includes studies of postpartum depression, fetal retardation, and placental endocrinology.

Internal Medicine

This Discipline has contributed to service developments, especially in renal disease and chest disease, with research programs in sleep disorders, especially in the elderly, placental endocrinology, and issues of fetal growth retardation. It has taken wide responsibility in stimulating a broad pragmatic approach to health services.

Surgical Sciences

This Discipline emphasizes oncology, with strong basic science research supported through philanthropic donations. For example, funds were raised to establish the Telethon Cancer Research Chair, which has provided much of the impetus to establishing the Hunter Oncology Service. The Chair of Surgical Oncology has established and evaluates a mobile mammography program. Other developments in Oncology include palliative care, with imaginative involvement of general practitioners, and preventive health programs strongly linked to Behavioral Sciences. Not all has been rosy and some clinicians have objected to the University's role as intrusive.

Psychiatry

This Discipline has developed a number of community outreach activities. These include support groups for the mentally ill and psychiatric residency postings in general practice. Unfortunately, current State government policy tends to separate institutional psychiatric care from general health care. This weakens patient care and education, and cooperation between Disciplines. It is, to our regret, a major failure in our cooperation with health services. The Discipline is sited at one of two main teaching hospitals and provides support there for oncology, palliative care, and clinical toxicology, thereby enriching education for both undergraduates and postgraduates. The Discipline is undertaking a population-based study of emotional sequelae of the earthquake that hit Newcastle in December 1989.

Health, Law, and Ethics

This is not a separate Discipline, but rather an educational interest group drawn from the faculty and others within the University and beyond. The undergraduate program in Health, Law, and Ethics is in Domain III and is assessed in all 5 years. The seminars, discussions, debates, and learning resources that make up the program deal with practical clinical dilemmas as they present to clinicians, many of whom join in the seminars. Others contribute from Departments of Law, Cultural and Curriculum Studies, and Philosophy, as well as from the legal profession and the clergy.

Over the last 2 years, there have been several further developments. These include a hospital bioethics committee at both major hospitals, ethics grand rounds, and conferences. A Masters program in Applied Ethics with medical bioethics as a major component will be operating in 1991. There have been recent grants from two Medical Defence Unions for visiting external scholars and curriculum improvements. All these developments provide a framework for consultation with the community at large on issues of ethical concern and public policy.

Medical Genetics

The definition of genetic predisposition to illness and susceptibility to risk factors is very likely in the future to provide a rigorous and quantifiable basis for preventive health care programs. The broad issues of genetic counselling, decisions on fertility and termination, and the ethical issues involved, made it essential for the faculty to develop a capacity in genetics. We have been closely involved in the recruitment of genetics staff through the Area Health Service. The group has chosen to be linked to Community Medicine as their academic base, and this augers well for future contributions to population health.

Medical Informatics

Again, this is not a formal Discipline but a small interest group that extends our capacity in the computer-based management of data. A Chair of Information Sciences elsewhere in the University will soon be filled and we shall make the appropriate linkage. A strand of the curriculum has just started, students are taught to undertake literature searches by computer and the basic principles of health information management systems. Staff appointed to the new John Hunter Hospital are to be trained in the use of information systems, a major feature in the hospital, and the faculty will play a part in its development. In time we may see students calling directly on individual and population-based databases as a learning resource, although we have learned already from the Hunter Health Development Unit that students need a lot of guidance to do that with discrimination.

Basic Science Disciplines

Even our basic science Disciplines have some dimension of community orientation. Physiology has major studies in exercise physiology in athletes and the aged, and had a founding role in the Academy of Sport. Medical biochemistry has assisted in rationalization of services and costs in clinical bio-chemistry. Pathology pursues population-based studies in viral infection, immunization strategies, and industrial chest disease in farmers. Anatomy has an interest in whiplash injury, rehabilitation, and pain management. The close cooperation between basic sciences and clinicians in the curriculum has enhanced these roles in research and clinical services.

V. Links to the Health Service

Maddison developed a good personal working relationship with the Regional Director of Health. There were, however, still major clashes over the matter of academic leadership for hospital departments and the faculty was kept at arms length by hospital boards with the Dean being positively excluded from membership at first. Nevertheless, the facilities of the hospitals, the community, and general practices were made available to the medical school, and clinicians generously committed their time to the curriculum, some accepting major administrative responsibilities. With the passage of time and the sharing of responsibilities in the hospitals, cooperation and goodwill have developed among individuals and among the faculty and the Health Service generally.

Following a government review in 1983, hospital services throughout the Hunter Area were rationalized. Although not spelled out at the time, the author of this review, Geoffrey Olsen, stated that the needs of the medical school were a high priority. A large new teaching hospital was proposed and will open in 1991. Named the John Hunter Hospital, as mentioned above, it is the main tertiary referral center for the Hunter Area for most specialties. The faculty's planning for the hospital has led it to a substantial leadership role in the Hunter Area Health Service. Current faculty roles are as follows:

- The Dean is a member of the Area Health Board and Chairman of the Appointments and Credentials Committee responsible for all hospital specialist appointments in the Region. This has facilitated the coordination of Area and University staff development. Other faculty members serve on key committees of the Hunter Area Board and this ensures a close correspondence between faculty developments and Area Health Service developments.
- The Dean and Deputy Dean are members of the Board of the Newcastle Mater Misericordiae Hospital, the other main teaching hospital, and faculty members provide medical services in the hospital.
- Faculty members serve on the Board of the Hunter Postgraduate Medical Institute, the body responsible for continuing medical education in the Region and a major vehicle for contact with the practicing community.
- The Professor of Medicine, Nicholas Saunders, is Chairman of the Postgraduate Medical Council of New South Wales. This is a newly estab-

lished organization responsible for coordinating placement of junior medical staff and for their early postgraduate education. His leadership in early postgraduate education in the Hunter Area enabled Newcastle to explore new approaches ahead of the rest of the State.

- The Professors in the four major clinical Disciplines have been appointed Chairmen of Departments in the new John Hunter Hospital and are members of the Commissioning Team. In the long-term this should assure a first class educational institution. In the short-term it is almost consuming our senior academic leadership and given the inevitable politics and compromise, forcing the faculty into political roles it does not always relish.
- The faculty and the Hunter Area Health Service have cooperated in a new pattern of senior appointments. Key leadership positions, such as Area Directors of services and Chairmen of departments in the new teaching hospital, are recruited and appointed concurrently as full University chairs. The first two appointments, Area Director of Pathology (Professor of Anatomical Pathology) and Director of Community Child and Family Health Services (Professor of Child Psychiatry), provide an opportunity for the University to play a role in the consolidation of health services. Further Chairs have been established in Medical Imaging, and Anesthesia and Intensive Care, and others are proposed in Medical Genetics, Geriatrics, Liaison Psychiatry, and Palliative Care. These chairs and the high quality of candidates they have attracted would have been impossible had the faculty not established its standing in health services and research.
- The Hunter Health Statistics Unit was originally set up jointly by the faculty of Mathematics and the then Hunter Regional Health Service and later the faculty of Medicine. At first there was concern that the faculty of Medicine might through an interpretive role, filter and distort the data! The Unit provides data in support of health planning and its quality is such that State and Commonwealth governments have commissioned a series of policy-related studies of demography, predictions of health needs, bed requirements, the use of diagnosis-related groups, and the evaluation of quality improvement programs. To reflect its wider scope the unit has been renamed the Hunter Health Development Unit. Future challenges include the development of a data system from general practice and community health services, and to link this with health surveys and the work of the Health Promotion Unit and with epidemiological studies of disease incidence. This will be helped by new electronic information systems based on the John Hunter Hospital and links between that hospital and General Practice through its Primary Care Unit. All this will take some years to set up.

VI. Postgraduate Education

Interest in innovation always seems to concentrate on the undergraduate program. However, as mentioned earlier, postgraduate education is equally important if the principles of the undergraduate curriculum are to be converted to practice. It is particularly difficult to do this for population health because the first experience of a new graduate occurs in the heat of acute clinical management and generally in a tertiary care teaching hospital. That experience can counter much that the new doctor learned during the undergraduate years.

Although Australian universities have no further formal responsibility for postgraduate education, individual faculty staff are prominent in the supervision of postgraduate training. The education of the graduate doctor is the responsibility of hospitals and specialty colleges including the Royal Australian College of General Practitioners. Although the latter attends to some issues of population health, by and large these have been ignored by other postgraduate colleges in the Australian system. Recent training fellowships in Clinical Epidemiology are a step in the right direction.

There are some promising developments in the postgraduate area in Australia and the Hunter Region:

Intern and Junior Medical Officer Education

In 1991 the Hunter Area Health Service will introduce a 2-year program that will continue many of the strands of the undergraduate program, including epidemiology, preventive care, the study of social issues in health, ethics, and critical reasoning. This is an experiment because only 1 year of internship is required for registration. If successful it may lead the way for the New South Wales Postgraduate Council to introduce this as a requirement for all interns.

Postgraduate University Education

The University is responsible for formal degree and diploma courses, not the vocational training referred to above. The community-based approach has influenced postgraduate teaching and research within the faculty. Degree and diploma programs are conducted by the Centre for Clinical Epidemiology and Biostatistics for specialist clinicians and health professionals, in epidemiology, biostatistics, health social sciences, economics, pharmacoepidemiology, occupational medicine, psychiatric epidemiology, and health promotion.

VII. National Developments in Health and Medical Education

In recent years there have been national developments that have a bearing on medical education and on some aspects of health services related to population health:

Doherty Commission on Medical Education and Workforce into the Twenty-First Century

This commission, set up by the Commonwealth Minister for Health, examined issues in the medical workforce and reviewed medical education. The latter became the main burden of the report (Doherty 1988). The Newcastle faculty made a detailed submission. Our recommendations and, more particularly, our experience in innovation were cited extensively throughout the report. The report recommended the strengthening of undergraduate education in general practice, continuity of education into the postgraduate years, training in communication skills, and education in the methods of public health and preventive care. It recommended the promotion of innovation in medical education, particularly problem-based learning and community orientation.

Formal follow-up of the report by the Government has been disappointingly slow, probably because the recommendations were more comprehensive than the Minister originally envisaged. A task force is examining issues of manpower planning and most medical schools are carefully studying the major initiatives recommended in the report. The Australian Medical Council is about to embark on a revision of its guidelines for undergraduate education and will, no doubt, draw extensively on the Doherty Commission Report.

Drug and Alcohol Education

Through its Drug Offensive Program the Australian Government has been active in the field of drug and alcohol education. Although the emphasis has been on illicit drug use, alcohol, which accounts for a significantly greater morbidity and mortality, is also prominent. After pressure from national advisory bodies, the government provided each faculty of Medicine in Australia with funding for the appointment of a staff member to be responsible for the development of drug and alcohol education in its undergraduate program. This initiative seems to have a substantial impact on curricula and should encourage Government to support further initiatives in public health education in the same way.

Australian Medical Council

The Australian Medical Council (AMC) was established in 1985, with one of its most important roles the accreditation of undergraduate medical education. The author is the Founding Chairman of the Accreditation Committee. Accreditations are delineating the patterns of medical education and its innovations. While innovators in medical education like to characterize all others as dead at the post, the reality is that most schools are strengthening their curriculum in communication skills, early clinical contact, and community rotations in general practice. Issues to be addressed by medical schools for the future include those in Aboriginal health, intercultural issues, ethics, the special health needs of women, and the needs of women entering medicine, of which there are an increasing proportion: 70% of the 1990 class at Newcastle.

The assessment teams represent a wide scope of experience and one member always has special expertise in Community Medicine since the Committee felt that this area could not otherwise be properly assessed. The need to develop faculty support of Community Medicine has been identified as a substantial issue. The problem has arisen because of the lack of a strong academic tradition in general practice and community medicine and the difficulty of developing a sense of collegiate identity among faculty practitioners broadly distributed throughout the community.

In the near future the guidelines for education, at presently largely borrowed from the British General Medical Council, will be rewritten. This process will involve broad consultation with the Deans and with other constituencies within the community. New Zealand, our nearest neighbor, has recently undertaken a similar review with broad community consultation through conferences and workshops. We shall have to see whether the AMC will bring its deliberations to the public as they did.

Reorganization of Higher Education

In Australia, the higher education sector has consisted of Universities and Colleges of Advanced Education (CAE). Starting in 1987 the Government has been amalgamating these two sectors into expanded Universities. This is a controversial move with substantial problems because of the Government's focus on cost-effectiveness and its reluctance to appreciate the need for funding the research infrastructure. Medical faculties are forewarned of reduced funding, being considered as over funded now. The extra resources and staff we have gathered through external grants may become crucial to our survival.

In Newcastle, the Hunter Institute of Higher Education, a CAE, was responsible for the education of nurses and other health professionals through its School of Health. In 1993 the faculty of Medicine will join with the School of Health, presenting us with opportunities for interprofessional education and a broader perspective on health issues.

The Better Health Commission

This Commission was set up to define national priorities for preventive health care. Stephen Leeder played a major role in this and in the subsequent committee to define targets and strategies. It was an important Government initiative in defining and coordinating preventive approaches to the population's health, and gives direction to policy, resource allocation, and research.

A National Health Strategy Review

This review, announced in late 1990, will examine public funding through Medicare, long a source of conflict between much of the profession and left-wing governments. It will also examine priorities in health care. The new Commonwealth Minister of Health and Welfare Services who set up this review has a strong interest in equity, social issues in health, and a just distribution of limited resources. This review may well reshape not only health care but also the priorities for research and education.

International Developments

It has been important for the faculty to develop an international perspective partly to keep in touch with centers with similar educational approaches, and partly to make sure we keep a high profile within Australia. This has come naturally from the interests of individuals and has been supported by participation in World Health Organization networks, and educational links to assist new medical schools. We have a regular stream of visitors to study our curriculum.

Are we stretching our energies and resources too far? We probably are. However, most of us feel that if we simply shut up shop and concentrate only on our local scene we will lose much creative stimulus. But, time spent abroad is time lost at home. The urgent calls to send strong delegations to international meetings are more seductive than the urging to evaluate our own program!

VIII. How Will Newcastle Sustain a Community Orientation?

Strategies to sustain a continuing community orientation will have to include the following:

- A sustained commitment to maintain, review, and revise the undergraduate curriculum. It is very easy to become a traditionalist of a new movement. It is also easy to introduce many new curriculum initiatives and lose track of what that does to our original intentions. We need constantly to question our methods and principles.
- It is crucial to develop research programs to meet the community's needs. All Disciplines must participate and in our experience they do. Interdisciplinary research is a particular strength in Newcastle and has been facilitated by our academic structure.

- There must be a dialogue with the community. Outside the health services we have done this only in part and have depended too much on the initiatives of individuals. Committees, especially in the health service, come naturally, but it needs extra effort and commitment to become involved outside standard health matters. The involvement of Newcastle students in the broad social issues of the city has been, with some exceptions, confined to elective periods, perhaps because our curriculum demands such a heavy commitment. A biennial conference in memory of David Maddison is aimed to further just such communication. We now look to our graduates to establish their own dialogue with the community. This will finally be the thing that matters.
- There must also be a dialogue internally. As we expand our commitments we all become so busy with subsets of the faculty's role that we can lose track of its whole. Retreats and consultations are just as important in the last as in the early stages of our growth.
- Close involvement in health services is essential. Maddison's recognition in Beersheva of the importance of close cooperation between the University and the Health Service has gradually been realized after many years of trust building and cooperation. We do run a substantial risk that this will become a professional priority rather than a priority for the community good. And we do risk our priorities being hijacked by those of the health service. These risks must be guarded against.
- We must seek links with appropriate departments in the rest of the University to broaden our perspective. Recent appointments to Chairs in Social Work and Sociology will help us to expand our students' experience of the social dimension of health—a dimension that has lost emphasis.
- The curriculum must be continually informed by an awareness of issues that emerge in the community. It will not do for us to be bound only to books and to theory. This awareness has given impetus to developments in a number of fields including community child and family care, drug and alcohol, medical genetics, child abuse, AIDS, aged care, and fertility. It has also led to proposals currently before the Commonwealth Government to set up in Newcastle two centers—one for the study of environmental toxicology, drawing on the challenge of industry, and another for a Drug Evaluation Unit, drawing on our strength in pharmacoepidemiology.
- We need to be alert to the hazards of external funds earmarked for specific purposes. These can beguile us off course. This is especially obvious in the health service. In the Australian health scene it is much easier to develop projects in the curative and technical field than in the public health and preventive fields.
- Program evaluation is crucial. We have had a number of initiatives but we have not been as persistent as we should. The Monitoring and Evaluation Committee provides us with concrete feedback from the course as it runs. The temptation to make changes in the curriculum based on student opinion without the benefit of a longer period of reflection must be re-

sisted. Evaluation related to outcome is much more difficult but it does provide that longer time scale. Unfortunately it is usually carried out in the years immediately following graduation, before students have assumed a mature role in the community. Community orientation must not become a pedagogic end in itself. Meetings about medical education tend to be high on philosophy and only moderately explicit on the realities of experience and outcome. If evaluation shows no evidence of better contribution to the populations' health then our curriculum initiatives will have been for naught.

- The national accreditation system must be sympathetic to a community orientation. Frequently, new innovations are halted for fear that the General Medical Council or the Australian Medical Council (AMC) might not approve. The reality is that the AMC's educational guidelines are broad and positively encourage a creative response to public's health needs. The new guidelines soon to be written are likely to do the same.

- The needs of our students and their career development are a constant challenge. We are now admitting a large number of women students: Our students show women perform better than men at least in the internship. Women will bring new qualities to the care of patients and we need to capitalize on that and to facilitate their careers. We are also pushing for career opportunities generally in public health, population health, and health promotion. As has been long recognized in developing countries, creative initiatives in the undergraduate curriculum come to nothing if there is no career path to carry forward the new skills.

Finally we must remind ourselves that we are all subject to the norms of our profession, the academic expectations of our peers, and to the imperatives of the means of career advancement. One long-term observer of our faculty recently questioned whether we were genuinely community-oriented if we did not concentrate our efforts and our research on the fundamental social origins of health and disease. It is very likely that our amalgamation with the School of Health and links to other social science faculties will facilitate attending to the deeper social issues of our population. Academically it may be our major challenge for the future, to do that rigorously, sympathetically, and with a tangible impact on the achievements of our graduates.

Appendix 1: Greater Newcastle Health Area

Demographic and Socioeconomic Profile[2]

The estimated resident population of the Greater Newcastle Health Area was 339,850 (as of June 1986). The population pyramid for the Health Area (Fig. 6.1) shows a peak occuring in the 15 to 29-year age group for both sexes.

---

[2]Compiled by Professor Richard F. Heller and Ms D.M. Lloyd. Based on data provided by Research and Planning, New South Wales Department of Health (Hunter Region), August 1987.

TABLE 6.1. Present population and projected population growth in the greater Newcastle health area, 1986–1991.[a]

Area	1986	1991	Projected population growth 1986–1991 %
Newcastle LGA	138,500	137,500	− 0.72
Lake Macquarie LGA	164,900	175,500	+ 6.43
Port Stephens LGA	36,300	43,000	+18.46
Greater Newcastle	339,700	356,000	+ 4.80
Hunter Region	486,250	512,950	+ 5.49

[a]Based on information from the New South Wales Department of Environment and Planning.

The average number of live births per 1000 females aged 15–44 years in 1984–85 was 63.3, which is low compared to the rest of the Hunter Region (79.5) and New South Wales (66.8). It is important to note that there are variations in the population sizes and growth rates between the three Local Government Areas (LGAs) that make up the Greater Newcastle Health Area (Table 6.1).

Port Stephens LGA has experienced rapid population growth over the last 10 years due to both a high birth rate and migration into the area. This trend will ensure that in the future Port Stephens will become a substantial population component of the Greater Newcastle Health Area. By contrast, there has been a lower growth rate for Lake Macquarie LGA, whereas Newcastle LGA has experienced negative growth over the last decade because of an ageing population and migration to other areas.

There is now a well-established inverse relationship between socioeconomic status and health. Table 6.2 shows selected socioeconomic indicators

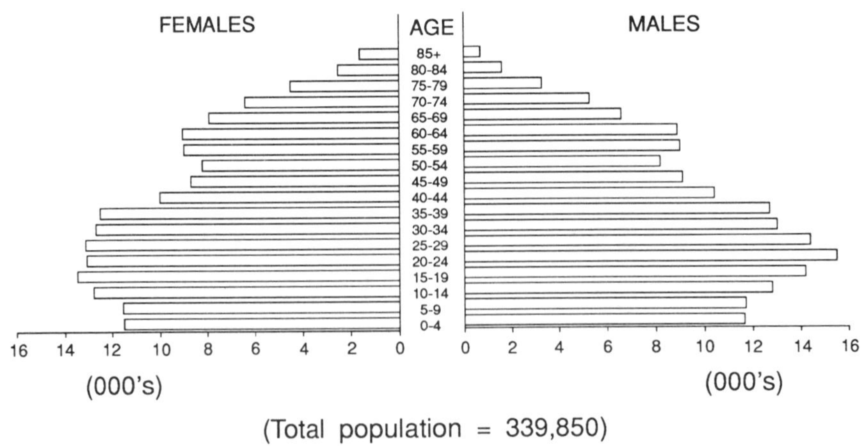

FIGURE 6.1. Estimated population pyramid of the greater Newcastle health area, 1986.

TABLE 6.2. Some socioeconomic indicators for the Greater Newcastle Health Area, 1981.

Indicator	GNHA	Hunter	NSW
Unemployment rate (%)[a]	12.5	12.0	10.5
Population with income <$1,000 p.a. (%)	3.2	3.5	3.3
Population with income $1,000–$12,000 p.a. (%)	54.5	54.6	54.9
Population with income >$26,000 p.a. (%)	1.8	1.9	2.4
Population in professional or admin. occupations (%)	16.9	15.5	18.5
Population in occupation of mining (%)	2.0	2.9	0.7
Aboriginals in population (%)	0.4	0.4	0.7
Foreign born in population (%)	11.7	10.3	20.3
Aged pensioners in population (%)	10.9	10.0	
Qualifications of potential labor force (% each category)			
Tertiary	5.5	5.5	7.5
Trade/other	20.0	18.5	18.0
None	63.5	65.0	62.5

[a]1985 figures.

for the Greater Newcastle Health Area that are relevant to health status. All these indicators are interrelated. For instance, members of our society who are aged pensioners or Aboriginal or unqualified are more likely to be poor. Those who are unemployed are more likely to have been unqualified, while those who are highly qualified are more likely to be employed and earning higher incomes.

These indicators provide an overall idea of the proportion of our society susceptible to or experiencing ill-health and, therefore, in greatest need of our health facilities and services. With regard to Australian society in general, we know that *unemployment* is associated with morbidity and chronic disability, as well as with mortality. Recent research has shown that ill-health is caused by the unemployment itself and not simply by chronic illness resulting in unemployment. Those who are *least educated and qualified* in our society report that they experience more ill-health than the rest of the population. Manual workers have more illnesses and die at younger ages compared to nonmanual workers. Differentials in the health status between the *more affluent and least affluent* members of population have been evident for many years. What is of great concern at present, however, is the widening gap between these two groups.

Aboriginal people experience more illnesses and are admitted to hospital more often than non-Aboriginals. They confront not only infectious diseases (in a similar manner to those in developing countries) but also life-style diseases common to all developed countries. *Aged pensioners* contend with the double disadvantage of old age and a low income, thus their health is often poor. The health status of *migrants* is often quite high when they arrive

TABLE 6.3. Major causes of mortality in the Greater Newcastle Health Area, 1979–1983.

Cause of mortality	Males	Females	Total	Total deaths (%)
	All ages			
Diseases of circulatory system	3682	3325	7007	53
Acute myocardial infarction	2018	1320	3338	25
Cerebrovascular disease	719	969	1688	13
Other	945	1036	1981	15
Malignant neoplasms	1704	1168	2872	22
Digestive organs	511	370	881	7
Lung	509	104	613	5
Breast	1	191	192	1
Other	683	503	1186	9
Diseases of the respiratory system	593	215	808	6
Chronic obstructive airways	283	53	336	3
Bronchitis, emphysema, asthma	140	47	187	1
Other	170	115	285	2
Accidents	502	226	728	5
Motor vehicle	323	108	431	3
Other	179	118	297	2
All other causes	1189	788	1977	14
Total	7670	5722	13392	100

in Australia, but social and economic stress, changing dietary patterns, and occupational health risks can bring about a deterioration over time.

Major Causes of Mortality[3]

A worthwhile point to consider regarding the major causes of death in the Health Area is how preventable are they? The major causes of death in the Greater Newcastle Health Area for all age groups are diseases of the circulatory system, with acute myocardial infarction (AMI) still being the greatest single cause. This pattern continues despite a reported Australia-wide decline in deaths from AMI since the late 1960s. Diseases of the circulatory system are followed by malignant neoplasms, diseases of the respiratory system, and accidents (both motor vehicle and other); together these account for 86% of all deaths in the Health Area (Table 6.3).

It may be enlightening to look at causes of death by age-group as well as by sex (Table 6.4).

It then becomes clear that for young people (up to 24 years of age) accidents, especially motor vehicle accidents, are a major cause of mortality. In the 25 to 44-year-old age group the cross-over takes place between ac-

---

[3]Compiled by Professor Richard F. Heller and Ms D.M. Lloyd. Based on data provided by the Hunter Health Statistics Unit and Research and Planning, New South Wales Department of Health (Hunter Region), October 1987.

TABLE 6.4. Major causes of mortality in the Greater Newcastle Health Area by age group and sex, 1979–1983.

Age group (years)	Cause of mortality[a]	Total deaths for each age group (%) Males	Females
0–14	Perinatal mortality	34.6	32.8
	Congenital anomalies	21.7	20.3
	Motor vehicle accidents	10.6	13.3
	Symptoms, signs, etc.	10.6	9.4
	Other accidents	5.1	
	Other malignant neoplasms		3.9
	Diseases of nervous system		3.9
15–24	Motor vehicle accidents	58.4	40.5
	Other accidents	10.9	12.2
	Suicide and self-inflicted	7.9	8.1
	Leukemia	3.0	
	Congenital anomalies		6.8
	Diseases of nervous system	3.0	5.4
25–44	Motor vehicle accidents	20.7	10.1
	Acute myocardial infarction	14.4	7.1
	Other accidents	13.1	
	Suicide and self-inflicted	9.5	7.1
	Cerebrovascular disease		7.7
	Malignant neoplasms of breast		7.1
	Other malignant neoplasms	6.6	
45–64	Acute myocardial infarction	33.2	21.4
	Other forms of heart disease	9.1	
	Malignant neoplasms of lung	8.0	
	Cerebrovascular disease	7.3	10.5
	Malignant neoplasms of breast		8.9
	Malignant neoplasms of genital organs		6.0
	Other malignant neoplasms	5.6	5.2
65+	Acute myocardial infarction	27.4	25.1
	Cerebrovascular disease	11.6	19.4
	Malignant neoplasms of lung	7.2	
	Other Ischemic heart disease	6.6	8.0
	Other forms of heart disease		7.4
	Chronic airways obstruction	5.2	
	Other malignant neoplasms		3.0

[a]Five leading causes for each age group and sex.

cidents, as a major cause of death, and heart disease. For the older age groups heart disease, particularly AMI, becomes dominant in both sexes. Many more males than females die of motor vehicle accidents in the 15 to 24 and 25 to 44-year-old age groups. Cerebrovascular disease becomes a major cause of death in females as they grow older.

The four major causes of mortality in the Hunter Health Area, as in the rest of Australia, are all noninfectious diseases related to our affluent lifestyle. All have behavioral and environmental risk factors that are modifiable.

TABLE 6.5. Major causes of mortality in the Greater Newcastle Health Area, 1979–1983, and associated behavioral and environmental risk factors.

Major cause of mortality % total deaths in GNHA	Behavioral and environmental risk factors
Diseases of the circulatory system (53%)	Smoking, hypertension, blood lipid levels,
Acute myocardial infarction (25%)	diet, exercise, relative weight
Cerebrovascular disease (13%)	Hypertension, diet(?), smoking(?), oral
	contraceptives plus smoking (young women)
Malignant neoplasms (22%)	Diet, alcohol, and smoking (upper alimentary
Digestive organs (7%)	tract)
Lung (5%)	Smoking, occupational exposures
Breast (1%)	Reproductive history, body weight, diet
Diseases of the respiratory system (6%)	Smoking, occupational exposures
Chronic airways obstruction (3%)	
Accidents (5%)	Alcohol consumption, driver's skill, vehicle
Motor vehicle (3%)	safety, road conditions

Consider the role of just one risk factor, smoking, in diseases such as AMI, cerebrovascular disease, lung cancer, malignant neoplasms of the upper digestive organs, and chronic airways obstruction (Table 6.5). Prevention is possible and worth considering in all these diseases to avoid not only the mortality but also the morbidity.

Appendix 2: The Objectives of the Newcastle Educational Program

The undergraduate educational program of the faculty of Medicine at the University of Newcastle is designed to ensure that, at its conclusion, the graduate can demonstrate the ability to

- engage in productive professional relationships and maintain those relationships to acquire, evaluate and communicate information;
- apply the processes of critical reasoning to medical care;
- apply his or her understanding of illness to its prevention, identification, and management, and to the promotion and maintenance of health;
- apply his or her understanding of the practice of medicine in a community or population context; and
- take responsibility for evaluating his or her own performance and implementing his own education.

These objectives assume a dynamic environment in which medicine will be practiced. In consequence the graduating student should be able to participate in change and to adapt to change.

Domain 1: Professional Skills

By the time of graduation students should demonstrate the ability to relate to, and function in an effective fashion with, patients and their families as well as with fellow professionals by

1.1. manifesting those personal characteristics essential for the practice of excellent medicine, including: (1) an awareness of their own assets, limitations, and responsiveness; (2) responsibility, thoroughness, reliability, and confidentiality; and (3) sensitivity to the needs of others and concern for other persons;

1.2. consistently displaying a deep regard for others, thereby showing that caring and comforting are held to be among the appropriate tasks for a medical practitioner;

1.3. showing that their approach to all patients reflects an understanding that the person who is ill is more important than the illness from which he suffers;

1.4. applying in an observable way both an understanding of the importance of the doctor/patient relationship, and its place in the provision of medical care at all levels;

1.5. showing (1) an enlightened involvement with patients, free from undue interference with communication created by the excessive use of psychological defense mechanisms, thus avoiding the demonstration of aloof and unfeeling detachment, undue aggression, and other unhelpful behaviors; (2) a recognition of those patients who display dependency or hostility to an extent that affects patient management and patient cooperation, and interacting appropriately with them; (3) an awareness of how their own personality affects their interaction with their patients and how their own anxieties and prejudices may alter patient attitudes and behavior; and (4) a capacity to accord with ethical principles that restrain practitioners from taking advantage of patients;

1.6. applying an awareness of the role of the physician in health/welfare professional teams and working cooperatively within them;

1.7. showing the establishment of effective communication and cooperation with a wide variety of patients, healthy members of the community, and other professionals;

1.8. applying an awareness of the potential conflicts imposed on them by their obligations to themselves and their families, to their patients, and the community they serve;

1.9. applying an understanding of the ethical basis of medical practice;

1.10. applying logical and probabilistic approaches to clinical problems, and displaying a tolerance for ambiguous situations by coping with uncertainty in the clinical context;

1.11. applying skills in interacting with patients to increase the probability of accurate diagnosis, patient satisfaction and compliance, and the patient's accurate recall of supplied information, and to decrease the anxiety associated with potentially threatening medical interventions;
1.12. obtaining a clinical history from a wide variety of patients, and eliciting clinical signs through the conduct of physical examination—skills that should be demonstrated with both adults and children;
1.13. writing an accurate clinical record on the basis of their own observations, recognizing and defining a clinical problem, and communicating their findings to others clearly and concisely (orally and/or in writing); and
1.14. carrying out the basic tasks required to be performed by all medical graduates during their preregistration postgraduation period.

Domain 2: Critical Reasoning

By the time of graduation students should demonstrate the ability to apply the processes of *scientific reasoning* by

2.1. making reliable observations of cellular, pathophysiological, and behavioral phenomena, extracting the relevant data from these observations, and integrating where appropriate the information provided from these three perspectives on human biology;
2.2. applying a critical appreciation of the techniques, procedures, goals, and results of biomedical research, and applying the various scientific methods in current use (particularly the hypothetico-deductive method) to assess the reliability and validity of observations, and the testing of hypotheses;
2.3. applying scientific principles to the study of the behavior of individuals, groups, and institutions;
2.4. locating biomedical information required for the understanding and management of medical problems, through the use of available educational resources;
2.5. assessing the veracity of conclusions based on reported data, including the interpretation of statistical treatment employed for the analysis of such data; and
2.6. interpreting and criticizing data from evaluation studies of medical services supplied to communities or populations.

Domain 3: Identification, Prevention, and Management of Illness

By the time of graduation students should demonstrate the ability to apply their understanding of *illness* and its *prevention and management*, by

3.1. applying an understanding of the mechanism and significance of health-related physical and behavioral events and adaptive responses to those events, both normal and abnormal, at levels ranging from the molecular to that of the community and wider environment;

3.2. applying an understanding of biological, psychological, social, developmental, and environmental mechanisms to the diagnosis, management, and prevention of illness;

3.3. applying a knowledge of the significance and limitations of the findings of standard laboratory and allied investigations;

3.4. planning and interpreting a program of investigations appropriate to the clinical problem presented by the patient, with due regard for patient comfort and safety and for economic factors;

3.5. applying the understanding implicit in 3.2, 3.3, and 3.4 to the diagnosis of a defined range of clinical problems;

3.6. applying an understanding of the principles of therapeutics, including the possible complications and human costs of treatment;

3.7. taking responsibility, under supervision, for the management of a defined range of common, acute, and chronic clinical conditions;

3.8. devising and implementing, under supervision, a management program appropriate for patients with chronic, intractable illness, including terminal disease;

3.9. carrying out the basic psychomotor tasks required to be performed by all medical graduates during their preregistration postgraduation period;

3.10. applying an understanding of the impact of illness on families, and the importance of family factors in prevention, treatment, and rehabilitation;

3.11. demonstrating a positive, consistent, and informed behavior toward promotion and maintenance of health, as well as the prevention of illness at both individual and population levels, and skill in educating patients, their families, and other health professionals for this purpose; and

3.12. applying an awareness that major changes in individual and community health are likely to depend as much or more on change in the behavior of people as on the manipulation of the physical environment.

Domain 4: Population Medicine

By the time of graduation students should demonstrate the ability to apply their understanding of the practice of *medicine in a community or population* by

4.1. applying an awareness of the importance of the practice of medicine in both community settings and hospital settings;

4.2. contributing to the identification and solution of community health problems and to the evaluation of the results of such interventions;

4.3. applying knowledge of the incidence and prevalence of disease in the Australian community;

4.4. applying an understanding of the organization of the Australian health care system, as exemplified by that existing in the Hunter Health Area at primary, secondary and tertiary care levels, from conception to death, including the care of the chronically sick of all ages, and including treatment, prevention, and the promotion and maintenance of health;

4.5. evaluating health care needs of individuals, groups, and communities, and evaluating the efficacy of health care delivery and the functioning of community health services;

4.6. applying an understanding of the impact of illness on families, and the importance of family factors in prevention, treatment, and rehabilitation;

4.7. applying a positive, consistent, and informed behavior toward promotion and maintenance of health, as well as the prevention of illness at both individual and population levels;

4.8. applying an awareness that major changes in individual and community health are likely to depend as much or more on change in the behavior of people as on the manipulation of the physical environment; and

4.9. applying an awareness of the role of the physician in health/welfare professional teams, and working cooperatively within them.

Domain 5: Self-Directed Learning

By the time of graduation students should demonstrate the ability to take responsibility for *evaluating* their *own performance, implementing their own education, and contributing to the education of others,* by

5.1. monitoring, granted appropriate consultation, their own progress in the acquisition of information and skills;

5.2. monitoring and evaluating, for the purpose of mutual education, the performance of their juniors and their peers;

5.3. engaging in a critical evaluation of the objectives and implementation of the faculty's education program;

5.4. being educationally prepared to undertake postgraduate training; and

5.5. demonstrating that medical education in its full sense is a lifelong activity and investing time in the maintenance and further development of their own knowledge and skills, above and beyond the pursuit of higher professional qualifications.

Acknowledgments. Vicki Shephard, a second year student of this Faculty, has undertaken much of the background research for this chapter. Barbara Wallis, Instructional Designer, and Kathy Byrne, Information Officer, assisted in editing. Typing through multiple drafts has been done by Vicki Caesar. The chapter has benefitted from discussions with many staff and students involved in the establishment of the school. Some I have mentioned by name but realize the hazards of picking out any from a team. Many others could equally have been mentioned for their contributions over the years. Space does not allow full recognition. Comments from them on early drafts helped to clarify history, philosophy, and experience. The author thanks them all.

References

Clarke, R.M., Leeder, S.R., and Maddison, D.C. 1981. Health orientation in medical education, Australia. *Prev Med* **10:**719–725.

Dickinson, J., Heller, R.F., Hensley, M.J., Kelman, R., Leeder, S.R., Lloyd, D., and Reid, A. 1985. Community medicine at Newcastle in the next five years. University of Newcastle (unpublished).

Doherty, R.L. (Chairman). 1988. Australian Medical Education and Workforce into the Twenty-first Century: Committee of Inquiry into Medical Education and Medical Workforce. Canberra: Australian Government Publishing Service.

Faculty of Medicine. 1976a. Working paper IV: Community Medicine. University of Newcastle.

Faculty of Medicine. 1976b. Working paper V: Towards a policy on student selection. University of Newcastle.

Faculty of Medicine. 1976c. Working paper VI: Undergraduate programme objectives. University of Newcastle.

Faculty of Medicine. 1977. Working paper XIV: Learning objectives for undergraduate education. University of Newcastle.

Faculty of Medicine. 1979. Working paper XVII: Revised undergraduate programme objectives. University of Newcastle.

Faculty of Medicine. 1980. The undergraduate programme: Volume 1. University of Newcastle.

Faculty of Medicine. 1983. The undergraduate programme: Volume 2. University of Newcastle.

Faculty of Medicine. 1986. The undergraduate programme: Volume 3. University of Newcastle.

Gordon, J.J., et al. 1989. Evaluating interns' performance using simulating patients in a casualty department. *Med J Aust* **151:**18–21.

Karmel, P. (Chairman). 1973. *Expansion of Medical Education. Report of the Committee on Medical Schools to the Australian Universities Commission.* Canberra: Australian Government Publishing Service.

Maddison, D.M. 1975. Medical school planning study tour. (Unpublished document). University of Newcastle.

Maddison, D.M. 1977. Curricular innovation: A tale of two cities. (Working group on educational strategies). Manila: World Health Organization, Western Pacific Regional Office.

Maddison, D.M. 1978. What's wrong with medical education? *Med Educ* **12:**97–102.

Powis, D.A., Neame, R.L.B., Bristow, T., and Murphy, L.B. 1988. The objective structured interview for medical student selection. *Br Med J* **296:**765–768.

Redman, S., and Hamilton, J.D. 1989. Community-based education in industrialised countries. University of Newcastle.
Saunders, N.A.S., et al. 1982. A clinical supervisor's rating form. *Medical Teacher* **4:**151–154.
Submissions to the Karmel Commission. 1972. Newcastle Chamber of Commerce, Royal Newcastle Hospital, University of Newcastle, Central Northern Medical Association.
White, K.L. 1986. Australia's Bicentennial Health Initiative. Canberra: Commonwealth Department of Health.

Discussion

Harvey Barkun

John Hamilton's chapter elicits a certain amount of jealousy simply because of the opportunity he describes of fashioning a medical school responsive to perceived needs in the latter part of the twentieth century. The ability to implement a new curriculum and employ new teaching methods has frequently presented almost insurmountable problems for established schools.

Newcastle obviously recognized the need for a faculty-based curriculum, and the absolute necessity to recruit leaders whose philosophy, coupled with credibility and leadership qualities, would permit implementation. Educational objectives and admission criteria were developed, and the school opened with a new approach to the training of general practitioners. Hamilton's description of the five domains of learning clearly lays out the very focused emphasis on the Community Base, on communications, and on ethical issues. The areas of Community Medicine, Behavioral Sciences, Health, Law, and Ethics are described in great detail, while Internal Medicine and the Surgical Sciences occupy much less space. Even the Basic Sciences have a Community orientation.

The Faculty of Medicine is highly involved in the structure and administration of Health Services at the hospital level and at the regional level. With such involvement goes the inevitable role of administration and the accompanying politics. Just two of the prices to be paid! In the realm of postgraduate medical education, the author bemoans the fact that given the hospital-based training programs in the management of acute illness in tertiary care institutions, trainees may unlearn the community orientation instilled in them during their undergraduate years. A relatively new undergraduate accreditation system and a recent Commission on medical human resources related to needs will hopefully maintain the momentum in curriculum innovation and community-based teaching. The future of Newcastle's innovations is far from assured. Diminishing funding and a Government bent on cost-effectiveness—in both the function and structure of the medical school—leave many questions unanswered. The author concludes with 12 cogent strategies that must be considered and implemented carefully if New-castle's plan is to be realized.

Hamilton's account is clear, well-documented, and vividly conveys the orientation, objectives, pitfalls, and evolution of the new medical school that has twinned community-orientation with problem-based learning—a path currently being followed by more and more Canadian faculties of Medicine. To McMaster, the patriarch, we must now add Sherbrooke, Dalhousie, Queen's, Montreal, and others to a greater or lesser degree. So-called traditional schools are modifying curriculums radically to meet community needs and fulfill their social responsibilities to these communities. Educational objectives in both undergraduate and postgraduate programs can be fashioned so as to honor the social contract. Hamilton states: "Finally, and most importantly, we need more information about whether the program works. Only two studies to date have attempted to explore whether graduates from New-castle are different from those of other medical schools in Australia." Therein lies the ultimate judgment. Until we devise measurements and criteria to make such judgments, we really don't know.

George I. Lythcott

The integral components of the curriculum crafted at Newcastle are not new. What is innovative is the integration of these into a community-learning experience with disease prevention and health promotion as hallmarks. Essential linkages that provide significant collaboration in teaching and research among the basic and clinical science departments, appropriate university departments outside the medical school, and with the health services are supported by a solid foundation of educational principles. Moreover, this new school has wisely committed itself to problem-solving methods of instruction. These are provided in a continuum for Newcastle students that extends from admission through graduation.

The decision to develop such educational initiatives in a new medical school certainly avoids many of the inevitable problems of similar attempts when academic departments are already firm in their profiles and agendas. Considering the objectives of the program and the nuances of its curriculum, and in order to maximize the opportunity to enhance the quality of its graduates, it follows that the criteria for the selection of new students are critical. The use of admission criteria other than academic achievement is not new. In specifics, however, the processes for admission to Newcastle are. Overt participation by individuals from the community in the selection process, the formal tests to assess motivation, empathy, and problem-solving skills and the opportunity for two personal applicant interviews in sharpening the final decision are, indeed, seductive.

Hamilton, with clarity, objectivity, and rare candor, has presented an account of the events and tortuous processes involved in the creation of a nontraditional medical school. Engaged, until my recent retirement, in the development of a new school with practically identical objectives in New York City, it was particularly instructive for me to have the opportunity to review the Newcastle experience. Having done so, my empathy is exceeded only by my admiration for what the group has accomplished. Let me, then, briefly comment on a few of the many points presented: the commitment to innovation, the curriculum and instruction, the admissions process, and, finally, evaluation of the program.

As the author points out, the commitment at the several levels of influence within and outside the school, in the development of a new model, is fundamental. Commitment at any level presumes, of course, an understanding and acceptance of both clearly defined objectives and a credible plan for implementation. The founding Dean wrote, "being given the mandate to construct an innovative program does not assure absolute freedom to carry it out" and he listed the most important constraints: the characteristics, attitudes, and expectations of the parent university, those of the local medical profession, the level of funding, and the characteristics and qualities of the existing health services. We could add a few more, from our experience in a state-supported institution, not the least of which are the local politicians.

While the jury is still out with respect to an evaluation of the new school at Newcastle, the leadership has taken a solid approach in addressing this important parameter. As an extension of its plans for evaluation, the group at Newcastle asks itself a fundamental question: How will we sustain a community orientation? The 12 strategies they embarked on to address this point are thoughtful and reflect keen insights into the realities. If maintained, they assure that the original orientation will be sustained.

One long-term observer of the Newcastle experience questioned whether or not they were genuinely community oriented if they did not concentrate their efforts and research on the fundamental social origins of health and disease. In response, Dean Hamilton ends his chapter with the acknowledgement that "This may be our major challenge for the future."

David H.H. Metcalfe

This is a fascinating account of what must be, by any standards, one of the success stories in medical education in the late twentieth century. The relative shortness of its history allows the author to explain this school's origins, and its growth from preexisting circumstances, in a way that is nearly impossible for older schools whose history is shrouded in the mists of time. We must remember that many of them too were responses to local needs and were often the achievement of philanthropists who appreciated them. The fact that in many cases they seem to have drifted away from meeting local needs is not necessarily only due to their preoccupations narrowing; the local needs have changed too. Newcastle is, in theory, just as vulnerable to such drift, over the long haul, but it has seen the danger and tried to put and keep in place mechanisms to prevent it.

Several points are of particular interest. The antipathy of a new University to taking on a medical school had its counterpart in the United Kingdom, when existing staff felt threatened by the disproportionate numbers of professors in the new faculty who could swamp the existing University bodies. Yet only 8 years later Newcastle University not only welcomed the new school but felt strong enough to propose innovative guidelines for the nature of its course. In the United Kingdom the new schools tried to avoid statements of any bias toward general or community practice lest it detracted from their power to recruit what they saw as high quality staff and students, since both the other Disciplines were (and are) seen as low caste. The quotation from the Karmel report spells out very clearly the contribution of these Disciplines to teaching Medicine as a whole. The capture of David Maddison as Dean, and his copllaboration with the Vice-Chancellor, Don George, were to ensure that development would be in the hands of one of the clearest thinkers in medical education of his time. His planning papers for the new school were models of enlightenment and inspiration.

Honeymoons always end, and once things start to move, feelings, even among erstwhile supporters, get ruffled. The "sitting tenants" will have had their own ideas about what the new school would be like, and what it would do for them, and when these expectations prove unfounded they feel betrayed. Newcastle was no exception. Professional conservatism was compounded by political conservatism; both distrust a "bottom up" needs-derived philosophy, whether of service, teaching, or research, and both prefer a "top down," "we know best" approach. It is naive to think that government support comes without strings. A community orientation in health care is bound to identify threats to health and failures to provide services that result from current and previous government policy (e.g., inadequate housing, employment, and pensions, and unhealthy environments) and which are seen to need government action. When the government is out of sympathy with such needs, the school that identifies with them is at risk.

Hamilton's description of curricular design is a fascinating and informative account of the achievement of a well thought out, objectively led system of learning to be taught to the students. The adoption of problem-based and vertically integrated learning has made the basic philosophy and the design case inevitable. One of the fascinating aspects is the delegation of responsibility to broad Disciplines rather than departments, and to a great extent thereby avoiding the territorial wars and "robber baron" syndromes prevalent elsewhere.

While linkages to the community that begat the school have been institutionalized, the school remains vulnerable to "top downism" unless materials provided by the Health Statistics Unit are used by delegates to the various committees described, to guide relevant actions.

Perhaps the most important part of the chapter is Section VIII in which Hamilton poses the question: "How will Newcastle sustain a community orientation?" He spells out the danger of regression to the mean, which has certainly characterized new schools in the United Kingdom, and sets out the requirements to defend against it: continuous review (stasis is regression), community/population-based research by all Disciplines (no retreat to the ivory tower, the wet lab must be relevant), viable (not token) links with the ordinary people in the community, in particular deferred student time for involvement with people, families, and groups there, avoidance of conflict with the health services when perceived needs are difficult to meet, openness to other University Disciplines (not just the "civilized" ones, but the "difficult" ones like sociology, economics, and politics, which are not above a bit of doctor-bashing), needs-led (e.g., AIDS, child abuse, and fertility) curricular development, and, lastly, wariness about funding with strings attached. He also points out the problem of national accreditation systems whose values are not community oriented, and of career progression criteria, in academia, that do not include the relevance of teaching and research to the people's needs.

We should be grateful to Hamilton for this lucid and well-organized account of an exciting endeavor and for the soberness of his recognition of the dangers of regression. Perhaps it could be summed up as "No medical school can ever achieve 'escape velocity'; energy must continuously be applied to combat gravity."

General Discussion

There was general agreement that Newcastle has had an enormous influence on undergraduate and postgraduate education in Australia and internationally. This contribution was termed truly inspirational and was distinguished from other plans and aspirations because it is a vision that has actually come to pass.

Two areas of concern were expressed by some:

- The outreach of the educational program into social problems of the community has an inherent danger of overmedicalizing the community (involving medical personnel where the problems might best be solved by nonmedically associated methods); and
- The development of a new hospital now under construction might be attended by a serious risk of the medical school's program regressing toward the conventional. However, the old hospital is literally crumbling and safeguards are now said to be in place to counter this possibility. Admiration was expressed, however, for the way in which the school has prevented development of powerful fiefdoms that might distort the original objectives of the school.

Other questions arose. As in any innovation in medical education or health services, the influence of the Hawthorne Effect needs to be kept in mind. Can the objectives of the Newcastle program be sustained over time? Do graduates relapse toward the attitudes of their more conventionally trained colleagues during the intern and residency years? Will it be necessary to extend the duration of medical education from 5 to 6 years as a number of other Australian schools have done? What are the longer term results of the career pathways, attainments, attitudes, and skills of Newcastle graduates compared to graduates of other schools? How widely can this model of medical education be spread?

7
Essential Institutional Competencies for Population-Based Education

DAVID H.H. METCALFE

I. Introduction

If a medical school is not turning out a mix of clinicians capable of meeting the wide variety of needs for medical care that characterizes all human populations, the relevance and validity of its teaching and research must be called into question, however distinguished that school may be. Its competence could be said to comprise the competencies of its graduates in meeting the entire population's medical care needs, either by clinical work or research. Institutional competence has to be addressed, therefore, in terms of the competencies bestowed on those it educates, and the way that task is addressed. The more hubristic its image the wider the scope it may claim for its graduates' distinguished contributions, but whether it aims to serve the world, its nation, region, or home town, it must relate its teaching and research to the whole range of problems encountered in whatever population it claims to serve. Where it is supported by public money there is an implied contract to provide for the population from whom the money comes. Meeting the needs of a defined population demands of a medical school teaching and research which addresses three "dimensions" of medicine: comprehensiveness, generality, and balance.

- *Comprehensiveness* means the whole range of medical care problems: all disease types (infective, degenerative, neoplastic, etc.) and all stages of natural history (at risk, preclinical, acute, chronic, and terminal).
- *Generality* means the medical care needs of the whole population: not just the rich, or the Caucasians, or the people who come to its clinics.
- *Balance* means the whole range of clinical skills: not only precise diagnosis, but prevention, acute and chronic disease management (not just treatment), rehabilitation, and terminal care.

It is not good enough to teach students how to diagnose the small number of "interesting" diseases for which a center of excellence has become a major national or international resource, without due attention to their treatment; let alone the diagnosis, management, and prevention of the whole range of illnesses they will encounter on completion of their training. They cannot all be liver transplanters!

This chapter presents three conceptual models in an attempt to define the competencies required by the mix of medical graduates needed to provide balanced, comprehensive care to the general public of the school's target population, whether local, regional, national, or international. The extent to which they hold such competencies reflects on the overall competence of their medical school.

These competencies are basic and need to be held by all doctors, but will be exercised in different proportions and different combinations depending on the situation in which the graduate works. The expertise related to individual specialties, whether secondary or tertiary, is to be added, at a suitable point in training, to this basic set. The basic set of competencies derived from these models is that of the primary care generalist for two reasons, one educational and one professional. The educational reason is that in most countries (but not all) primary care generalists currently have a shorter postgraduate training than specialists, and so have to have the basic competencies well-established at graduation. The professional reason is that the more specialized the task, the more the specialist depends on the work of other doctors. If that division of responsibility is to be technically and economically efficient, the specialists must understand the others' work and respect their expertise, just as much as they expect their expertise to be respected. Since students are exposed to many more specialists, who become powerful role models, than generalists, the latter respect can usually be taken for granted, whereas respect for the generalist cannot.

The models are related to each other. The first illustrates the way in which medical care services are related to the society they serve and reflect their internal characteristics. The second illustrates the distribution of different levels of health in such a society and attempts to define the different medical tasks at or between given levels. The third illustrates the range of skills needed to perform those tasks in relationship to both medical and social and cultural pressures. They could be used by the faculty as a template against which to check their teaching about needs, tasks, and skills, and to establish a frame of reference whereby their students could understand the relevance of what they are being taught. Like all two-dimensional models these are very limited, and may be challenged as simplistic. They are not offered as a definitive description of the interactions that they depict, but as a starting point, or agenda, for deeper consideration.

II. The First Model: A Society and Its Hospitals: The Amoeba and the Box

Figure 7.1 displays the characteristics of any population in the Western world (and many in the third world too), of primary care and of hospital-based specialist medicine. All the characteristics noted in the "society" area have

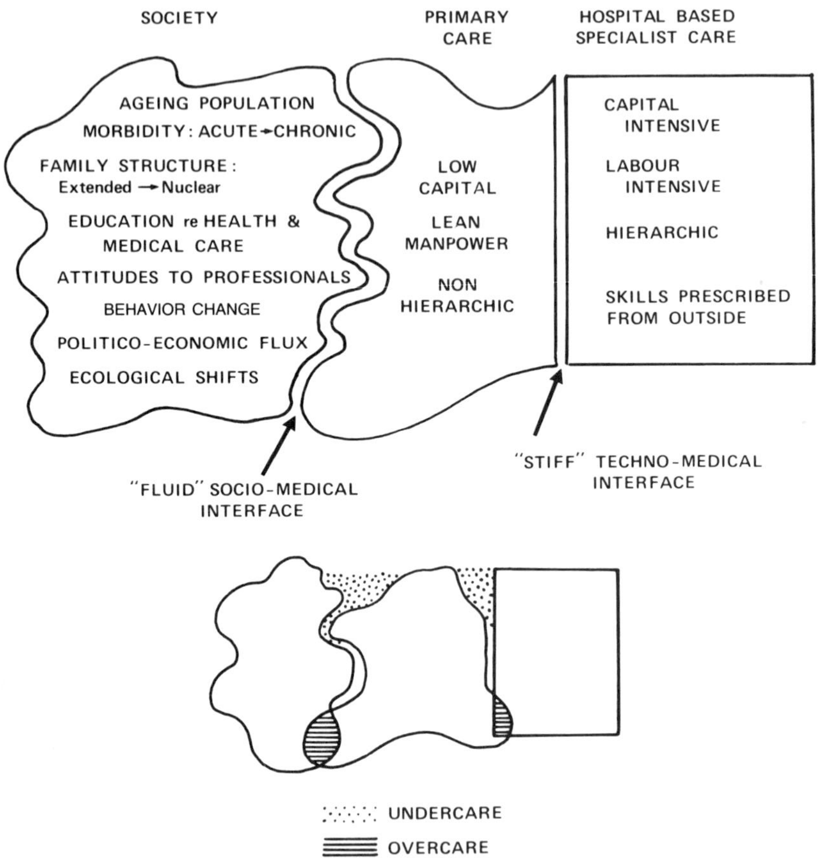

FIGURE 7.1. The first model. Characteristics of primary care and of hospital-based specialist medicine. The ideal (top): The reality (bottom).

direct effects on the patterns of disease and the way people present for, and comply with, care; there are of course other characteristics. Society is drawn like an amoeba because it is always changing, pushing out pseudopodia here (taking some more responsibility for its health, or transferring demand to "alternative" therapists) and drawing them in there (demanding care for "new" perceived needs, e.g., screening). The rate of change of these, and other parameters, is high and probably higher than we realize. Some can be documented in numerical terms, as, for example, the proportion of those over 65 years old or the number unemployed or homeless. Others have been, and continue to be, subjects of specific epidemiological, sociological, and anthropological research. Others are informally recognized by clinical experience. Of the research disciplines mentioned, however, only epidemiology gets any recognition in most medical schools.

All the characteristics noted in the "hospital box" reduce flexibility. Once capital has been invested in large buildings and sophisticated equipment neither of which are readily resalable, it cannot be quickly redeployed. Hospitals have large staffs [83% of the million employees of the National Health Service (NHS) in the United Kingdom are hospital-based] so task change requiring role change requires huge retraining. Moreover both professional and technical hospital staff are deployed in strictly regulated hierarchies. Not only would change have to be negotiated all the way down each hierarchy, but those at the top have got there by being good at doing the job in the old way and are unlikely to relish change. Lastly, professional advancement is controlled by examinations set by professional bodies outside the hospital concerned (e.g., the Royal Colleges in the United Kingdom). With all the difficulties examiners face in balancing validity with reliability, once an examination has been shown to be reasonably valid, fairly discriminating, and as reliable as possible (because reliability is in effect "fairness" and candidates' livelihoods depend upon it) it tends to stay stable. Thus while the examinations stay the same, the task for which they are testing competence may have changed. Learning is always directed to passing the next examination rather than to performing the task for which it tries to assess competence. Indeed the way tasks are tackled can come to reflect the ethos of the examination more than clinical effectiveness and efficiency. These are not pejorative statements; in a high intensity operation like a general hospital stability is essential. As long as the task remains the same (the diagnosis and treatment of acute illness or acute phases of chronic illness in referred patients) stability is an asset. However the relatively inflexible and stable nature of hospital-based specialist medicine presents a sharp contrast to the ever changing medical care needs of the "social amoeba."

If, between the "amoeba" and the "box" however, there is a properly trained and resourced primary care sector, the mismatch is neutralized. Primary care is low on capital investment, lean on manpower, and aims to be nonhierarchical and informal in its intra- and interprofessional relationships. Increasingly, however, it has established examinations to assure competence, with the concomitant problems outlined above. Indeed, validity is even harder to attain with regard to the protean nature of primary care, where skills and attitudes are relatively more important than knowledge per se, but much more difficult to test reliably. Primary care therefore has characteristics that allow flexibility; the task can be varied as the problems encountered and the way they are expressed change. Theoretically, therefore, primary care maintains a fluid, responsive "sociomedical" interface with the society in which it works, and a stiffer "technomedical" interface with its back-up hospital-based specialist care. Paradoxically, in the last 30 years the hospital task has not changed significantly while the technology with which it carries it out has changed almost out of recognition. Primary care on the other hand has seen major changes in its task without very noticeable changes in the technology that it uses.

This is the model of a rational health service. The effectiveness of such a service will be reduced by incompetence at either interface, where there may be overcare or undercare. At the sociomedical interface undercare may represent failures in accessibility, availability, or preventive outreach; people are not getting services from which they could benefit. Overcare results from the medicalization of nonmedical, that is nonillness, distress: bereavement treated by antidepressants, anxiety by tranquilizers, and somatization by invasive investigation. These are the results of applying a crude medical model: "Distress is the product of disease; diagnosis and treatment are required." Dysfunction at the sociomedical interface is a failure of primary care doctors' skill and application and must reflect the fact that their medical education was almost entirely in the hospital "box."

At the technomedical interface, undercare may represent failure to refer, failure to accept, or politicoeconomic factors reflected in rationing, whether by waiting list, or ability to pay. Overcare results from collusion between primary and secondary care doctors (and patients sometimes) to "play games" with the care of patients whose needs are difficult to meet in conventional terms. As a result they are subjected to unnecessary investigation, and sometimes treatment, at great cost and some risk. Overcare here too may represent an educational failure, particularly in the need to establish explicit objectives for care, and in the teaching of ethics.

Using this model the faculty should ask themselves the following types of questions: "Do our students know enough about the sociomedical interface? For example, do they understand the forces acting on people which affect their decision whether or not to enter care? Do they understand the justification for unmandated "outreach" programs? Do our students know enough about the technomedical interface? Do they understand the dynamics of referral and the handing over and receiving of responsibility, or the costs to the patient of crossing it?" They could use this model to justify to students instruction from psychologists and sociologists about topics such as health beliefs and locus of control, and from ethicists about mandates and permissions.

Clearly effective primary care demands appropriate education, some of which must be in the field and specifically addressed to the tasks to be done at both interfaces. The competencies required to discharge those tasks, and therefore the educational objectives of such a learning opportunity, will be discussed later, but it is worth reiterating that a proper understanding of society, its needs, and the sociomedical interface demand cognizance with, and respect for, epidemiological, sociological, psychological, and anthropological research methods. It should also be noted that the epidemiology of a defined population provides data on probability, a necessary, but not sufficient, component of the diagnostic process.

III. The Second Model: A Society and Its Health Status: A Cellular Model

The human life cycle is characterized by changing vulnerabilities to disease; few if any people lead a disease-free life and die simply of old age. Most people are well most of the time, or take brief excursions into minor short-term illness that may or may not need treatment to cure it or ameliorate its effects. Sooner or later most people succumb to a major acute illness from which, with treatment, they may make a complete recovery (e.g., appendicitis or pneumonia) or which turns out to be the initial phase of a chronic disease (e.g., myocardial infarction announcing ischemic heart disease). Others may slip into a chronic disease without a dramatic acute presentation (e.g., hypertension, osteoarthritis, or psoriasis).

Although chronic disease is, by definition, incurable, subjectively it is experienced at four levels of effect:

- *Impairment* (pathophysiology) without impact on function;
- *Disability*, where the impairment results in some reduced function that, however, does not reduce or limit necessary or desired activities;
- *Handicap*, where the disability impacts on activities which are essential or highly desired; and
- Lastly people may become *terminally ill*.

Figure 7.2 represents these levels of health as "cells" separated by "membranes." Since in the real world complete health, however defined, is never available to everyone in a population, a "healthy population" can be defined as one in which as many people as possible are in the "right" cells. Well people are not treated as ill, people with acute major illnesses are not treated as minor problems, and handicap is not permitted when it could be reduced to disability. Like all two-dimensional models this picture has its limitations. A person might of course go straight from acute major illness to terminal care (e.g., brain tumor) or from being well to being irretrievably handicapped (e.g., stroke), but, in general, medical care personnel should be organized, trained, and resourced to achieve correct categorization, and to resist the "downward" progression.

This model suggests that the medical task has two interrelated but different components. *Within* the "cells," doctors provide mainly disease-centered care with the objective of reversing, halting, or at least slowing down the pathological process and preventing predictable complications; they are all exercising technical skills and are providing treatment. *Between* the "cells," doctors and patients negotiate the passage of the "membranes" from one health state to another; they are exercising interpersonal skills and providing management. The dynamics of these negotiations can be intense. Obviously no patient finds it easy to accept the change in status from perceived normal

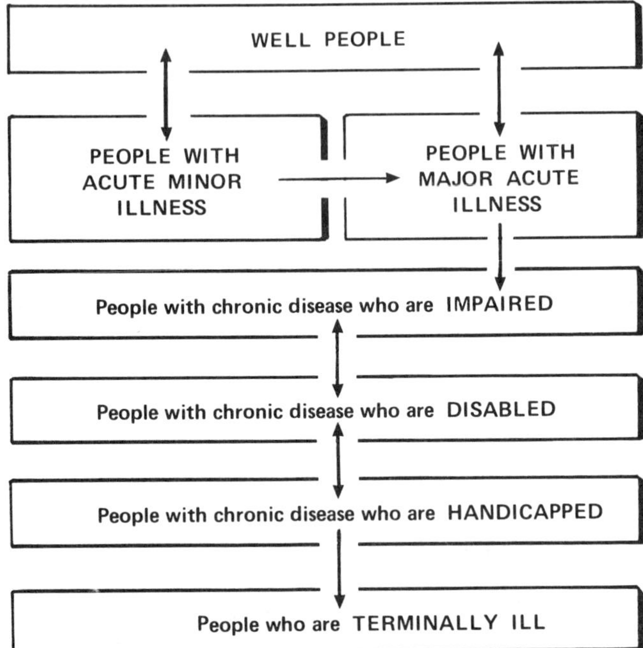

FIGURE 7.2. The second model. Four levels of health.

health to the possession of (or by) a chronic degenerative disease and may have to be persuaded to accept the reality and the life changes entailed. Nor is this easy for the doctor when the patient is well-known. The "downward" transition may not only be an admission of relative medical impotence, but within a good doctor–patient relationship the distress is shared. But "upward" transitions can have their stresses too; patients often need permission to be better, and encouragement to extricate themselves from the safe "womb" of medical care. Doctors are sometimes loath to relinquish control, or anxious about the autonomous patient's risk-taking behavior.

These two task components differ in two other ways. First, in the diagnosis and treatment of disease (the "intracellular" task) the patient is largely passive, and the immediate focus is not so much the sick person as the diseased system, organ, or tissue. In the establishment and improvement of health status (the "intercellular" task) the patient is the main operative, and the target is his or her personal and social function. Second, in the "intracellular" task the objective can be, and usually is, implicit; medicine fights disease. In the "intercellular" task the objectives have to be made explicit for two reasons. First, so that both protagonists agree on their desirability, relevance, and practicability and, second, so that progress toward them can be monitored. "Patient centeredness" and explicit objectives are unfamiliar concepts in the care, teaching, and research provided in centers of excellence, because essentially they are the optimum site for "intracellular" care.

There are other secondary differences that have implications for care, teaching, and research. In the acute illness situation the clinician is unquestionably in a leading role; it is the doctor who has the highest levels of skill in diagnosis and treatment. The other disciplines are called on, as and when necessary, to make their specific contributions, in short bursts of high intensity activity, in close proximity, and therefore easy communication range, to the doctor, the patient, and each other. The classic example would be in the operating theater where the surgeon is supported by anesthetists, technicians, and nurses in various highly skilled but well-defined roles, all of whom are involved in very intense activity, communicating easily, and sharing professional objectives.

Assumptions about objectives, obedience, and willingness that are safe or fairly safe in "intracellular" care are not reliable in long-term "intercellular" care in the community. As an example, consider a person felled by a "stroke;" unconscious and in great danger he is admitted to hospital. His airway has to be maintained, cerebral perfusion optimized, hypostatic pneumonia and bedsores avoided, and nutrition provided to a nonautonomous patient. Doctors, nurses, and physiotherapists know what they have to do, why they have to do it, and how. It does not need to be spelled out. In their mind's eye they see the wedge of neural tissue served by the blocked end-artery, and the zone of edema and therefore temporary dysfunction around it; secondarily they concern themselves with the functions that the ill person cannot carry out, such as movement, nutrition, respiration, evacuation. The team can provide high quality treatment of the disease process in the protective controlled environment of the hospital. This is not to say, of course, that there are no other considerations. Both the humane concerns for the dignity of the patient and the comfort of the family, when life support technology is involved, and the social responsibility with regard to the costs involved, will not be far from a good clinician's mind even in the most intense phases of "intracellular" activity. There may be acute conflict in the doctor's mind, or within the team, between the technical imperatives and the human and social responsibilities involved.

A week or two later the conscious but hemiparetic person is back at home hoping, with his family and his primary care doctor, for further improvement in neurological function. His disease process is stable, his hypertension controlled, and complications avoided. The "intracellular" task has been completed, now the "intercellular" task must be addressed in order to move him from handicap to mere disability. There are three main jobs to be done. His environment must be modified, with appliances or even rehousing, so that his disabilities do not stop him dressing, toileting, and eating, nor taking part in family and social activities. His remaining functions must be enhanced: his good leg and arm must be strengthened, his hemianopia explained to him and neutralized by suitable teaching, and his speech defects minimized, or if necessary, by-passed by signaling. His self-image and outlook must be rebuilt, and the care needed from the family must be supported, encouraged, and demonstrated. These jobs require a wide range of skills: social work, physiotherapy, occupational therapy, speech therapy, and nursing, respectively. The doctor's role is to explain to the patient what can be done and secure from him agreement and commitment to the process of care, setting sensible objectives. The doctor can then call on the other professionals, but they have to establish their own relationship with the patient, and *modus operandi*. They will set their own professional objectives for their interventions, and their input will be intermittent, done in isolation, and over the long haul. The doctor does not necessarily call the shots; whoever identifies an unmet need, or who can provide most restoration of function, or give most relief from distress, at any one time, "leads" the team and has the right to call on one or more of the others for help or support.

In terms of this model, for a medical school to contribute to the health of a defined population, the appropriate compartmentalization of people with different health status, the collective faculty must know, and be able to demonstrate, the epidemiological distribution of people in the various "cells." From that it could work out the needs, both in terms of volume and activities, for the "intracellular" care for which it is superbly qualified by its research and the concentration of expertise to teach. But it must also research, demonstrate, and teach the skills of "intercellular" care: interpersonal negotiation, objective setting, and care sharing, and the shift from disease-centered treatment to person-centered management.

The teaching hospital is not well placed to do this for two reasons. First, it is there to provide effective "intracellular" care; to undertake "intercellular" care would impose opportunity costs in terms of throughput and case-mix. Second, its protective and therapeutic environment (i.e., warmth, cleanliness, proper nourishment, and supportive professional input from nurses, physiotherapists, and others) is taken for granted by the student as his or her working environment, and not seen as part of the treatment plan. This in turn may inculcate arrogance toward the other professionals; without a leadership role in these circumstances they can easily be seen as "menials," working *for* doctors rather than *with* them.

Even if hospital-based specialists concentrate properly on "intracellular" disease-centered diagnosis and treatment, they should know about their patients' needs for "intercellular" care and the skills required to provide it. This knowledge and understanding are not readily available within the center of excellence; it should be acquired in the world outside.

Furthermore, it is only in the world outside that preventive care, especially primary and secondary, can be demonstrated. This falls into three distinct categories:

- First, there is traditional "public health," concerned with environmental control and immunization;
- Second, there is the "new" preventive medicine, directed at the degenerative diseases, based on life-style modification to reduce exposure to

causative factors. This raises questions of mandate and requires communication and negotiating skills. It may also promote the call for social action, since poverty, joblessness, and poor housing stand indicted of causing ill-health and complicating care;
- Third, and seldom seen as personally or clinically rewarding, is the most important task for the first contact doctor of using high clinical skills in history-taking and physical examination *reliably to exclude* significant illness and thus maintaining the competence of the health/ill-health membrane or the sociomedical interface.

Using this model, the faculty should ask themselves: "Do our students understand the differences in needs and tasks between the 'intracellular' and 'intercellular' transactions of care?" "Are they aware of the different sorts of clinical objectives applicable in each health level 'cell'?" "Have we ensured that, as well as learning sufficient communication skills to elicit the information required in the 'intracellular' situation, they have learned those needed for the negotiating component of the 'intercellular' task?" "Furthermore, have they acquired appropriate attitudes, particularly in the areas of power and control?" They could use this model to justify to their students the need to learn from other health professionals such as occupational therapists and physiotherapists about setting and achieving realistic objectives for the management of chronic illness, and from social or clinical psychologists about counseling and negotiation.

However clearly needs, and the tasks that derive from them, have been defined, those tasks have to be carried out within the cultures in which the doctor and the patient operate. Culture, in this sense, can be taken to center on their value systems. Value systems in turn represent (perhaps as a dynamic equilibrium rather than a static one) the compromise between conflicting forces, for example, altruism and selfishness, or technical ambition and compassion. Competence in those tasks can be acquired only if the cultural milieu is recognized and understood.

IV. The Third Model: A Society and Its Doctors: A Role Map

There are two axes of tension in medical care. One axis is between reductionism characterized by focusing down and down until the basic components of dysfunction are revealed and targeted for intervention, and "holism" characterized by treating the "case" as a person in equilibrium with his or her physical, social, and psychological environments. The other axis is between the provision of protection at the cost of dependency and loss of autonomy, and the maintenance of autonomy and independence at the cost of risk and unprotectedness. Figure 7.3 draws these at rightangles to provide a 2 × 2 matrix or map on which medical tasks are plotted. The horizontal

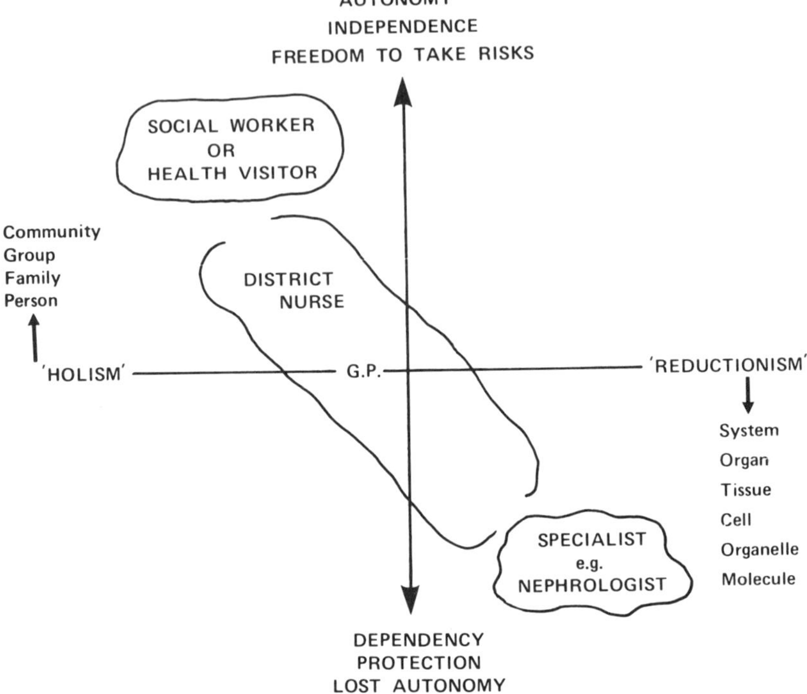

FIGURE 7.3. The third model. Plot of medical tasks. Horizontal axis, tension between person-centered and disease-centered care. Vertical axis, tension between patient power and doctor power.

(holism versus reductionism) axis could be said to represent the tension between "person-centered" and "disease-centered" care. The vertical (dependence versus independence) axis could be said to represent the tension between "doctor power" and "patient power," or "who calls the shots."

The tertiary care specialist, for example a nephrologist or oncologist, works mainly in the bottom right-hand corner. His or her patients need a lot of protection, are highly dependent, and (usually) gladly give up autonomy in exchange for help and expected benefit. He or she deploys enormous expertise and sophisticated resources in order to meet the patients' deep and intense needs at the tissue, cellular, or even molecular level. The bottom right-hand corner is where most benefit can be provided from the exhibition of this expertise and resource.

"Community health workers," for example, public health nurses, health visitors, or social workers, work mainly in the top left-hand corner. Their professional objectives are to protect or enhance their clients' independence and autonomy, and they accept risk-taking behavior, provided it represents informed choice. Their objectives have regard to the functional relationships and obligations between the clients and their families, workmates, and social groups. In their work, detailed knowledge of pathophysiology and its treatment are less important than their interpersonal skills and attitudes toward their clients. Obviously these stereotypes are overdrawn; social workers have to work in the bottom left-hand corner when they take a child into care. Both oncologist and nephrologist concern themselves with their patient's social well-being, working into the top right-hand corner. But these "excursions" represent secondary and occasional concerns rather than the prime focus of their professional work.

Between these two "polar" positions, however, there is a wide range of need to be met. Not only do people with different diseases have different needs for care, but an individual's needs may vary from time-to-time as the natural history of his or her disease progresses. For example, a diabetic may need major review of his therapy to avoid slipping toward ketoacidosis; a few weeks later that poverty stricken and homeless person needs help in getting a proper diet for his, now stable, diabetes. The patient is the same person, but the focus of care has shifted "up left." A patient with rheumatoid arthritis needs to be able to go on using her word processor so fixed finger flexion and ulnar deviation must be fought off; at a later date her sky-high sedimentation rate becomes the focus of treatment; care has shifted "down right."

These are the tasks of the primary care physician working in the community that comprises the patients' physical, social, and psychological environments. He or she needs two sorts of competence: to be at the right point on the map at the right time (not ignoring the rising tide of ketones for the sake of ameliorating poverty, nor fussing with small variations in a low sedimentation rate instead of titrating management against function) and to have the right skills to help the patient at that point on the map.

The competencies described for the primary care physician are, it must be emphasized, basically *clinical*. They are essentially concerned with the ability to exclude or identify illness and to provide initial treatment and, where necessary, long-term management. Some aspects of the latter may overlap the competencies of social workers or health visitors, and indeed such an overlap enhances teamwork because it informs referral and provides a basis for mutual respect. Similarly, diagnosis and initial treatment may overlap the competencies of specialists, and this too should enhance cooperation and mutual respect. Good care at any point from top left to bottom right depends on different competencies; it is unproductive to stratify these in terms of "hard" or "soft," "difficult" or "easy," or "important" or "unimportant." A social worker might not have the scientific bent of the nephrologist but the nephrologist might not have the communication skills and interpersonal sensitivity on which the social worker relies.

Again, it is obvious that student learning confined to the bottom right-hand corner cannot contribute to competencies needed elsewhere in the matrix. Even though the primary care physician has the greatest need to learn in more areas (perhaps exchanging depth for breadth, and some quanta of knowledge for a wider range of skills) any specialist who provides ambulatory care for his patients with a chronic disease must learn some things "upward and to the left" of his or her core skills if he or she is to provide effective, economical, and acceptable care. "Admitting privileges," apart from their financial advantages, are seen from inside the hospital as a strong stimulus for maintaining and improving the technical competence (for "intracellular" and "down right" care). From outside they could be seen as deflecting from the acquisition or maintenance of the competence needed at the sociomedical interface (for "intercellular" and "up left" care).

The one crucial skill that can be properly demonstrated to students *only* in the primary care setting (which of course includes the accident and emergency department) is the reliable **exclusion** of serious illness at first presentation. This requires high levels of core clinical skills and considerably more intellectual intensity than the recognition of the "classical" presentation of common important diseases, which research has shown to be mainly by pattern recognition. It requires a knowledge of probabilities, and the use of clinical logic in the face of uncertainty. Most of the core skills might be learned in the bottom right-hand corner but their use for exclusion cannot be demonstrated there. That can best be done where people present for first contact care, which is well up into the left-hand upper corner.

Using this model the faculty should ask themselves: "Could our students make an accurate assessment of where, on the 'up left' to 'down right' track the patient's most important needs lie, at any particular time?" and "Do they have a sufficient range of skills, and flexibility in deploying them, to adjust their performance according to the patient's position on that track?" This could be summed up as: "Will they be at the right point on the track and, if there, will they be able to cope?" The faculty could use this model to justify to students the need to learn outside the hospital from primary care doctors who are "there." Students need to learn for themselves by observing and interacting with people who, although having an illness, are living out their lives in their own physical, social, and psychological environments.

V. Observations

Where "excellence" has come to mean "scientific precision" the medical school and its teaching hospital is well placed to extend the frontiers of medical science. Its concentration of intellectual power and laboratory resources tend to become focused on particular medical problems, whether those are neonatology, medical oncology, transplant surgery, or the demyelinating diseases. Indeed, most institutions define their special interests in a variety of categorical terms: by age group, treatment mode, or disease type. In so doing, the school, department, or unit quickly attracts a supply of both cases and workers in its chosen field; they come from far and wide. Exciting, rewarding, and stimulating as this work is, it needs to be kept under educational supervision if it is not to skew further the learning experience of the institution's students, few of whom will devote themselves, in the long run, to this particular topic. Overspecialization has obvious effects on the case mix on which students are taught and sometimes on the content of didactic teaching. It has more subtle ill-effects in the warping of their sense of probability and the "importance" that they attach to different sorts of illness and care. High-powered research can lead to tunnel vision, not only in terms of relevance to society's needs, but also in terms of effectiveness. Consider the investment in cancer research, with its limited effectiveness in terms of cure, compared to the cost-effectiveness of the eradication of small-pox. These are dangerous biases to impart to the medical neophyte.

Nevertheless, tertiary care and fundamental research should be based in medical schools and their associated teaching hospitals rather than hived off into special institutions for two reasons. Firstly, they have stimulus value by generating a climate of general clinical inquisitiveness and a respect for methodological rigor that will pervade the whole establishment; and secondly, being based in an institution that has to respond to more mundane needs, tunnel vision is minimized. The humility of the top-level researcher, whether clinical or in the basic sciences, who can say to students and junior doctors "I don't know, but I will try to find out" should be a powerful antidote to the hubris and arrogance unfortunately found elsewhere in such establishments.

In a properly balanced medical school, bioscience, clinical, and social researchers should work alongside each other and enjoy equal respect. These would be the preconditions for interaction, from which at least two benefits would accrue. At the theoretical level a better understanding of the proper balance between validity and reliability; and at the practical level the ability to mount concerted attacks on major medical care problems. A good example needing input from all three categories would be non-insulin dependent diabetes. To provide a forum in which researchers from one discipline could, constructively, ask those from another "Why do that?" or "What is it for?" might improve relevance and reduce the large number of publications which are never cited.

VI. Lessons

The mission of every medical school is to produce doctors who will care for people's medical care needs. Those needs vary from the mundane to the exotic, and in volume from rare events to huge problems. They will have to be met by different mixes of preventive, acute, chronic, and terminal care, and therefore by doctors with differing but complementary competencies. The "grounded theory" for those competencies used to come mainly from clinicians in the field, but more recently from medical scientists in laboratories—yet another sort of doctor. This "retreat" to the laboratory (and its reductionist *modus operandi*) has had several effects that bear on the medical schools' effectiveness in the primary mission described above:

- The range of research methods has been narrowed, with concomitant skew in the applicability of the discoveries that have been made. The elegance and immediacy of laboratory-based bioscience have always been more glamorous than dispersed and long-term disciplines like epidemiology. Its technology confers an aura of precision to which the disciplines of "human enquiry," sociology, psychology, and anthropology could not aspire even if they wanted to. Numeracy has been such a powerful component of scientific enquiry that quantitative research has established a supremacy that in part may be spurious; reliability is often bought at the expense of validity; quantitative research often provides the "frame" but not the "picture." Qualitative observations such as case studies, once the mainstream of medical enquiry, have become devalued with some loss to clinical understanding and hypothesis generation. The educational consequences of this shift in research values will be to make the graduate tend to trust evidence from the laboratory and distrust the evidence of his or her own eyes and ears when attacking clinical problems. This in turn will raise doctors' dependency on technical services, with serious implications for both medical care costs and geographic distribution of doctors.
- Problems are selected for investigation on the grounds of their intellectual challenge, or the availability of funding that, too frequently, mirrors public concern manipulated by interested bodies, rather than their impact on society as a whole.
- The laboratory offers a "clean" and controllable workspace compared to the pragmatic messiness of real world clinical practice, but only so long as human subjects are kept out of it or, if they have to be used, rendered passive and nonautonomous by removal from their natural habitat.
- Basic sciences, by definition, primarily ask: "What happens?" and "How does it happen?" with more excitement and elan than "What can we do about it?" Hence the preponderance of improvements in the precision (and noninvasiveness) of the diagnosis, over improvements in the effectiveness of interventions. Even less effort is made to answer the question "Why does it happen?" Why do some people get diseases when others, apparently exposed to the same risk, don't?
- Major success in a defined area can be claimed as contributing to "world health" and therefore used as an excuse for ignoring mundane problems in local populations. The biggest cause of premature death on the world scene is in fact starvation, but few tertiary care teaching hospitals evince much interest in that!
- Publications and grant-earning capacity are much easier to measure as the "output" of a medical school than the quality (effectiveness, efficiency, and acceptability) of care given to its own patients and provided by its

graduates when they reach clinical maturity. This bias extends also to the difference between the value given to teaching quality and that given to research production.

Thus in some (very prestigious) schools, the production of medical scientists and research results have become the main concerns, instead of being by-products of a broad-based approach to the primary mission of producing competent doctors to care for the full range of the population's health problems. This works to the disadvantage of their local populations and the graduates who will provide day-to-day care for the populations that they find themselves serving.

What can be done? One of the remarkable features of institutions that see themselves as the custodians of medical education is their antipathy toward educational theory and practice, and the scarcity within them of professional educational expertise. The ability of faculties, disciplines, or individuals to describe their educational objectives in terms of knowledge, skills, and attitudes is very limited in many medical schools. Not only should such explicit objectives be required for each component of the curriculum, but they should each be justified in two ways. First, they should be derived from, and clearly related to, the clinical performance expected of a new graduate as an intern, or to the foundation on which higher skills are to be built later, but which must be in place at graduation. Second, they should make it clear how these objectives differ from, and relate to, those of other departments. Explicit, justified objectives like these would allow governing bodies to review the range of competencies to which each department's teaching was directed, and compare them to those required to meet a population's needs. They would also allow them to identify gaps that needed to be filled, and unnecessary duplication that is wasteful. To help in these tasks, every medical school should have some professional educationalists at the center of its organization.

Once explicit, justified objectives are agreed, rational and economic choices of learning content and teaching methods can be made. Objectives derived from an understanding of the population's needs and the competencies required to meet them will dictate that much learning must take place outside the current "center of excellence," and in the patient's natural environment, the community. They will also dictate that teaching there must be provided by two groups of professionals who currently have low status in most medical schools; primary care doctors and social and behavioral scientists. The former will have two major teaching responsibilities: diagnostic logic used *ab initio*, including the rational management of uncertainty, and the interpersonal skills needed for negotiation in the "intercellular" role described in the second model. The social and behavioral scientists will have the responsibility of helping students to understand the ways in which the wide range of human experience affects health and care seeking behavior. Topics that they would teach about include health belief systems in different ethnic and cultural groups, self and body image, and the effects of socioeconomic factors on behavior, health, and use of services.

Proper academic recognition of both primary care clinicians and social scientists will in turn hinge on their contributions to research, for which they must be properly resourced. The difficulty here lies in the unfamiliarity of their sort of research to the leading exponents of reductionist bioscience, who occupy the high ground and dispense the resources in most institutions. Both the questions they address and the methods they use seem strange to those whose research horizons are defined by the walls of the laboratory or the tertiary care ward, but it is these people who have the power within medical establishments. Not only are the researchers in these new fields more likely to want skilled interviewers than particle counters or DNA probes, and longer times in which to carry out prospective studies, but the results produced will not have the elegant precision of bioscience enquiry. Each looks on the other's "laboratory" with incomprehension. Eventually what is beginning to be called "new paradigm" research, in fields such as psycho-neuroimmunology, may bridge this gap, but the fierce rearguard actions that characterize the passing of an established paradigm could well delay such progress for longer than we can afford.

These three steps, setting explicit justifiable objectives, bringing in primary care and social science teachers, and establishing a better balanced research agenda, are vulnerable not only to the forces of reaction, but also to the relative shortage of people with the necessary skills to make them work. Denied status and resource in the centers of excellence they have developed in other ways and adopted other values, among which rigorous research is relatively rare. In some cases this is because they have seen a lot of research in which "rigor" has been characterized by reliability at the expense of validity.

VII. Actions Needed

Governing bodies and funding agencies will have to be persuaded that the reductionist bioscience paradigm is falling victim to the law of diminishing returns, and that they have a responsibility to society at large to open up new fields in the attempt to define the successor paradigm.

They will have to accept that medical learning must take place in a wide variety of sites in addition to the traditional venue of the teaching hospital. Some of that learning will be self-directed and independent, probably using problem-based methods, but much will require teaching from health care professionals and social scientists who understand the needs to be met at these unconventional but important sites. The models described, and the questions for the faculty derived from them, should inform choices of what is to be taught, where, and by whom.

This will, however, present two problems. The first, removal of curricular time and, therefore, resources, from the conventional power bases of medical education will generate resistance and conflict that will have to be dealt with. Evidence that their school's graduates do not have the competencies required to meet a wide range of needs will be a necessary but not sufficient weapon in that struggle! The second problem is that there is a grave shortage of teachers in primary care and the social sciences involved with medicine who are distinguished in research and therefore recognizable in terms of the usual criteria for appointment to high academic rank. Even if new opportunities are created for them to acquire the skills it will take too long for them to achieve the necessary distinction in the usual way.

Two approaches to solving the latter problem can be discerned. The first is to restore the balance in kudos between teaching and research; many members of these "new" disciplines have learned to teach well, even though they have not invested equal time in learning to do research to underpin that teaching. It would then be justifiable to appoint people who can teach well but whose achievement is limited, as it is at present to appoint people who can do good research but who teach badly. The second is to establish, possibly at international level, a special training institution for people from these disciplines, where they could be taught the necessary academic skills intensively, rather than learning them slowly by experience. Successful graduation from such an institution would have to be accepted as the equivalent, for appointment, as a suitable volume of completed research.

Without such urgent action, medicine may turn inward on itself, first to the teaching hospital ward, and second to the research laboratory. If it does it will lose, and deserve to lose, the public's confidence, respect, and support.

Discussion

Roger J. Bulger

Generalizing about medical education across national boundaries is difficult and hazardous, and I shall restrict my commentary to the United States, leaving it to others to assess the relevance of these comments to their countries.

Metcalfe has developed three interesting and, I think, provocative and potentially useful "models" to inform thinking about educational reform in medicine and the necessary evolution of institutional competencies to achieve that reform. But his models may also inform misplaced emphases in the care setting.

My comments fall into three areas, but are offered on the understanding that I agree with most of the basic thrust of what Metcalfe says. Furthermore early on, he clearly points out that his models cannot express everything that needs to be said on the subject. What he has done courageously is to lay out a conceptual framework, that enables us to organize our discussions, debates, and arguments around the main issues. In brief summary, my major areas of modest disagreement with Metcalfe follow:

- He overstates the importance of what is taught in medical school and what is conditioned by external societal forces and conditions in terms of fixing major health-related matters. Medical school faculty will not cure malnutrition and homelessness by curricular alterations, only society can do that. In fact, payment patterns are more likely to influence and determine specialty choice than is the nature of the undergraduate curriculum, especially in view of the growing debt burden being accumulated by most medical students. On the other hand, this perspective is not a reason to justify not altering the medical school experience so as to bring it more into line with societal objectives.
- He misses or understates the importance of specialization. In the United States, biomedical-reductionism has led to specialized science, which in turn has led to specialization and a proliferation of clinician-specialists, not necessarily researchers. Even our most prominent research-rich institutions turn out mostly clinicians, rather than mostly researchers and academicians; the problem is that the clinicians are specialist clinicians rather than generalists. The basis of the problem, therefore, lies in the control of our schools by specialists. We all too often have 12 or 13 clinical specialty schools, rather than a single medical school. These 12 or 13 clinical departments (or postgraduate "schools" of specialty medicine) are each headed by a chief who feels a greater allegiance to specialty colleagues across the nation than to school colleagues across the hall.

  Thus, the hospital is not so much the problem as specialization is; and specialization is moving out of the hospital. Thus, if our hospitals become Emergency Rooms and Intensive Care Units with most specialty hi-tech interventions being done on an ambulatory basis, one can envision that teaching can shift to the clinic but remain specialty driven and, therefore, almost as unsatisfactory as it is currently.
- The paradigm shifts are already on us and cannot be ignored. George Engle's biopsychosocial model (1977) has been argued forcefully for many years, but has made little headway in replacing the Newtonian bastions of biomedical reductionism within our traditional faculties.

  The additive impact of post-Newtonian physics, relativity with its attendant awareness that the observer alters the experiment, chaos theories, and postmodern uncertainty has been to raise serious questions about biomedical traditionalism and its capacity to dominate our enterprise without modification. More people understand and think in terms of Kuhn's historical construct (1970) of scientific paradigmatic differences and shifts. There is an appreciation that the biomolecular paradigm has to take some significant account of the epidemiologic, population-based paradigm. The broadening of the scientific paradigm to include the concepts of the new physics seems to make the biopsychosocial paradigm easier to consider.

- Finally, Metcalfe fails to mention the increasing role of health services research and the growing awareness of cultural, anthropological, moral, ethical, and legal dimensions to health care. Science leads to technology, much of which does not work; our educational programs and institutional role-modeling have failed to take adequate account of these factors.

My conclusions then would be to:

- Establish units for generating information about the relevant population and develop research into unmet needs and challenges for the academic health center. This kind of information must be consistently fed back to faculty and students.
- Develop faculty from among existing faculty cadres—many of whom already have tenure—whose purpose will be to implement the new paradigms, to practice in the ambulatory mode, teach continuity of care, focus on the generalist-education of medical students, and become involved in health services research.
- Reorient teaching to the community, which means deemphasizing hospital/specialty orientation—break the hammer lock of specialists on schools. How to achieve this is one of the central questions. Clinical chiefs can be reeducated; they can learn and some are doing so, perhaps better than critics think.
- Reallocate resources over time so that each medical school could have a critical mass of faculty in sociology, anthropology, economics, epidemiology, ethics, law—a core of faculty, hopefully several with the MD degree—buttressed by the rest of the university. *This* is why the modern medical school is at a university and should be. University presidents should take an interest.
- Teach, learn, and practice with other health professions. But recognize that students are flocking to the specialties for better pay, higher prestige, and sometimes better hours. Whatever is done with the curriculum, students will not choose primary care careers until society shows greater respect for generalists.

References

Engle, G.L., 1977. The need for a new medical model: A challenge for biomedicine. *Science* **196**:129–136.

Kuhn, T.S., 1970. *The Structure of Scientific Revolutions* 2nd ed., Chicago: University of Chicago Press.

Victor R. Neufeld

Metcalfe has given us a fresh and invigorating set of ideas on how medical schools can enhance their contributions to the central institutional mission: "to produce doctors who will care for people's medical care needs." The three models described in this chapter speak for themselves. I will comment on two other sections: the three "dimensions" of medicine described in the "introductory" section, and the "actions needed," at the end. Finally, I will comment on institutional capabilities that need to be identified and strengthened, for universities to contribute to the health of populations.

Three Dimensions of Medicine

The three terms used by Metcalfe capture important ideas although I might quarrel slightly with the choice of word "dimension" to "label" the idea. These three concepts can help us assess the extent to which our academic institutions are, in fact, contributing to improvements in the health of the communities served. My suggestion is that we translate these "dimensions" into questions, each of which calls for some kind of specific evidence about the institution. The questions might be posed as follows:

- *Comprehensiveness*: Does the medical school, in its academic (research and education) programs, address the full range of important health problems that affect the population it serves?
- *Generality*: Is there a defined population (community) to which the institution has a committed relationship, and is the institution involved through its academic and service programs with the full range of subgroups within that population?
- *Balance*: Are the full range of competencies required for "population-oriented" future physicians emphasized in the institution's education programs?

I believe these physician competencies go beyond just "clinical skills," and include the knowledge, skills, and behaviors involved in performing such roles as educator, researcher, and team player; they also should include the abilities in identifying, analyzing, and managing the problems of "populations," and not just of individuals.

If these questions appeared, for example, in the list given to an accreditation team, the institutions under scrutiny would need to provide evidence of various kinds, including

- An analysis of the "content" of the curriculum;
- A look at the mix, number, and range of researchers; and
- An analysis of the "content" of the topics represented in the research profile of the institution.

Recommended Actions

Metcalfe's recommendations can be summarized as follows:

- Improving medical education by writing and using clearer objectives, by involving education specialists, by broadening the range of settings where learning occurs, and by using more effective methods of learning.

- Strengthening the contribution of primary care physicians, and of social and behavioral scientists to the academic programs of the medical school.
- Broadening the research agenda of the institution to achieve a better balance among the disciplines required to understand the health of populations.

These are helpful recommendations. An additional comment is that the "targets" of these recommended actions should be not only (and perhaps not even primarily) "governing bodies and funding agencies." I suggest that the main targets must be the medical schools themselves, for the most part using the already available resources, energy, and talents in the institution. It is too easy to say, "we could make these changes if only we had extra resources." Strategies must be developed to achieve institutional change within the current resource constraints, and with the colleagues now "on board."

Another Look at Institutional Capacities

It is increasingly evident that to improve the health ("quality of life") of populations, universities, communities, and governments must join together to achieve this goal; this idea is shown in Figure 7.4. The distinctive contributions of universities to this partnership include the preparation of graduates with the appropriate competencies, the creation of new knowledge relevant to important societal problems, and the development of new models. Institutions committed to demonstrating these products will require a distinctive set of institutional "capacities," such as those listed in the diagram. Other capacities could be added: for example, "partnership skills"—the capacity to listen to and work with community groups and government agencies.

Peter Richards

The suggested mission of turning out a diverse bunch of doctors capable of meeting the wide variety of needs for medical care is a suitable objective for a medical school. Not that graduates should emerge immediately "capable" at graduation but that they should have the basic skills and, among them, the breadth of vision and interest to prepare to meet many of those diverse needs. Few medical schools can realistically expect to cover the medical needs of "all" human populations, because needs vary substantially in different places and there is much to be said for each locality concentrating primarily on its own environment.

The key competence required whatever the situation is indeed "to be at the right point on the map at the right time . . . and to have the right skills to help the patient at that point on the map." In other words, to be able to decide correctly what is wrong or may become wrong if not prevented, and to know what to do about it, either oneself or by referring efficiently and effectively on.

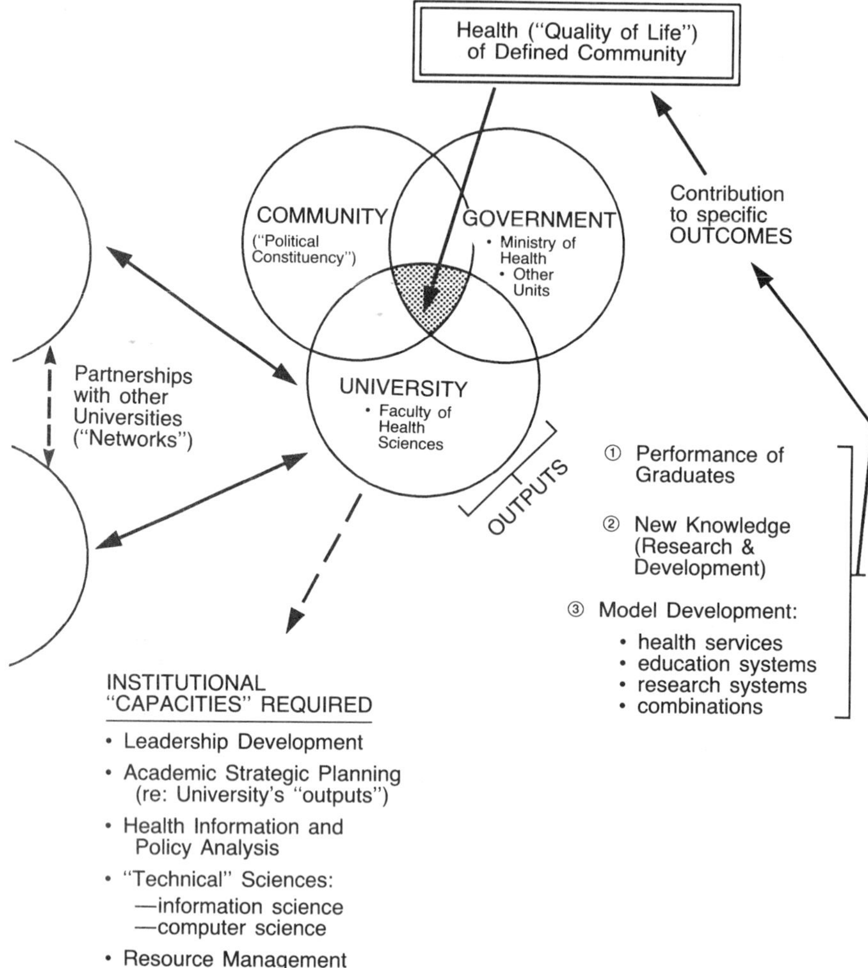

FIGURE 7.4. Universities as contributors to health and social development.

The map is larger than it used to be. The danger is that it will become too detailed. It is the relationships between areas that matter most—how it all fits together. Intelligent map reading requires a good grasp of the principles of both physical geography (anatomy, physiology, biochemistry, and pathology) and of human geography (psychology and sociology) if the map is to be used not only for finding out where the patient is but how he came to be there and where he is likely to go, and whether it is a person or population whose position is being charted, full understanding of the problem and its resolution may well call on those basic skills of statistics and computer science that long since made geography a numerate study rather than a catalogue of landmarks, natural resources, and products.

A theoretical knowledge of how to read a map does not always show where the patient is: after all, it may be foggy (for example, as a result of difficult or inexpert communication) and frequently is. Orienteering (clinical skills) certainly requires the map but it also requires the use of ears, tongue, eyes, nose, and hands, the ability to learn from experience, and to make choices between alternatives on incomplete data. Finding the way ahead (management of the problem) and taking the patient along require additional knowledge of the terrain (pharmacology and therapeutics) together with empathy, explanation, reassurance, teamwork, and, sometimes, stamina. It is no use, like the proverbial Irishman when asked the way, to say that you would not start from here; the starting point may well be inconvenient and the environment may be unfriendly but that is how it is. Doctors can neither alter the map, like landscape contractors, nor change the weather, like witches, but they can appreciate the importance of environment and do their best on the one hand to find suitable experts who may be able to modify it and on the other, help and encourage the patient to adapt to difficult circumstances.

These "basically clinical" skills happen to be those needed by primary care physicians. They are not taught, however, *because* postgraduate training for that specialty is shorter than for others. They are taught because they are the foundation of all good practice and they bond emerging doctors with patients and populations.

These skills are best developed in "the first presentation" situation of general practice although the hospital outpatient clinic should not be discounted, for the second presentation is often not radically different from the first and is also instructive in revealing the outcome of variable diagnostic skills at first encounter. The most educational situation of all is the patient's home. Here, on the one hand, diagnosis amid domestic confusion and concern is doubly difficult, yet on the other, the extent to which environment is responsible for ill-health or will materially complicate its management is clearly displayed.

While clinical logic and courage of diagnostic convictions are vital in the first encounter situation, to ensure rapid reassurance and to avoid unnecessary, expensive, and inconvenient investigation, it not only seeks "reliable exclusion" of "significant disease" but preferably a positive diagnosis of the perceived ill-health, significant to the patient if not serious to the doctor.

Further development of this clinical logic is a proper task for the medical school and teaching hospital where the whole environment should, as pointed out, be one of burning clinical inquisitiveness and "respect for methodological rigor." But having said that, the author is right to call for checks and balances to assure proper perspective in relation to the spectrum of ill-health, to society's needs and to cost-effective practice. He also points to the value of the mixture of highly specialized, research-oriented practice, and more general service in the university hospital where the great medical scientist accustomed to his well-controlled and relatively tidy research is faced with the everyday clinical conundrums that reduce all thinking cl'ni-cians to size.

The medical school and its main hospital are the control center of the educational process. The control center should not, however, be seen as the center of the world. In research, perspectives of what needs to be known and how it can be discovered must widen; not everything that matters can be measured and not everything that can be measured matters. Health needs cannot always be precisely defined. In service, the public as much as the profession needs weaning off a high technology approach to low technology problems. In education, the traditional principle of a patient-centered, basic clinical education needs to be given wider perspective than before. This provides the common core of medical skills and attitudes required before the diverse specialization begins, whatever the system of health care delivery and audit. The old mold has much to offer; it needs cleaning up and using better.

General Discussion

There was wide agreement that population-based perspectives, concepts, and skills are most attractive to students when introduced during the care of *individual patients* and, to the extent feasible, by knowledgeable clinical teachers. A wide variety of dimensions can be explored beyond the narrowly defined biomedical; these include family, occupational, environmental, economic, and social factors.

It was suggested that we guard against homogeneity in the analysis of health problems and needs. Diversity should be encouraged in designing strategies for investigating problems and implementing changes presumed to improve the population's health, and for evaluating the latter. Since 80–90% of medical interventions are unsupported by objective evidence that they do more good than harm, there is ample scope for innovation and evaluation. Small-scale community-based research, service, and teaching projects provide experience and create opportunities to link with and learn from other medical schools attempting similar changes. There are now numerous national networks evolving that have as their objectives the development of strategies for understanding and improving the population's health and health care.

A variety of institutional models for providing opportunities to learn population-based concepts and skills could be tried. Effective collaboration between schools of medicine and public health was observed to be very much the exception in the United States; their separation and isolation from one another were deplored on numerous occasions. Indeed, the absence of a population perspective in medical schools in the United States was widely attributed to this unhappy split some 75 years ago. Canada and Australia no longer have schools of public health, the United Kingdom has 3, and the United States has 26. Career paths for clinicians with training in epidemiology (clinical epidemiology) were now said to be more attractive in North America and Australia than in the United Kingdom.

8
Essential Population-Based Competencies for Undergraduate and Postgraduate Medical Students

Robert D. Cohen

I. Introduction

This chapter is written from the standpoint of an academic clinician. Its perspective is therefore likely to differ from that which might be advanced by an epidemiologist, community physician, or other expert in population-based medicine. But perhaps this is no bad thing, for all fields benefit from external scrutiny from nonexperts, and in addition it is possible that any recommendations emerging might be closer to the practicable than those that might be advanced by experts in the field almost inevitably tinged with missionary zeal! On the other hand, the writer is disadvantaged by his own lack of expertise in population medicine and apologizes in advance for the *faux-pas* that will inevitably be committed. The attitudes expressed have been largely derived from exercising substantial responsibilities for organization of undergraduate medical education at my own medical school, together with a more nationally oriented role in postgraduate education in internal medicine in the United Kingdom.

II. Definitions

The term "population-based" means exactly what it says and is assumed to exclude competencies that deal with many interactions between physicians and their individual patients, e.g., communication skills, many of the skills required in obtaining a history and making a physical examination—a caring approach and the technical skills needed for many diagnostic and therapeutic procedures. However, interpretation of clinical and investigative findings and decisions on clinical management are in the last analysis heavily dependent, implicitly or explicitly, on knowledge derived from the study of populations. Population-based activities may occur in both primary and secondary care settings, and on a local, national, or international basis. The term 'competency' covers two levels of achievement—"understanding" and "skill." *Skill* will be used to imply expert practical knowledge—a statistician performing a complex analysis of data from a study that hopefully he or she has had a hand in designing is exercising a skill. On the other hand a clinician who appreciates in broad terms the principles of statistical analysis and the pitfalls of study design may be said to have an *understanding*, which although essential for his or her professional competency, falls far short of a skill. "Community Physician" is a term that, in the United Kingdom, denotes physicians whose prime responsibility is to monitor the health needs of the local community and organize and evaluate health services for the community, especially in the ambulatory care, preventive, and health maintenance spheres. They have relatively little or no direct clinical involvement at the individual patient level. They are entirely distinct from General Practitioners (Family Doctors).

III. Why Teach Population-Based Competencies to All Students?

The majority of undergraduate medical students will eventually fill clinical roles, either in primary or secondary care, a minority will enter pathology or other investigational fields or full-time research, and a small number will become epidemiologists or community physicians specializing in the organization of health services. For this last group much of the present subject matter will be the daily content of their vocation. It is for the remainder that we have to give principal consideration.

For undergraduates, there is widespread agreement that the objective of training should be educational rather than vocational, and therefore based on acquisition of principles and methods of learning, which will serve as a basis for their as yet undetermined future career direction. Acquisition of skills should at this stage be the minimum needed to be able to enter the intern year. That there is such agreement is at its lowest level dictated by the clear educational disadvantages of cluttering up the undergraduate curriculum with matters that might better be included in the postgraduate period as part of vocational training. At a more positive level the approaches to problem-solving, continued self-education, and interpersonal communication need to be firmly inculcated at the outset of medical education. Clearly, the teaching of population-based competencies in the undergraduate period must be constrained by these principles and for the most part should be at the level of understanding rather than skills.

The necessary range of understanding of population-based medicine is dictated principally by the related problems that will be confronted in subsequent clinical practice. The range includes the following five main elements:

- Descriptive epidemiology;
- Statistical analysis;
- The organization of health and related services;
- Preventive medicine approaches; and
- Evaluation and audit.

A more detailed examination of each of these elements follows.

Descriptive Epidemiology

All clinicians must have information on the *importance* in the community of the illnesses in which they profess expertise. Without such information they cannot organize the services for which they are responsible optimally, have no sound case with which to bid for resources, and have no means of assessing temporal trends, whether these are due to their interventions or not. They must therefore understand the methods and pitfalls of collection of mortality and morbidity statistics, of the concepts of incidence and prevalence, and of analysis by age, sex, social class, housing variables, and ethnicity. They must also know how to access expertise in relevant data collection and analysis. Estimation of the importance, or burden, of a disease of course requires not only data of the above nature, but information on the effect of the disease on life-style, and economic, social, and personal well-being. Appreciation is therefore needed of some of the indices used to estimate these aspects, e.g., work lost, dependency.

Statistical Analysis

All clinicians, whether involved in research or not, have to update continually by reading medical and scientific literature, attending conferences and courses, receiving promotional literature, and many other methods. None of these educational methods can be properly effective without an understanding of statistical principles—and perhaps even one or two skills. The potential damage done to patients by uncritical assessment of alleged new advances is too serious to contemplate too minimalistic an approach to this subject. In addition to the importance for continuing education, statistical understanding is of course essential for most analysis of one's practice and for research design and execution both in the biomedical and health services fields. There are also some types of individual patient interaction that require the mobilization of population-related skills; explanation to the patient of the natural history of his disorder and the likely outcome of therapy depend on knowledge of studies of groups of patients. Frequently diagnosis rests on some type of pattern recognition, of which the fundamental roots are statistical.

I would regard the acquisition of *understanding* of the following concepts and techniques as an essential objective of undergraduate medical education:

- Biological variability;
- Normal and nonnormal distributions;
- The meaning of P values and confidence intervals;
- Concepts of parametric and nonparametric statistics;
- Comparison of group data;
- Regression analysis;
- Correlation: difference between correlation and regression;
- Analysis of variance;
- χ^2 analysis;
- Pattern and cluster recognition;
- Type I and Type II errors;
- Statistical power;
- Trial design: prospective and retrospective studies, randomization, and "blinding";
- Criteria for causal relationships; and
- Risk factors and risk analysis.

Knowledge of the Organization and Availability of Health and Health Related Services

All undergraduate medical students must have an overview of the way health services are organized at a national and local level. Health services of course comprise not only primary and secondary medical services for the acute and chronic sick, but other critical components of health support. These include nursing, both hospital and community-based, social work, physiotherapy, occupational therapy, health education, child welfare and well-women clinics, screening services, social services for the elderly, handicapped, chronically sick, and many specific "disease-oriented" patient support groups. The student must understand how to measure the *need* for such services and the importance of setting the need against the availability. He or she must be aware of the gross inequalities that exist within and between nations in the matching of availability to need. Lastly, students must be informed of their future statutory responsibilities for notification of births, deaths, and certain specified illness, and of the mechanisms for exercising these responsibilities.

Preventive Medicine Approaches

The student should understand the basic principles of selection and implementation of health screening initiatives, the techniques and psychology of mounting campaigns to change harmful aspects of life-style, e.g., alcohol, smoking, and inappropriate nutrition. He or she should appreciate the issues underlying the implementation of immunization programs, including the factors determining their uptake. Safety at work in the United Kingdom is monitored by a statutory body, the Health and Safety Executive, which is concerned with all types of physical and toxic hazards in the workplace—the student should be aware of the operation of this and similar national bodies and their powers.

Evaluation and Audit

Students must understand both the critical importance of the evaluation of health care, and the numerous difficulties and pitfalls in its execution. They must appreciate the differences between evaluation based on intermediate or overall outcomes, on the one hand, and economic evaluation, on the other, including cost–benefit analysis. They should be introduced to the ethical and political implications of economic analyses. They must participate in and learn the structure and purposes of clinical audit procedures in the services to which they are attached.

These five subjects constitute the range of *understanding* in population-based medicine that I believe to be appropriate for a graduating medical student. But merely stating this range leaves many questions unanswered:

- What depth of understanding should be aimed at?
- Who should teach it and by what methods and when?
- To what extent have medical schools already incorporated such teaching into their curricula and how are they assessed?
- What ways are there of ensuring that proper attention is given to this material?

IV. Mechanisms and Practicalities in Undergraduate Education

The Depth of Understanding

The major practical determinant is the competition for time in the medical undergraduate curriculum. I have no personal doubt that since the majority of students will eventually end up in clinical practice the most important priority of the undergraduate medical course is the training in individual patient-based medicine, i.e., the competencies that are for the most part non-population based, except for the implicit and explicit statistical element in diagnosis and therapeutic decisions. There are many reasons for this. The *first* and most important is that the principal ethic of medical practice is based on providing the best available care for the individual patient. Though this ethic frequently brings clinicians into conflict with administrators, managers, economists, specialists in community medicine, and politicians, it has to be sustained, not only because of its intrinsic rectitude, but because in the long term, only by sustaining this approach will better services be made available for the population as a whole—the history of the development of renal transplantation services is a good example of this. The *second* reason for the concentration on non-population-based subjects is that it is the idea of service to individual patients that attracts most students into medicine; at this stage in their careers it is psychologically as harmful to overemphasize the population-based aspects as it is to overfill their brains with unnecessary details of topographical anatomy. *Third*, doctor–patient interactions and skills are, with the possible exception of statistics, much more difficult conceptually than the population-based subjects listed above, and it is therefore necessary to spend more time on these.

My purpose in stating this viewpoint forcibly is not in any way to demote the importance of the agenda outlined in the previous section, but to determine what I would personally regard as a proper sense of balance in time allocation in the curriculum. As indicated earlier, medical schools are having to deal with the overcrowding of the undergraduate curricula by concentrating on the educational rather than the vocational. One approach to this concentration adopted by many schools is to consider which aspects of the course should be compulsory and which should be elective; for the latter category the student has to choose a relatively small number of electives out of a considerable range of options. It is clear that a formal course in population-based medicine should be compulsory; its length should, however, be *influenced* by the fact that due to the all-pervasive nature of the subject matter there will be innumerable occasions in the rest of the course when population-based topics are discussed, and that they will have an inevitable role in the postgraduate training to follow. The formal course in population-based medicine will, *inter alia*, draw attention to the fundamental statistical roots of diagnosis and therapeutic decision making; this point should be reinforced in clinical attachments by the staff repeatedly drawing attention to this background to their clinical practice.

Who Should Teach it and by What Methods and When?

There is no real doubt that the teachers of formal courses should be mainly professional epidemiologists, statisticians, and community physicians. Their efforts should be leavened and illuminated by contributions from clinicians who have particularly embraced population-based methodology in their practice, clinical administration, or research.

The methods require rather more thought. Disembodied lectures on statistics, the organization of health services, etc., are likely to be hypnotically dull and poorly attended. Three approaches seem well suited to overcome this problem: (1) to graft statistical exercises on to class practicals undertaken in basic medical science, with subsequent discussion on a seminar basis, (2) to use population-based topics for student projects, and (3) to prescribe a number of exercises in which the student is required to comment critically on selected papers on population-based topics or which employ population-based approaches.

These exercises may be undertaken at different times throughout the course. During clinical attachments a particularly appropriate exercise is for the student to take a specific episode from the medical history of one patient and to determine in depth, using the literature, the scientific bases for each of the diagnostic, investigative, and therapeutic decisions made during this episode; the rationales will of course be heavily dependent on population-based studies. In addition, clinical attachments to general medical and some other services provide admirable opportunities for observing the organization and use of various community services. Especially in socially deprived areas, much of the discussion toward the end of many patients' stay in hospital is directed toward the facilitating of discharge by the mobilization of these services; a common event is for the social worker or occupational therapist to visit the patient's home before discharge to assess the situation. Excellent insights are provided by the student attached to the patient accompanying the relevant health worker on these visits; student attitudes and interests are frequently strongly influenced by these experiences. Attachments to general practitioners, which are the rule in the United Kingdom in undergraduate medical education, also provide experience in these areas and in the application of preventive programs. Necessary coherence to the overall program may be provided by compulsory short attachments to the Department of Epidemiology/Community Medicine. In my own school this attachment is based on miniproject work, seminars, interactive handouts, visits to Health Centers, self-learning exercises, and provision of detailed information on health-care-related demography and health care resources of the health District in which the school is located.

What Ways Are There of Ensuring That Proper Attention Is Given to This Material?

In the United Kingdom the statutory responsibility for ensuring proper standards of medical education is in the hands of the General Medical Council (GMC). This body consists of approximately 90 members, some elected by various sections of the medical profession and others nominated by various bodies, notably universities with medical schools. There are approximately 10 lay members, including some representing various patient organizations. About every 10 years the education Committee of the General Medical Council publishes a revision of its Recommendations on Basic Medical Education. University Medical Schools are expected to keep within these guidelines, but they are couched in such terms as to permit much flexibility and a good deal of experimentation in the arrangement of the course, of Departments within Medical Schools, and, indeed, in course content. The wide range of curriculums among medical schools in the United Kingdom indicates that substantial advantage is taken of this flexibility.

Within these guidelines Universities develop their own course and assessment requirements for undergraduate medical teaching, which are far more detailed than the GMC guidelines. The assent of the Education Committee of the GMC is obtained for any major development, such as the implementation of a completely new curriculum. The GMC monitors adherence to its guidelines both by approval of curriculums as above and also by sending teams of inspectors to attend university examinations in medicine to report both on the conduct of the examinations and the standards of proficiency needed to pass. The GMC's ultimate sanction is to refuse to recognize a university's medical qualification for the purpose of Registration as a qualified medical practitioner.

The last GMC guidelines on Basic Medical Education were issued in 1980 (Recommendations on Basic Medical Education 1980); the Council is currently working on a revision. The guidance is in two parts, Part A—a definition of the extent of knowledge and skill required at graduation, and Part B—a more detailed commentary. The statements respecting population-based topics in Part A are as follows:

- The student must acquire knowledge and understanding of "the organization and provision of health care in the community and in hospital, the identification of the need for it, and the economic, ethical, and practical constraints within which it operates"; and
- The student must develop appropriate attitudes to the practice of medicine, which include "the ability to assess the reliability of evidence and the relevance of scientific knowledge, to reach conclusions by logical deduction or by experiment and to evaluate critically methods and standards of medical practice."

This may appear to be an extraordinary short statement, but it amounts to about 10–15% of the whole statement in Part A, and must be regarded in the light of the need to set a broad guideline rather than to prescribe and in the light of the commentary in Part B.

Part B refers again to the need for knowledge of organization of health services, and of the role of other health professions and of health education in the promotion of health and the prevention of disease. Its specific comments on the teaching of Community, Social, and Preventive Medicine include the following:

- Systematic instruction or demonstration in the responsibilities of community medicine;
- The uses of epidemiology in establishing the social and environmental and other causes of disease;
- The principles of occupational medicine;
- Simple health care economics;
- The planning and organization of medical care and policies for the prevention of disease and the promotion of health.
- Teaching of prevention and community medicine may include instruction on the effects of malnutrition and on the social as well as the medical consequences of drug, alcohol, and tobacco abuse.

- The relevance of community medicine to other clinical subjects should be illustrated by integrating some of the teaching of this topic with that of other branches of clinical medicine.

Taking a specific example of interpretation of the GMC guidelines by Medical Schools, the University of London Syllabus has many elements in common with this commentary, but adds specific detail in terms of the instruction concerning evaluation of health care, methods of collecting routine statistics, screening, and the relative contribution of genetic and environmental factors to disease.

To What Extent Have Medical Schools Already Incorporated Population-Based Studies in Their Curriculums and How Are They Assessed?

So far as the United Kingdom is concerned, all schools have Departments of Epidemiology/Community Medicine responsible for teaching population-based subjects. In many the teaching of statistics is part of their remit, but some schools have separate Departments of Medical Statistics. At the lowest level it would be impossible not to pay substantial attention to these subjects because neither universities nor ultimately the GMC would permit this. Furthermore, competence in these subjects is assessed, both informally in course and by examinations. In my own school statistics is formally assessed at the end of the second year, and the other aspects of population-based studies during the final examinations, by multiple choice questions, compulsory questions in the written examination in medicine, and an oral examination.

I do not believe for one moment that all our graduates possess the range and depth of understanding outlined earlier as desirable. But nor do they achieve such standard uniformity in other fields of study. It is indeed possible to compensate in our examinations for a poor performance in population-based topics by a good performance in other areas and vice versa. One could argue that there is no point in setting educational goals unless a minimum standard is achieved in all cases, and this might be construed as a powerful argument either against the use of compensation in this way in determining the results of examinations or, alternatively, against the idea of "final" examinations.

This is not the place to become embroiled in arguments about the relative merits of "final" examination or "in course assessments," but I would strongly support the use of compensation. Medical students vary very much in their particular natural aptitudes. The purpose of education should be to allow individual aptitudes to develop, not to produce a series of look-alike (and correspondingly dull) clones who have acquired a series of relatively uniform standards in both clinical topics and population-based studies.

The issue brings me directly to the following possible recommendation which has been suggested by the Conference: "In order to reassure the public, every medical school should demonstrate through practical examination or other methods of assessment that each undergraduate and postgraduate has specified population-based competencies in addition to those traditionally encompassed by the medical curriculum." It should be clear from what I have said that I cannot wholly agree with such a recommendation. My own view is that the public might be best reassured if they knew (1) that most (not all) graduates from medical school had some understanding of population-based matters and that (2) medical schools were encouraging the development of the many diverse talents possessed by their future physicians. As medicine becomes more complex conceptually, philosophically, and technologically, the more will medical schools have to adopt this more liberal approach.

It must be remembered that the undergraduate phase is only the start of medical education. There are innumerable future opportunities for gaining understanding—if necessary—in a topic at which a particular student did not shine when an undergraduate. The author is very conscious of the fact that 35 years ago neither he nor his classmates received formal instruction in any of the topics in population-based medicine that I have outlined above as necessary components of the undergraduate medical curriculum. This was at a time when population-based medicine was at least as important as it is now. What knowledge in this field my classmates and myself have gained since then has been by "osmosis," *force-majeure*, and bitter experience. This method of learning is inefficient and haphazard, and I am delighted that a proper place has now been given to these matters in modern undergraduate curriculums. However, I doubt whether a case could be convincingly made that either we or the public have been irreversibly disadvantaged by our original educational deficiencies! I make this point to emphasize that all is not lost if a minority of the class graduates with less than adequate knowledge of population-based studies (or with similar gaps in a small number of most other topics). The long-term dangers to the public of enforcing uniformity far outweigh the advantages.

In a recent paper the Dean of the Harvard Medical School suggests that as much as 40% of the undergraduate curriculum should be devoted to optional subjects of some special interest to the students selecting them (Tosteson 1990). This is considerably more liberal than is the case in the majority of medical schools in the United Kingdom, but I believe it to be a welcome and inevitable development, which should rekindle the enthusiasm of medical students demoralized by factual and material overburden. Those responsible for the overburden are, of course, none other than those teaching staff who are incapable of perceiving that their own subject may be unsuitable as core material for this stage of medical training; on occasion, insistence on a greater share of the available core time is dictated by reasons other than purely educational. When admitting a topic to a share of the scarce core time the claims of the population-based sciences need no less scrutiny than do those of anatomists, physiologists, biochemists, physicians, surgeons, and pathologists. Indeed, we have to ask if 60/40 represents a reasonable core/option split at the moment, what will be the situation in 20, 50, or 100 years? It is possible that in the distant future the whole concept of unified undergraduate medical education will simply break down and our successors will in fact have to train two or three distinct types of doctors from day one of the medical curriculum, each with needs for different knowledge, skills, and attitudes. If this were to come about, then the only one of the population-based competencies enunciated above for the present undergraduate curriculum that would with undoubted certainty be core material for each different type of medical trainee would be statistics.

V. Population-Based Competencies in Postgraduate Medical Education

Requirements and Opportunities

Graduation is followed by an intern year, which is the effective start of both practice and in-service training. In the United Kingdom this is the last year of medical training that is under the direct control of the universities. The problem with all in-service training is to ensure that the exigencies of providing the service do not relegate the training element to a secondary feature of the post. From the viewpoint of population-based medicine, the most obvious benefit gained from the intern period is practical knowledge of the organization of services both within the hospital and in the community, and how to use them for the benefit of individual patients. An obvious example is the intern's responsibility for arranging discharge of an elderly woman who lives alone and who requires support from several types of social services if she is to maintain an individual noninstitutionalized existence. Intern posts are so demanding in service terms in the United Kingdom that there is usually little time for formal educational exercises. It is within the power of the universities to disallow a particular post for intern training if it believes the educational content is insufficient; but the practical situation is that the Universities apply this sanction only if the post becomes physically and mentally intolerable in terms of service workload.

It is in subsequent years that there is potentially more opportunity for educational development. A common pattern is for the trainee to undertake a rotation of posts at Resident (Senior House Office or Registrar in the United Kingdom) level during which he or she selects an ultimate career pathway. There is a special pathway of vocational training in the United Kingdom for those wishing to enter general practice; this includes some elements of hospital-based practice. The major hurdle in hospital practice in the United Kingdom, which has to be overcome in open competition, is to enter the Higher Training level, which will eventually lead to accreditation in a specialty; this is roughly equivalent to Board Certification in the United States.

In the United Kingdom, both the general postgraduate period and the Higher Training period are under the overall coordination of the General Medical Council (Recommendations on the Training of Specialists 1987) but are in effect controlled by the national professional bodies (The Royal College of Physicians, Surgeons, etc.), not the Medical Schools. The Royal Colleges, jointly or otherwise, lay down guidelines, inspect training posts, and approve or disapprove them.

As a starting point for considering postgraduate training in population-based aspects of medicine I have examined the Higher Training (Training Manual, Joint Committee on Higher Medical Training, United Kingdom, 1989–1990) programs of all the medical (as opposed to surgical, pathological, obstetric, psychiatric, etc.) specialties in the United Kingdom to determine what recommendations are made in this respect.

Nearly all the programs are in clinically orientated fields of medicine. Training in one or more aspects of population-based medicine is required experience in 11 of the 41 programs. Such training is explicitly mentioned as optional or acceptable experience in a further seven programs. There is no explicit mention in the 23 remaining programs. These figures exclude the programs in Adult and Pediatric Community Health, which are obviously principally directed toward population medicine.

The situation as regards encouragement of training in population-based medicine is certainly, therefore, very uneven among those fields under the purview of the Joint Committee on Higher Medical Training, and it is probably at least as uneven in those fields supervised by the other Higher Training Committees. It is of interest that precisely this issue was raised in respect of epidemiology at a meeting of the Medical Higher Training Committee in 1989. As a result all its individual Specialist Advisory Committees were formally requested to consider whether their programs provided adequate training in epidemiology. It should be noted that notwithstanding the lack of explicit direction on population-based studies in most programs, a large number of trainees receive training in epidemiological and/or statistical methods during the periods when they are undertaking research, which may be during either the general postgraduate training period or the Higher Training phases, or in both. Since demonstration of capacity to carry out effective research is *de facto* almost a necessary condition in most fields for overcoming the hurdle to Higher Training and for achieving career consultant appointments, the vast majority of trainees undertake research to meet this requirement; and it can be assumed, therefore, that most postgraduates inevitably receive some training in statistics at least, though the depth of understanding achieved is clearly very variable. Epidemiological training is far less often achieved in this incidental fashion, and depends on the research topic chosen. Other channels by which unscheduled experience in these areas is achieved are exposure to presentation of population-based material at conferences related to the trainees own field, and at grand rounds.

A most important educational experience is participation in local exercises in defining workload and service needs mounted in order to bid for an appropriate share of resources. This is particularly pertinent in the United Kingdom, where the overall envelope of financial resources for health care within the National Health Service is both finite and defined. Once the maximal possible share has been achieved locally to finance a given specialty, the only further approaches possible if the provision is still unsatisfactory are charitable appeals and political activity. The physician-in-training has to learn to marshall the facts in a way that will stand up to scientific and political scrutiny when these approaches are made. For this purpose he or she needs direct involvement with experts in population-based studies. One particularly onerous consequence of this situation is that the physician frequently has to act as "gate-keeper" for new and successful but highly expensive investigations or therapies, defining which groups of patients shall and which shall not have access to these facilities. In the National Health Service this decision is not made on the basis of the patients' ability to pay, either directly or through health insurance. Thus the whole responsibility falls on the physician. This responsibility requires the most careful application of population-based methods to determine the characteristics of patients who are most likely to benefit by these techniques; clearly many issues other than purely medical ones are involved. All these nonscheduled exposures together may constitute a very significant contribution to training in population-based competencies and may make a lasting impact on the attitudes of newly appointed consultants to their future practice. Nevertheless it can be argued that it is too haphazard and that more formal training should be included regularly either in general postgraduate or Higher Training or both. It is therefore necessary to consider what practical mechanisms exist for generating this change.

Mechanisms for Change

Probably the most practical way of achieving sufficient understanding of the population-based techniques to be able to fulfill the responsibilities of a career physician is to add to the in-service experience a short period of formal secondment to a training course in these techniques. Perhaps the most relevant appropriate timing would be in the Higher Training period, in which the trainee could attend appropriate courses organized by the National Society concerned with the trainee's specialty. In the United Kingdom posts for Higher Training are not approved unless they schedule time for private study and research; this principle could be extended to cover courses in population aspects of the specialty, which need last no longer than 7 to 10 days. The course content would be largely epidemiological and statistical; it would differ from that which might be taught in the undergraduate curriculum in its specific application to the specialty concerned.

Medical Audit and Evaluation

Medical audit procedures are much more extensively developed in North America than in the United Kingdom. Nevertheless rapid developments are taking place in the United Kingdom. The need for population-based skills in many types of audit is obvious—a simple example is comparison of results of one's own practice with published series. It is of crucial importance that postgraduate trainees participate in exercises of this nature on their own services. Clinical audit procedures are of course much better developed in some fields than in others. Notably effective examples are the systems developed for comparison of performance in Intensive Therapy Units; the attention of trainees in many fields could with profit be directed to one of these systems (e.g., APACHE II). In addition to purely clinical audit, they must also participate in economic and efficiency audit procedures. The opportunity for postgraduates to learn and be involved in these various types of audit procedures should be an essential condition for the approval of a post for training purposes.

Evaluation studies are closely related to audit. Simple description of the outcomes of health services systems are obviously much enhanced by making formal comparisons between the costs and benefits of alternative systems. But there is one form of evaluation in which trainees need to learn a very specific lesson. This is the evaluation of new technologies, which are often very sophisticated and very expensive.

A common situation is the emergence of a new technology that has the potential to replace that currently in use. The expense of the new technology leads to demands from those responsible for the distribution of resources—including, among others, politicians and Government agencies—for a comparative evaluation study to assess the new against the current technology. Unless the timing of this study is chosen with extreme care, such studies have an extraordinarily high chance of failure. This is because not only is the new technology still in the process of evolution during the period of the study, but it is quite likely that the current technology is also changing. The upshot is that the results of the study are either uninterpretable or are completely obsolete by the time they become available. Yet cohorts of keen young population-based doctors, goaded on by resource managers and politicians, embark on these studies, determined to evaluate the unevaluable! They thereby waste their own time and public money. The physician in training should learn of these fundamental traps in evaluation studies. He or she should also learn of the alternative approach—the consensus development conference—which is cheap, pretty unscientific, but often gets rather close to the true answer. The author expresses this view with some feeling since he has been involved (e.g., Cohen 1979, 1980), either as participant or scrutineer, in at least three Government or Government Agency-inspired formal evaluation exercises of new technologies, the outcomes of which have been of little value, for the reasons discussed above.

V. Conclusions and Recommendations

- Certain population-based competencies have been defined that doctors should acquire (see Section III);
- By the time of graduation, most doctors should have an understanding of these defined competencies. This *understanding* should guide and illuminate their subsequent clinical practice, but they do not need the *expert skills* required by population-based specialists;
- A major factor in determining the level of understanding which should be aimed at is the urgent need to restrict the core requirement of the curriculum;
- Certain population-based competencies are critical to the running of effective clinical practice at a senior level and to fulfillment, so far as is possible, of the ethical obligations of doctors to individual patients;
- Evidence from the United Kingdom suggests that provision in postgraduate training for acquisition and reinforcement of population-based competencies is haphazard, and varies greatly among specialties;
- It is suggested that in addition to in-service experience of the deployment of population-based approaches in clinical practice, each postgraduate undergoing specialist training should attend a course in population medicine as applied to his or her specialty;
- It is suggested that these courses should be organized by the national specialist societies;
- All postgraduate trainees should participate in the routine audit procedures of their services. This should be a condition of approval of the post for training purposes; and
- Postgraduate trainees should be made aware of the advantages and pitfalls of evaluation exercises.

References

Cohen, R.D. 1979. Evaluation of computer systems in medicine. In: *Proceed Med Informatics, Berlin, 1979*. Barker, B., Cremy, F., Uberla, K., and Wagner, F. (Eds.). Berlin: Springer-Verlag, pp. 931–937.

Cohen, R.D. 1980. Computing in the National Health Service. *Royal Soc Health J* **100**:113–117.

Recommendations on Basic Medical Education. 1980. London: United Kingdom General Medical Council.

Recommendations on the Training of Specialists. 1987. London: United Kingdom General Medical Council.

Training Manual. 1989–1990. London: United Kingdom Joint Committee on Higher Medical Training.

Tosteson, D.C. 1990. New pathways in general medical education. *N Engl J Med* **322**:234–238.

Discussion

Jo Ivey Boufford

I see two main goals for educational interventions to develop core competencies in population-based medicine: first to provide all physicians with a new and broader context for the practice of comprehensive 1:1 clinical medicine, and, second, to provide a specific set of skills for all physicians unique to the understanding and practice of population medicine.

The first and more difficult goal requires the introduction of a new way of thinking about medicine and its role in assuring health and, by extension, of physicians and their roles. In the 1:1 clinical encounter, physicians are concerned with the assessment, diagnosis, and treatment of an individual patient's specific problem. Exploration of the context in which the patient lives is limited by each physician's definition of his or her role in promoting the patient's well-being.

To use stereotypes for a moment, the superspecialist consultant in the hospital may be satisfied with making a diagnosis and outlining the accepted treatment plan for the affected organ system, being concerned little if at all about the psychological impact of the diagnosis, the social reality of the patient's adhering to the prescribed plan, or the influence of family structure, home environment, or financial well-being on the patient's health status. The primary care physician, however, is likely to be confronted with this wider set of concerns at one time or another during a longer term relationship with the patient. In defining this broader role for the primary care physician in supporting the patient's health and well-being, he or she more or less effectively attempts to take this larger set of factors into consideration in managing the patient.

As an advocate for preparing all physicians to see patients in a context that is broad enough to make them effective practitioners, I would see many of the understandings and skills that the author has described as core competencies in population-based medicine, as, instead, fundamental to the clinical training of all physicians. I would include the following items from Cohen's list in this broader category:

- Information on the effect of the disease on the life style, economic, social, and personal well-being of the patient;
- Explanation to the patient of the natural history of his or her disorder and the likely outcome of therapy—I would identify as "clinical trials" or "clinical research" the research with groups of patients that Cohen identifies as population medicine;
- How the organization and availability of health services affect the patient's discharge planning and overall therapeutic program;

- Preventive medicine and patient education at the individual patient level; and
- Medical audit and quality assurance skills.

Many of the recent critiques of and recommendations for change in United States medical education have focused on the need for all physicians in training to acquire these understandings and skills during their education. Progress is being made, albeit slowly, but these understandings and skills are not, to my mind, unique to population medicine, nor should their teaching be the unique responsibility of this group of faculty.

However, when we do ask the physician to go further and broaden the context for viewing the individual patient to include consideration of the immediate community from which the patient comes or, by extension, the population at large, we confront a change in the way of thinking that is fundamental and difficult. This involves a shift from the *numerator* focus, i.e.,the individual patient for the physician, or the user of services for the institutional provider, to the *denominator*, i.e., both patients and nonpatients, users and nonusers who live in or are part of a defined community. I agree with Cohen that the clinical encounter is the most powerful model in medical teaching. Thus, it would seem logical to begin by using the population perspective to broaden the context in which the patient is viewed, and, therefore, as a means of enriching the clinical orientation that is fundamental to the way the majority of medicine is taught.

With this idea in mind, I would characterize the core competencies for population medicine as the understanding and skills needed to assess, diagnose, and treat the community's health problems, using much the same paradigm as for the individual patient but with differing data sources, a different professional literature, different specialist consultants (the epidemiologists), and different interventions, both curative and preventive, aimed at population groups. Like the clinical model, these skills would include the issue of communication and partnership with the community in such a process.

The following items from Cohen's list would be consistent with such a view of core skills unique to population medicine:

- How population health data are collected and the problems with these measures;
- The types and power of statistical tests for significance;
- The general organization, availability, and effectiveness of health services in influencing community health status;
- Preventive medicine strategies focused at the level of the community's health; and
- Design of population level interventions and evaluation of their effectiveness that also require special skills.

Faculty development is fundamental in any effort to integrate population orientation into undergraduate or postgraduate medical education. Such efforts must provide the basic science and, especially, the clinical teachers with both the new mind set—thinking in the population context—and with the data they will need to effectively present this context in the course of their teaching about patient problems—in earlier years, through clinical correlation lectures and problem-based learning and, later, and most important, during clinical clerkships and residency years. This effort must be a major responsibility of the population medicine Faculty with the support of institutional leadership.

For teaching the specific skills, I would like to see Cohen's basic statistical teaching package introduced as part of a general course on interpreting the medical literature, with broader applicability to all the specialties. The epidemiological perspective can be introduced here and be further explored later, reinforced by the "population orientation" in the clinical encounters described above. I think the specific teaching of population-based medicine—epidemiological techniques, the specifics of population assessment, diagnosis, intervention, and evaluation, the organization of the delivery systems, etc., is best presented in the senior year after the student is exposed to the realities of the health care system, has concerns, questions, and is looking outward to the broader community. A teaching model involving practical experience in the community could be most effective.

There are models in the United States for teaching population-based medicine in graduate medical education—the Residency Program in Social Medicine at Montefiore Hospital and Medical Center in New York is one example. There are, however, significant barriers to such efforts in traditional departments and in the residency accrediting bodies, though recent shifts by the more powerful Residency Review Committees, most notably Internal Medicine, toward requirements for greater primary care training certainly open the door for integration of a population medicine orientation.

If we are clear about what population medicine is and pragmatic about how to integrate it into the educational experience, I think we can be optimistic about achieving a valuable change in the orientation of all physicians.

Paula L. Stillman

In his chapter, the author succinctly presents the case for including essential population-based competencies in undergraduate and postgraduate medical education. He defines the scope of population-based medicine as including descriptive epidemiology, statistical analysis, organization of health and related services, preventive medicine approaches, and evaluation and audit. These are all critical competencies that should be incorporated into the undergraduate and postgraduate medical curriculum. Our perspectives diverge, however, on the extent of "understanding" to be achieved in each area and some of the specific recommendations on how these should be taught.

Descriptive Epidemiology

Cohen states that descriptive epidemiology includes an understanding of "morbidity and mortality statistics, . . . incidence and prevalence, . . . and an analysis of illness by age, sex, social class," etc. as well as "how to access expertise in relevant data collection and analysis." He elaborates that the student should also know about the effect of disease on life-style and on economic and social well-being. This content outline is reasonable. The undergraduate student must understand these terms and principles. However, if a few diseases were chosen as prototypic examples to illustrate these principles, this understanding would take on additional relevance. For example, a student might learn about chronic lung disease as a result of environmental or industrial hazards. He or she could review group data on morbidity and mortality, incidence and prevalence, and effects of different variables on the course and prognosis of a patient with this problem. He or she might make a home visit to a patient with this condition, obtain a history on the patient, and inquire how this condition as affected the patient's life-style, well-being, and ability to work. Additionally, the student could explore the effect of a patient's illness on the family, inquire about what is or is not being done to decrease the risks to other people, discuss access to health services, etc.

Statistical Analysis

Physicians must be able to critically review and critique medical literature. They do not have to be able to perform the actual statistical calculations but rather should understand the statistics involved and the limitations of the conclusions. They must also be aware of statistical versus practical or clinical significance. I, therefore, have no argument with the statistical concepts that Cohen lists as being essential for undergraduate medical education. I would urge, however, presenting students with two articles drawing conflicting conclusions about the same subject or intervention for the purpose of encouraging active discussion about the strengths and weaknesses of each study and its conclusions.

Knowledge of the Organization and Availability of Health and Health-Related Service

Cohen suggests that all medical students must have an "overview of the way health services are organized" and that the student "must understand the need for such services and the importance of setting the need against the availability." Although there can be a core of didactic teaching in this area, the content is probably best learned by first-hand experience. Each student should have an opportunity to visit a nursing home and, if possible, be exposed to two facilities—one excellent and one substandard. Students should also attend a community disease-oriented support group and be exposed to individuals sharing experiences, problems, and solutions in an environment that is safe for discussion of potentially emotionally charged issues. For students to understand the "need" for various community services, they must be exposed to the purpose and scope of such services and decide on their utility.

Preventive Medicine Approaches

Cohen writes that "the student should understand the basic principles of selection and implementation of health screening initiatives, the techniques and psychology of mounting campaigns to change harmful aspects of life style." Besides this "understanding," I would propose that the student know the screening procedures with the highest yield for each age group and sex. Early on in their training, students can participate in health screening initiatives by conducting free blood pressure screening at a shopping mall or visiting an elementary school and checking the children's vision and hearing. Patient education and counseling about health promotion and disease prevention should be included in each patient interaction that the student has throughout medical school. The student should have an opportunity to practice these skills multiple times until he or she becomes comfortable in applying the principles of negotiation and counseling. This might initially involve "role-playing" exercises in a safe situation with critique and feedback by the faculty and then progress to interactions with simulated patients. Finally, these skills should be used with real patients. To appreciate the difficulty of counseling patients to stop harmful behaviors such as alcohol abuse, the students might attend a meeting of Alcoholics Anonymous.

Evaluation and Audit

The final core competency discussed in this chapter is the understanding of "the critical importance of the evaluation of health care . . . and cost–benefit analysis." I propose that each student might accomplish this by reviewing the literature and developing audit criteria for at least one diagnostic condition. Students must be made aware of the costs of health care. This might be accomplished by including costs on order forms for laboratory and diagnostic studies. Many of our current students essentially have no knowledge about the costs of the tests that are ordered for a given patient.

How Do We Ensure That This Material Is Placed into the Curriculum?

When Cohen discusses the competition among various disciplines for time in the undergraduate medical curriculum, I feel that he makes an artificial schism between training students in "individual patient-based medicine" and the competencies that are population-based. Many competencies can be claimed by both. To provide excellent care to an individual patient, the student must be able to critically review literature regarding new therapeutic modalities, be aware of risk factors, and be knowledgeable about community resources. The student must be capable of interacting positively with a patient in an effort to change harmful behavior; he or she must be aware of health hazards. I do not believe the author is maximizing curricular time by suggesting that the content of population-based medicine be taught as a separate formal course. How much more relevant this material would be if it could be integrated with existing courses in physical diagnosis, pathophysiology, etc. Equally important, to provide optimum learning for our students, our clinical faculty must be educated in population-based medicine and encouraged to integrate these principles into their clinical teaching activities with students beginning with their first days in medical school. The students' learning should be active and participatory and, whenever possible, the content should be anchored into a clinically relevant situation.

Finally, I would disagree with Cohen's support of the principle of compensation, i.e., it is all right for a student to compensate on an examination for poor performance in population-based topics by good performance in other areas. I would suggest that a core curriculum in population-based medicine can and should be defined for every student. If this information is essential to becoming a good physician, academic advancement should not be permitted until this material is mastered.

Postgraduate Medical Training

Almost all of the suggestions made in Cohen's chapter regarding undergraduate medical education are applicable to postgraduate training. However, I would propose that the population-based principles not be segregated into "a short period of formal . . . training . . . in these techniques," as suggested by the author, but rather integrated into patient care experiences.

Conclusion

I agree with content of population-based medicine as defined by Cohen for both undergraduate and postgraduate medical training but believe that, whenever possible, this material can best be learned when it is integrated into existing course work and the learning should be active. Interactions with patients and community experiences are both essential.

John Wade

The author has described the essential population-based competencies for undergraduate and postgraduate medical students. He defines these to be acquired and the level of understanding of these competencies required for future practice. This knowledge and these skills are applied to a current standard curriculum.

It is my impression that many Canadian medical schools have evolving curriculums based on the Report on the General Professional Education of the Physician (GPEP 1984). The curriculum of many medical schools is moving in the direction of being student-oriented, problem-based, integrated, taught in the community, and liberally sprinkled with electives. Some faculties have begun to strengthen their community medicine departments and some have developed working relationships with governments to utilize the Canadian Claims Data Base and to define the health status of the population to be served.

In Manitoba we have begun to introduce community medicine in the early years as small groups focus on societal problems (e.g., disabled, native health, the health care system). In the clerkship the students must complete an 8-week rotation in community–family medicine outside of urban Winnipeg. Part of the rotation requires every student to write a paper describing a community health problem; the satisfactory completion of the paper is necessary for graduation.

Students also participate in summer research (the B.Sc. Medicine Program) in community medicine or work in the Northern Health Unit.

Postgraduate Community Medicine

The Royal College of Physicians and Surgeons of Canada now grants its Fellowship in Community Medicine. This is a growing residency program with about 12 positions in Manitoba. The postgraduate programs in community health are rapidly growing and provide opportunities for physicians (family practitioners or specialists) to obtain skills in population-based medicine. While biomedical science and clinical medicine are increasingly difficult to combine, there is a growing group of physicians obtaining the skills to do excellent population-based research while practicing as active clinicians.

Reference

Panel on the General Professional Education of the Physician and College Preparation for Medicine. 1984. *Physicians for the Twenty-first Century: The GPEP Report*. Washington, D.C.: Association of American Medical Colleges.

General Discussion

On the question of "compensation" by which graduates might substitute strength and competencies in one discipline for weakness or even ignorance of another there were differences of opinion. On balance, the opinion was against compensation. In other words, all medical graduates should have an understanding of the population perspective, and most should have some of the essential skills.

The extent of patient dissatisfaction as a consequence of current modes of educating physicians was discussed. The consensus favored the view that this was most likely to be expressed in relation to individual patients rather than as neglect of the community, but the situation undoubtedly differs within and among countries.

All agreed that medical education should be nonvocational; all believed that medical schools should strive to equip graduates with effective attitudes and skills for life-time self-learning. The dimensions of population medicine and epidemiology were discussed as including many of the competencies to be acquired. There was wide agreement that these should be considerably broader than those outlined in the original contribution.

There was agreement that the final recommendations from the conference should be unambiguous, capable of attainment, and encumbered by threats.

9
Balancing Perspectives

KERR L. WHITE and JULIA E. CONNELLY

For 3 days the participants in the Turnberry Conference debated the points raised in the eight preceding chapters by the authors, discussants, and others. All were agreed that while medical education had adapted well to biomedical advances during the past half century other aspects of the medical schools' mission now require further substantial shifts in perspectives, priorities, and educational venues. The central task before the group was to develop principles, definitions, and recommendations that would facilitate change. This chapter summarizes the results of these deliberations and is advanced as a communique. It comes from a group of colleagues committed to building on medicine's remarkable biotechnical achievements, and to maintaining those professional ideals and aspirations directed at providing compassionate, science-based, effective, and appropriate services. We commend these ideas to other similarly dedicated colleagues with the hope that they will find them worth considering, adopting, or adapting.

I. Background

Most contemporary medical schools in Canada, the United Kingdom, the United States, and Australia have seriously neglected many aspects of the population's health. Their top priorities are caring for the sickest individuals and biomedical research into disease processes. As a consequence, their faculties and students have lost sight of the health and health care problems that are commonly encountered by most members of all societies. To redress the serious imbalances that now exist in medical education, research, and services, medical schools will need to increase their recognition of the central importance of social, behavioral, and environmental determinants of disease, health status, and health care.

To varying degrees in all four countries there is growing public dissatisfaction with health care arrangements, and by implication, with many aspects of medicine's leadership. Governments, the media, the public, and the medical profession have each contributed to the present disarray but much of academic medicine's reluctance to change its priorities and preoccupations is attracting insistent scrutiny. Responses of too many medical schools and affiliated institutions to individual and collective health problems increasingly are perceived as inadequate. Sources of societal and professional dissatisfaction vary within and among countries but include such factors as escalating costs, inequities in accessibility to needed care (e.g., long waiting lists, incomplete insurance coverage, imbalances between generalists and specialists), failure of many physicians individually, and the profession collectively, to listen to patients' and the public's concerns, imbalances between use of high technology and early care (e.g., expensive neonatal care of low birthweight infants while rates escalate for teen pregnancies and infant mortality), wide variations within and among countries for many procedures and in the quality and outcomes of care, increases in tort liabilities and malpractice suits, and concerns about patient autonomy.

Substantial changes, initiated by governments, are afoot in all four countries. Commissions in most Canadian provinces are advancing proposals for major changes in manpower and educational priorities. Substantial shifts in financing and organization of the National Health Service in the United Kingdom will have important implications for medical education and its funding. Following extensive reviews of medical and public health education in Australia, the Federal government has launched a major review of its health services. A spate of commissions, boards, Congressional hearings, and other manifestations of alarm about deteriorating health services in the United States have yet to demonstrate a consensus about the root problems. The level of concern is high enough in these four countries to warrant academic medicine's leadership examining the assumptions and values that guide their institutions. How do medical schools determine their collective activities, establish priorities, and implement goals and objectives for education, research, and patient care? How do medical schools individually and collectively view their responsibilities for the public's health? How can physicians most effectively address the health and health care problems of the populations they serve? The situation is sufficiently critical to recognize this as an opportune time for initiating fundamental changes in the ways academic medicine goes about meeting its societal obligations. There is an urgent need to devise generic responses to the ubiquitous contemporary distress surrounding the health affairs of our four nations. There is an urgent need to embrace new and broader perspectives as guides in educating physicians competent to cope with the full range of problems that affects the public's health.

The relationship between the medical school and the population it serves is governed by an implicit *social contract*—a concept central to the ideals of Western democracies. This contract should be maintained by consensus based on terms that are clearly understood and openly accepted by all parties. The obligations incurred by medical schools are in part based on the public's direct or indirect financial support of medical education, including their willingness to provide generous compensation and unique privileges for the faculty. The strongest argument for change, however, may be a moral one. Change is required because it is the just response of a profession with deep moral traditions. When the social contract is periodically renegotiated, society's interests are *always* accommodated. Current unrest on the part of both the public and the profession may have resulted from an unraveling of the medical schools' unwritten contract with society. The central issue concerns the nature of the relationship between the medical school, its affiliated institutions, faculty, and the population served. What is the nature and extent of medicine's responsibility and what knowledge, skills, and attitudes ("competencies") should the medical school's faculty and its undergraduates and postgraduates possess? In turn, what should medical schools expect from society by way of cooperation and understanding, as well as through the provision of adequate material and financial resources?

Financial, legal, cultural, philosophic, and moral grounds support the conclusion that, as a matter of urgency, all medical schools should acknowledge the existence of the implicit contract with the populations they serve and proceed to make it more explicit. The character and dimensions of their responsibilities should be considered and agreed to by the entire faculty, and widely publicized. Of greater importance, the conclusions should be manifested in the actions of each school as it organizes, in concert with its affiliated institutions, to educate students (undergraduate, and where feasible postgraduate), conduct research (fundamental, clinical, and health services), and provide patient care. Once these matters are determined goals, objectives, priorities, and the faculty's collective activities can be determined within a balanced framework.

For most of the twentieth century, the medical school's endeavor has embraced two dominant preoccupations. The first is clinically based and focuses on the care of individual patients, one at a time. The second is laboratory based and concerned with cellular and molecular disease processes. Biomedical research and technological development are essential for teaching and for providing graduates with a set of indispensable competencies to meet individual patient needs for medical care. At the end of this century this component has a high profile, is demonstrably productive, widely understood, and, with some exceptions, well-resourced. These successes, however, have been accompanied by serious educational imbalances. Among these are the domination of narrowly defined biomedical aspects of disease in individual patients to the exclusion of other equally important considerations bearing on the patient's care and well-being. A third domain of the medical school's endeavor uses knowledge and experiences derived from population-based approaches. These are essential for providing graduates another set of competencies to facilitate understanding other vital determinants that affect the natural history and management of each patient's illness, as well as the disease process.

II. Issues and Definitions

Effective implementation of the *social contract* has two components. One defines a *point of view* to guide development of the medical school's goals and objectives. The other describes a set of *scientific means* for implementing the goals and objectives. All medical schools should proceed to balance the individual patient–physician and the biomedical perspectives by embracing the *population perspective*. Such a move would restore a viewpoint that was a part of medicine's mission until the beginning of this century. One perspective is not "right" or "wrong," "good" or "bad," "soft" or "hard"—all three are essential for fulfilling medicine's mission. Medical schools should also recruit and develop faculty members, especially clinicians, with the necessary skills for applying *population medicine* (or in the United Kingdom "the new public health"). The ideas underlying these two components are of much greater importance than the terms or definitions but the following are offered:

- *Population Perspective*: The capacity to appreciate the determinants, ranges, and variations of health status and disease in the entire community.

This perspective is employed when considering the problems of both individual patients and groups. It enables physicians to understand the contributions they, their institutions, and their professional colleagues can make to improve the health of populations, i.e., the public's health. Incorporation of the *Population Perspective* augments the individual and biotechnical perspectives. Terms such as population health, health of populations, and public health also employ the population perspective as an organizing concept.

- *Population Medicine*: The application of those concepts and methods embodied in such largely quantitative disciplines as epidemiology, economics, demography, and statistics, and in such behavioral sciences as cultural anthropology, sociology, and social psychology.

Research, clinical practice, and institutional policies employing the knowledge and skills of these disciplines are directed at responding to the population's health problems. Population-based medicine is an analogous term.

To improve the public's health, all faculty members and students should understand both components. While all need to be knowledgeable about the *Population Perspective*, not all will be equally skilled in the disciplines of *Population Medicine*, although many may wish to be. However, if each medical school is to fulfill its direct and indirect obligations for improving the public's health, the institution as a whole must be seen to be employing both components. If medical schools collectively succeed in meeting their responsibilities to the population they serve, they will have major impacts on such vital issues as the population's health status, maintenance of a trusting relationship between doctors and patients, negotiations surrounding the privileges and prerogatives of the medical profession, and the flow of funds to support education and much needed fundamental, clinical, and health services research.

Opinions may differ about the levels of understanding and the specific skills to be acquired by all undergraduate and postgraduate students but to provide some guidance, in addition to the viewpoints and suggestions in the preceding chapters, an outline of desirable population-based competencies is provided in the Appendix at the end of this chapter. Professor David Metcalfe has provided a clinical example to illustrate an educational application of both the *population perspective* and *population medicine* in the context of an individual patient's problem:

In many populations breast cancer is the commonest and greatest cause of lost years of life for women. There is little evidence of increasing effectiveness of treatment; the standardized mortality rate is rising regardless of 5-year survival; and there is no evidence of an increase in the number of women who live long enough to die of something else.

There is no consensus among specialists as to the optimum treatment; it varies from "lumpectomy" to extensive radical mastectomy, with or without adjuvant therapy; indeed some specialists allow women to choose the treatment mode themselves. Women still delay, on average, for four-and-a-half months after finding a lump before presenting for care, and far fewer than the 80% needed to make mammography screening effective, present themselves for this test.

How does teaching and research address this appalling set of problems? In particular:

- What research and teaching addressing the problem of late entry and rejection of screening seek to find out about women's feelings associated with this condition and their effect on behavior? Does this include attention to issues such as self-image, body-image, sexuality, health beliefs, locus of control, and lay perceptions of breast cancer and its treatment? Does it include the effects of social class, age, and ethnicity? Are issues such as direct and opportunity costs to patients and their families, barriers to care (inequity), and the thrust of health education and publicity addressed?
- What research and teaching focus on the identification of the oncogene and its activators, and what consideration is given to the social and ethical implications of the ability to identify women at risk?
- What research and teaching are there about the impact of unmandated outreach programs, the anxiety generated by the invitation, the wait for results, and the elimination of "false positives"?
- What teaching and evaluation are there about communication, counseling, and consultation skills focussing on a woman's fears of and feelings about breast cancer? What research and teaching are there about restoring sexuality and sexual function after mastectomy, and organization of follow-up without keeping the woman in the sick role? How are students taught to help the woman with metastatic disease? How are students taught to conduct palliative and terminal care?
- What research is being done to evaluate modes of treatment? What end points are being used, and at what intervals? Are there failure criteria for chemo-

therapy and radiotherapy? What research is being done into surgeons' and oncologists' decision-making to illuminate the unjustifiably wide range of procedures undertaken? How are functional capacity and quality of life assessed?

Without clear and positive answers to these sorts of questions society will have to infer that the medical faculty is not satisfactorily addressing one of the major health problems in the population surrounding the medical school.

III. Objectives

The principal goal of medical education, and therefore of the medical school, is to provide a balanced medical education that produces graduates, in appropriate ratios, competent to meet the population's health care needs. The school's "population," therefore, is, in the last analysis, the people for whom its graduates, together with graduates from other medical schools, care. There is a clear need, therefore, for each medical school to clarify and acknowledge the dimensions of the population for which it assumes responsibility; it is this population with whom the faculty negotiates the implicit social contract and for whom it promulgates the medical school's mission statement.

The medical school's commitment to improving the population's health should be addressed at three levels:

- *Individual Patient–Physician Level*: All graduates should understand the natural history of each patient's disease, possible methods of prevention and health promotion, as well as the management of the individual's illness in relationship to psychological, social, occupational, and environmental factors in its genesis, and in the contexts of treatment and management, and the community resources to be invoked.

  For example, graduates should know the relative importance of conditions in both small populations (1000 to 3000 persons) served by primary care generalists (general practitioners, family physicians, etc.) and in large populations (100,000 to 1,000,000 or more), and the nation. These are frequently expressed in measures based, for example, on age, sex, and occupational prevalence, functional states, and extent of unmet need. Graduates should also know the indications, potential risks, benefits, and costs of diagnostic and therapeutic interventions. Faculty with clinical responsibilities should encourage understanding and application of this knowledge in concert with colleagues from the population-based disciplines.
- *Institutional Level*: All medical schools and their affiliated institutions should assume responsibility for addressing the health needs of a general population. Fulfilling these societal obligations is best accomplished when each medical school and its affiliated institutions assumes responsibility for an explicit *catchment area* or *defined population*. These can be determined by geography or through enrollment in group practices, clinics, health maintenance organizations, and the like.

Where two or more medical schools exist in close proximity, especially in densely populated metropolitan areas without any formal regionalization scheme, responsibility for potential populations will need to be negotiated. Those schools whose faculties believe they have national and global missions should also promote active dissemination of the population perspective; they too will need to define a population for whose health status they recognize responsibility.

To teach and investigate many aspects of *population medicine*, especially such components as primary medical care, disease prevention, and health promotion, requires each medical school to establish contractual or other agreements with a variety of community-based health institutions, ambulatory clinics, and practice-based sites. Appropriate teachers in such settings will require faculty appointments. These educational consortia and networks should enjoy administrative, financial, and material resources on a par with those accorded tertiary care services.

Achievment of change will, for the most part, be gradual and the patterns and stages will vary by country and by medical school. When both the broadened perspective and the means for investigating the health of populations are included in renewed versions of the social contract between medical schools and the public, and are embodied in clear mission statements, what benefits might ensue? Among the projected outcomes of these innovations are the following: preparation of balanced ratios of generalists and specialists competent to respond to the public's perceived needs and those determined objectively by health surveys; greater pursuit of investigator-initiated and institution-sponsored clinical, epidemiological, and health services research into the health problems of the population served; effective collaboration with other health professionals and institutions, and with health departments; provision of responsive patient care that recognizes the full range of a population's health problems; and the development of many more effective, sensitive, and satisfactory interventions to prevent and treat disease and to promote health.

IV. Recommendations

To achieve these goals there is a need to establish clear expectations that govern institutional performance and that can be subjected to objective and external monitoring and public scrutiny. To this end, and recognizing that adjustments in terminology will be required for each of the four countries, the following five *recommendations* are offered:

- *Goals and Objectives*: Each medical school should develop and publicize a *Mission Statement* of goals and objectives that defines its commitment to both individuals and populations. This statement should reflect clear recognition and understanding of the nature and intent of the contract that exists with the population it serves, however defined. The statement should cover undergraduate, and where feasible postgraduate, education, research, and service. Arrangements should be defined for implementing these goals and objectives with representatives of the population to be served. The statement should include strategies for evaluating progress towards the institution's goals and objectives using population-based and individual outcomes.

- *Faculty Development*: Each medical school should establish methods to ensure that each faculty member understands the distribution of health problems in the population served.
- *Education*: Each medical school should establish methods to ensure that each graduate has acquired knowledge, skills, and attitudes that reflect appropriate applications of individual patient-physician, biomedical, and population-based perspectives.
- *Educational Resources*: Each medical school should assemble an adequate breadth of resources (faculty and facilities) to ensure that all students have a balanced experience with the full range of health problems in the population served, and have opportunities to work with other health professionals and agencies.
- *Health Intelligence*: Each medical school should establish a unit or links with an organization capable of transforming raw "data" bearing on health and health services into usable "information." In turn this "information" needs to be interpreted, in social, political, and other contexts, as "intelligence" to guide the faculty and Dean in establishing institutional priorities for education, research, and service. The unit should have strong ties to clinical departments, and to governmental and other community agencies, including health departments.

V. Implementation

Implementation of these recommendations is most likely to be accelerated through the mechanisms of institutional accreditation, examinations, certification, and especially through the process of licensure, preferably done nationally on completion of all postgraduate (residency, registrar) training. Some countries may wish to consider national, state, or provincial legislation to ensure effective implementation of these or similar concepts that are responsive to the public's and the profession's mounting dissatisfaction. Early introduction of these recommendations, suitably modified for each country, into academic, organizational, professional, and governmental settings accompanied by prompt discussion of them can result in their adoption.

Appendex: Proposed Competencies

I. *The graduate should demonstrate*

- A balanced *understanding* of the individual patient-physician, biomedical, and *population perspectives* needed to practice medicine and respond to the health care needs of the population served, however defined; and
- The *knowledge*, *skills*, and *attitudes* required to integrate the concepts and methods of *Population Medicine* into clinical practice and to address the health care needs of the population served.

II. *The graduate should demonstrate an understanding* of the Population Perspective by

- Describing the origin, nature, and implications of the *social contract*;
- Acknowledging responsibility for addressing the health and health care needs of a general population, however defined;
- Describing methods and means by which all physicians, generalists as well as specialists, can incorporate the population perspective into their teaching, research, and service responsibilities;
- Documenting a full appreciation of the fact that diseases experienced by patients who consult physicians and are admitted to teaching hospitals do not represent the full spectrum of human illness that exists in general populations and cannot be used to describe or understand the health and health care needs of the general population.

III. *The graduate should demonstrate knowledge* of the capacities provided by Population Medicine to

- Identify and define general and special populations;
- Identify, measure, and assess areas of concern about health and health care in a defined population;
- Understand why these areas are of concern for a particular population;
- Recognize the importance of the individual's and the population's perspectives of health and health care problems;
- Obtain available evidence to describe the distribution of two or three major health problems by, for example, demographic characteristics, socioeconomic status, occupation, housing, severity, and availability of health care and related social services in the general population served by the medical school, e.g., perinatal mortality, dependency with aging, spread of AIDS;
- Identify available national, regional, and local data sources to determine the health problems of general populations;
- Assess the validity and reliability of these sources;
- Assess statistically the credibility of health-related data and information;

- Use evidence from population-based disciplines other than those currently embraced by medicine, e.g., cultural anthropology, demography, economics, sociology, and social psychology, in understanding and managing the health problems of individuals and populations; and
- Use probabilistic thinking and quantitative evidence in decision-making at the health services and individual patient levels.

IV. *The graduate should demonstrate the skills of Population Medicine to*

- Critically evaluate scientific literature;
- Design a study of an important health problem in a general population (*vide supra*) that includes a statement of the question asked or the hypothesis to be tested, a description of feasible methods for collecting, tabulating, evaluating, and analyzing the data; and
- Devise a plan or strategy for dealing with the problem above, and a design for evaluating the outcome of the strategy proposed.

V. *The graduate should demonstrate attitudes* that reflect the need for individual physicians and the profession generally to

- Understand and address the health and health care needs of the entire population;
- Understand that auditing the effectiveness of health care will help to improve the care of both individuals and populations;
- Retain an open mind until credible evidence from any source is thoughtfully and critically evaluated; and
- Appreciate that the public's opinion and interest are important and need to be listened to.

A set of competencies required of graduates in the Population Medicine component of one medical school is to be found in Appendix 2 of Chapter 6.

Conference Participants

DAVID AXELROD, M.D., Commissioner, New York State Department of Health, Albany, NY, USA

HARVEY BARKUN, M.D., Executive Director, Association of Canadian Medical Colleges, Ottawa, Canada

SIR DOUGLAS BLACK, M.D., Past President, Royal College of Physicians, Reading, England*

MAXINE E. BLEICH, President, Ventures in Education, New York, NY, USA

SIR CHRISTOPHER BOOTH, M.D., Past President, The Royal Sociey of Medicine, London, England*

MARKLEY H. BOYER, M.D., Professor of Community Medicine, School of Medicine, Tufts University, Boston, MA, USA

JO IVEY BOUFFORD, M.D., Visiting Fellow, King's Fund College, London, Clinical Associate Professor of Pediatrics and of Epidemiology and Social Medicine, Albert Einstein College of Medicine (Former President, New York Health and Hospitals Corporation), New York, NY, USA

ROGER J. BULGER, M.D., President, Association of Academic Health Centers, Washington, D.C., USA

RUTH E. BULGER, Ph.D. Director, Division of Health Sciences Policy, Institute of Medicine, National Academy of Science, Washington, D.C., USA

RT. HON. LORD BUTTERFIELD, M.D., (Retired Vice-Chancellor and Regius Professor of Medicine, University of Cambridge), Cambridge, England

ROBERT. D. COHEN, M.D., Professor of Medicine, London Hospital Medical College, London, England

JULIA E. CONNELLY, M.D., Associate Professor of Medicine, School of Medicine, University of Virginia, Charlottesville, VA, USA*

DAVID S. GREER, M.D., Dean and Professor of Community Health, School of Medicine, Brown University, Providence, RI, USA*

JOHN D. HAMILTON, M.D., Dean and Professor of Medicine, Faculty of Medicine, University of Newcastle, Newcastle, Australia

THOMAS S. INUI, M.D., Professor and Head, General Internal Medicine and Professor of Health Services, School of Medicine, University of Washington, Seattle, WA, USA*

HARRY S. JONAS, M.D., Director, Division of Undergraduate Medical Education, American Medical Association, Chicago, IL, USA

ARTHUR KAUFMAN, M.D., Professor of Family, Community, and Emergency Medicine, School of Medicine, University of New Mexico, Albuquerque, NM, USA

GEORGE I. LYTHCOTT, M.D., Retired Dean, City University of New York Medical School, New York, NY, USA

ARTHUR J. MAHON, ESQ., President, The Royal Society of Medicine Foundation Inc., and Vice Chairman, Board of Overseers, Cornell Medical College, New York, NY, USA

MICHAEL G. MARMOT, M.B., Ph.D., Professor of Community Medicine, University College and Middlesex School of Medicine, London, England

WILLIAM D. MATTERN, M.D. Associate Dean and Professor of Medicine, University of North Carolina, Chapel Hill, NC, USA

LIONEL E. McLEOD, M.D., Vice-President, Medical Services, University Hospital, University of British Columbia, Vancouver, Canada*

IAN R. McWHINNEY, M.D., Professor of Family Medicine, Faculty of Medicine, University of Western Ontario, London, Canada

THOMAS H. MEIKLE, Jr., M.D., President, Josiah Macy Jr. Foundation, New York, NY, USA*

DAVID H.H. METCALFE, M.B., B.S., Professor and Chairman, Department of General Practice, University of Manchester Medical School, Manchester, U.K.*

VICTOR R. NEUFELD, M.D., Director, Centre for International Health, and Professor of Medicine and Clinical Epidemiology, Faculty of Health Sciences, McMaster University, Hamilton, Canada*

WILLIAM G. O'REILLY, Executive Director, The Royal Society of Medicine Foundation Inc., New York, NY, USA*

PETER RICHARDS, M.D., Ph.D., Dean and Professor of Medicine, St. Mary's Hospital Medical School; Pro Rector (Medicine), Imperial College of Science, Technology, and Medicine, London, England

MUTYA SAN AGUSTIN, M.D., Director, Department of Ambulatory Medicine, North Central Bronx Hospital/Montefiore Medical Center; Associate Professor, Pediatrics, Albert Einstein College of Medicine, Bronx, New York, NY, USA*

DAVID A. SHAW, M.D., Dean and Professor of Neurology, University of Newcastle Medical School, Newcastle-upon-Tyne, U.K.

ROBERT A. SPASOFF, M.D., Professor and Chairman, Department of Epidemiology and Community Medicine, Faculty of Medicine, University of Ottawa, Ottawa, Canada*

PAULA L. STILLMAN, M.D., Curriculum Dean and Professor of Pediatrics, University of Massachusetts Medical School, Worcester, MA, USA

JOHN WADE, M.D., Director, The Manitoba Health Services Commission (Former Dean and Professor of Anaesthesiology, Faculty of Medicine, University of Manitoba), Winnipeg, Canada

MAMORU WATANABE, M.D., Dean and Professor of Medicine, Faculty of Medicine, University of Calgary, Calgary, Canada

KERR L. WHITE, M.D., Retired Deputy Director for Health Sciences, The Rockefeller Foundation, New York, Charlottesville, VA, USA*

SIR DAVID INNES WILLIAMS, M.D., President, The Royal Society of Medicine, London, England

ANTHONY B. ZWI, M.B., Lecturer, Department of Community Medicine, University College and Middlesex School of Medicine, London, England

* Members of the Planning Committee

Name Index

Subject Index